SOCIAL BRAIN, DISTRIBUTED MIND

PROCEEDINGS OF THE BRITISH ACADEMY · 158

SOCIAL BRAIN, DISTRIBUTED MIND

Edited by
ROBIN DUNBAR
CLIVE GAMBLE
JOHN GOWLETT

Published for THE BRITISH ACADEMY
by OXFORD UNIVERSITY PRESS

Oxford University Press, Great Clarendon Street, Oxford OX2 6DP

Oxford New York

Auckland Cape Town Dar es Salaam Hong Kong Karachi
Kuala Lumpur Madrid Melbourne Mexico City Nairobi
New Delhi Shanghai Taipei Toronto

With offices in

Argentina Austria Brazil Chile Czech Republic France Greece
Guatemala Hungary Italy Japan Poland Portugal Singapore
South Korea Switzerland Thailand Turkey Ukraine Vietnam

Published in the United States
by Oxford University Press Inc., New York

British Library Cataloguing in Publication Data
Data available

Library of Congress Cataloging in Publication Data
Data available

Typeset by New Leaf Design, Scarborough, North Yorkshire
Printed in Great Britain
on acid-free paper by
CPI Antony Rowe
Chippenham, Wiltshire

ISBN 978–0–19–726452–2
ISSN 0068–1202

Contents

Illustrations

Notes on Contributors

Katherine Andrews graduated with a first class honours degree in Zoology from the University of Dundee, then studied social behaviour of feral goats on the Isle of Rum before commencing a postgraduate degree in primate social networks at the University of Liverpool. This research was supervised by Professor Dunbar as a part of the British Academy Centenary Research Project. She now works for the open access publishers, BioMed Central.

Holly Arrow is Associate Professor of Psychology and a member of the Institute for Cognitive and Decision Sciences at the University of Oregon. She has two primary research interests. The first is the formation and development of small groups. The theoretical framework can be found in *Small groups as complex systems: formation, coordination, development, and adaptation* (2000, with Joseph McGrath and Jennifer Berdahl). The second is the psychology of war, in particular the evolution of social capacities that help men and women cope with the challenges to survival and reproductive success posed by war. This includes computational modelling as a strategy for theory development (in collaboration with Oleg Smirnov, John Orbell and Doug Kennett), and experimental work investigating gender differences in cognitive and behavioural responses to inter-group conflict and competition.

Lawrence Barham is Professor of Archaeology at the School of Archaeology, Classics and Egyptology, University of Liverpool, UK. The chapter in this volume reflects his long-term interest in the development of human behavioural diversity in the period between 400,000 and 130,000 years ago, with a focus on south-central Africa. He is co-author (with Peter Mitchell) of *The first Africans* (2008) and has published books and articles on the Middle Stone Age (Mode 3) of Zambia.

Alan Barnard is Professor of the Anthropology of Southern Africa at the University of Edinburgh. His field research is mainly with San or Bushmen in Botswana and Namibia. Recent books include *Hunter-gatherers in history, archaeology and anthropology* (edited, 2004), *Social anthropology* (2nd edn, 2006), *Anthropology and the Bushman* (2007), and the *Encyclopedia of social and cultural anthropology* (2nd edition, edited with Jonathan Spencer, 2009).

Yonas Beyene is actively engaged in archaeological research in Ethiopia, specifically in the paleoanthroplogical sites of Fejej and Konso in southern Ethiopia and the Middle Awash, and Chorora sites in the Afar Rift. He earned his PhD in prehistoric archaeology from the Museum National d'Histoire Naturelle, Paris, France, 1986–1991. He was Senior Expert in Archaeology at the National Museum of Ethiopia, then became Head of the Department of Archaeology and Anthropology and, later, the Department of Archaeology and Paleontology in the Authority for Research and Conservation of Cultural Heritage (ARCCH), Ethiopia. He teaches African Archaeology in the Addis Ababa University Archaeology Unit on part-time basis.

John Chapman, is a Reader in Archaeology at Durham University. He took a PhD at the London Institute of Archaeology ('The Vin: a culture of South East Europe', 1981). His appointment at the University of Newcastle upon Tyne led to two major interdisciplinary fieldwork projects 'The Neothermal Dalmatia Project' (now Croatia) and 'The Upper Tizsa Project' (Hungary). He developed the sub-field of fragmentation in archaeology with two books (*Fragmentation in archaeology*, 2000; *Parts and wholes*, 2006). He edited the *European Journal of Archaeology* (1996–2003) for the European Association of Archaeologists and is currently Vice-President of the UK Prehistoric Society.

Paul Connerton read Modern History at Oxford and English Literature at Cambridge. He has held a Research Fellowship at Gonville and Caius College Cambridge, a Visiting Fellowship at the Humanities Research Centre in the Australian National University and a Simon Senior Research Fellowship in the University of Manchester. His publications include *The tragedy of enlightenment: an essay on the Frankfurt School* (Cambridge University Press, 1980), *How societies remember* (Cambridge University Press, 1989) and *How modernity forgets* (Cambridge University Press, 2009).

Fiona Coward is based in the Geography Department at Royal Holloway University of London. Her research interests centre around the evolution of the human brain and behaviour, with particular reference to how our ancestors' social and ecological relationships with other plant and animal species, elements of the physical landscape and material culture impacted on the course of human evolution. Her work on relational archaeologies investigates how these more-than-human entities are integrated into identity and social networks, and used in social performance and interactions.

Terrence Deacon received a PhD from Harvard University in 1984 and has served on the faculties of Harvard University, Harvard Medical School, Boston University, and the University of California, Berkeley, where he is currently Professor of Anthropology and Neuroscience. His research combines human evolutionary biology and neuroscience with a focus on the evolution of human language capacity and cognition. His work extends from laboratory-based cellular-molecular neurobiology to semiotic theory and struggles with the special challenge of explaining emergent processes in biology and cognitive neuroscience. Many of these interests are explored in his book, *The symbolic species: the coevolution of language and the brain* (Norton, 1997) and are further developed in a new book *Homunculus: the emergence of mind from matter* (Norton, in press) which explores the relationship between thermodynamics, self-organization and evolutionary processes.

Robin Dunbar is currently Professor of Evolutionary Anthropology at the University of Oxford, and was elected a Fellow of the British Academy in 1998. His principal research interests focus on social evolution in mammals (with particular reference to ungulates, primates and humans). He is co-Director of the British Academy's Centenary Research Project 'Lucy to Language: The Archaeology of the Social Brain'—a collaborative multidisciplinary project involving staff in evolutionary and social psychology, archaeology, evolutionary and social anthropology and history at seven UK universities. He is involved in several other collaborative multi-institutional research projects with computer and information scientists applying the 'social brain' concept to the design of mobile technology. Among his books are *The trouble with science* (1995), *Grooming gossip and the evolution of language* (1996), *Primate conservation biology* (2000), *Human evolutionary psychology* (2002), *The human story* (2004), and the edited volumes *The evolution of culture* (1999) and *The Oxford handbook of evolutionary psychology* (2007).

Daniel Finkel is pursuing his PhD in Anthropology at the University of Connecticut, where he studies human evolution as it relates to music, religion/ritual and social cognition. He holds degrees from the University of Pennsylvania (BA, Biological Basis of Behavior) and the Siegal College of Judaic Studies (MA, Judaic Studies in Jewish Education). He is an alumnus of the National Outdoor Leadership School's Outdoor Educator Program, and was a Covenant Fellow.

Clive Gamble joined the Department of Geography at Royal Holloway University of London in 2004 where he is a Research Professor in the Centre for Quaternary Research. Previously he founded the Centre for the Archaeology of Human Origins at Southampton University. He has undertaken research into the evolution of human society concentrating in particular on the Palaeolithic. He is currently co-director of the British Academy Centenary Project (2003–10) 'From Lucy to Language: The Archaeology of the Social Brain' and a member of NERC's RESET consortium (2008–13) that investigates human adaptations to abrupt environmental transitions during the Pleistocene. Among recent projects he was Chair of the NERC-funded programme 'Environmental Factors and Chronology in Human Evolution and Dispersal' (EFCHED), completed in 2006. His recent publications include *Origins and revolutions: human identity in earliest prehistory* (Cambridge University Press 2007); *The individual hominid in context* (Routledge 2005, edited with Martin Porr); 'Climate change and evolving human diversity in Europe during the last glacial' (with W. Davies, P. Pettitt and M. Richards 2004, *Philosophical Transactions of the Royal Society* B 359: 243–54); *The Palaeolithic societies of Europe* (Cambridge University Press 1999). He was elected a Fellow of the British Academy in 2000 and is currently a Vice-President of the Society of Antiquaries of London.

Bisserka Gaydarska is an Honorary Research Fellow in Durham University Department of Archaeology. Her specializations are Balkan prehistory, GIS, artefact fragmentation and landscape archeology. After graduating from Sofia University, she took her PhD at Durham: *Landscape, material culture and society in South East Bulgaria* was published in 2007, the year after she co-authored *Parts and wholes: fragmentation in prehistoric context* with John Chapman. She has studied the prehistoric exploitation of salt in Bulgaria, Romania and Ukraine, and studied figurine collections in Romania and Bulgaria. Her current project involves a re-assessment of the value of intra-site surface artefact collections.

John Gowlett is Professor of Archaeology at the University of Liverpool. He has worked in East Africa at intervals since 1972, excavating early sites at Kilombe, Kariandusi and Chesowanja in Kenya. The latter site stimulated his long-lasting interest in early fire. Social and technical questions of early fire were reopened for him by research at Beeches Pit in East Anglia, UK. Very recently, he has resumed research in the central Rift Valley of Kenya in a collaborative project with D. Curnoe, J. Brink, I. Onjala and others. His related main interests are the concepts underlying the evolution of early technologies. He is co-Director of the British Academy Centenary Project 'Lucy to Language', in which he has written recently with Stephen Lycett on questions surrounding the Acheulean tradition.

Matt Grove is a postdoctoral researcher at the Institute of Cognitive and Evolutionary Anthropology, University of Oxford, and a Junior Golding Research Fellow of Brasenose College, Oxford. Funded by the British Academy Centenary Research Project, 'Lucy to Language: The Archaeology of the Social Brain', his research centres upon the reconstruction of prehistoric mobility patterns and social systems through the application of quantitative and computational methodologies to archaeological data. The research presented here forms part of an attempt to build a basic evolutionary geometry of hunter-gatherer mobility.

Julie Hui is a graduate student of Biological Anthropology at the University of California, Berkeley. Her research interests include the interaction between evolution and behaviour, computer simulations of evolutionary mechanisms, and self-organization in evolution.

Carl Knappett teaches in the Department of Art at the University of Toronto, where he holds the Walter Graham/Homer Thompson Chair in Aegean Prehistory. He works on Bronze Age material culture in the Aegean and east Mediterranean, focusing on Minoan pottery from a wide range of sites, among them Akrotiri Thera, Knossos, Malia, Myrtos Pyrgos and Palaikastro. He is also interested in material culture studies, cognitive archaeology and network theory. His publications include *Thinking through material culture: an interdisciplinary perspective* (University of Pennsylvania Press 2005) and *Knossos: protopalatial deposits in Early Magazine A and the South-west Houses* (with Colin Macdonald, 2007, British School at Athens Suppl. vol. no. 41).

Robert Layton is Professor of Anthropology at Durham University (UK) and a member of the department's Evolutionary Anthropology Research Group. His research interests include social evolution and social change. He has carried out field research on land tenure, foraging practices and religion with a number of Australian Aboriginal communities, as well as an extended project originating in his PhD research to study social change on the Plateau of Levier (Eastern France), including the history of collective land ownership, producer cooperatives and mutual aid. Publications include: *Anthropology and history in Franche-Comté: a critique of social theory* (Oxford University Press, 2000), *Order and anarchy: civil society,* *social disorder and war* (Cambridge University Press, 2006), 'Representing and translating people's place in the landscape of northern Australia' (in A. James, J. Hockey and A. Dawson [eds] *After writing culture: epistemology and praxis in contemporary anthropology*. Routledge, 1997).

Julia Lehmann is a senior lecturer at Roehampton University, London. Her main research interest is concerned with questions related to the evolution of sociality and the factors influencing social organization in mammals, including humans. In her most recent research she tackles questions about primate social networks and the dynamics of social relationships.

Steven Mithen is Professor of Early Prehistory and Dean of the Faculty of Science at the University of Reading. His research interests focus on the evolution of the human mind, language and music, and on Late Pleistocene and Early Holocene hunter-gatherers and farmers. Since 1987 he has been directing a field project in the Hebridean Islands of Western Scotland to explore Mesolithic settlement, and is currently co-directing the excavation of the Pre-Pottery Neolithic A settlement of WF16 in Wadi Faynan, southern Jordan. Steven is also the lead PI on the interdisciplinary project 'Water, Life and Civilisation' (see www.waterlife civilisation.org) that is exploring the impact of changes in the hydrological climate in human communities in the Near East between 20,000 BP and AD 2100. His recent books include *After the ice* (2003), *The singing Neanderthals* (2005) and *The early prehistory of Wadi Faynan* (edited with Bill Finlayson, 2007).

Sean O'Hara is a member of the Evolutionary Psychology and Behavioural Ecology Research Group at the University of Liverpool. He has interests in the evolution of sociality, with specific focus on humans and non-human primates, including behavioural ecology and the cognitive bases of social behaviour. He lectures on cognition, primate behavioural ecology and human evolutionary psychology. His research on the chimpanzees in Budongo Forest, Uganda, dates back to the mid-1990s and he is a former assistant director of the research centre there.

Dwight W. Read received his PhD at UCLA in mathematics, doing research on properties of abstract algebras. He is a Professor of Anthropology and of Statistics and publishes in all the subdisciplines that comprise a four-field anthropology (transition from biological to cultural evolution, theory and method of artefact classification, mathematical representation of cultural constructs, especially kinship terminologies). His current research focuses on the interrelationship between the material and the ideational domains in human societies. He had a Visiting Scientist affiliation with the IBM Los Angeles Research Center from 1986 to 1989. He has edited two Special Issues of the *Journal of Quantitative Anthropology* ('Computer-based Solutions to Anthropological Problems' [1990] and 'Formal Methods in Anthropology: Past Successes and New Directions' [1993]) and a Special Issue of the *Journal of Artificial Societies and Social Simulation* ('Computer Simulation in Anthropology'). He has developed a major computer program (*Kinship Algebraic Expert System*, or *KAES*) that constructs a formal (algebraic) model for the logic underlying the structure of a kinship terminology. He has developed an agent-based model that incorporates cultural knowledge in decision-making by agents and is currently working on an agent-based model for the evolutionary origin of vervet monkey warning cries viewed as a proto-language.

Sam G. B. Roberts is a postdoctoral researcher at the Institute of Cognitive and Evolutionary Anthropology, University of Oxford. His research is funded by the EPSRC and ESRC as part of the 'Developing Theory for Evolving Socio-Cognitive Systems' (TESS) project. His research interests lie in exploring social relationships and social cognition in human and non-human primates from an evolutionary perspective. For his PhD, he examined social cognition in free-ranging and captive primates. His postdoctoral work focuses on the structure and dynamics of human social networks, with an emphasis on understanding the time and cognitive constraints that may act to limit network size. He is also interested in how social relationships are maintained over time and how they are affected by new communication technologies (e.g. email, mobile phones, social network sites).

Mark Rowlands is Professor of Philosophy at the University of Miami. He is the author of a dozen books tranlsated into more than twenty languages. These include *The body in mind* (Cambridge University Press, 1999); *The nature of consciousness* (Cambridge University Press, 2001); and *Body language* (MIT Press, 2006). His autobiography, *The philosopher and the wolf* was published by Granta in 2008.

Richard Sosis is an associate professor of anthropology and director of the Evolution, Cognition, and Culture Program at the University of Connecticut. His work has focused on the evolution of cooperation and the adaptive significance of religious behaviour, with particular interest in the relationship between ritual and intra-group cooperation. To explore these issues, he has conducted fieldwork with remote cooperative fishers in the Federated States of Micronesia and with various communities throughout Israel, including Ultra-Orthodox Jews and members of secular and religious kibbutzim.

Paul Swartwout is a doctoral student in the Department of Anthropology at the University of Connecticut. He received his BS in Evolution and Ecology from the Ohio State University in 2007. He is interested in the evolutionary anthropology of religion, human behavioural ecology and social information use in humans and animals.

Anna Wallette is an assistant professor of history at Lund University, Sweden. Her research focuses mainly on the historiography of the Old Norse Sagas and the Viking Age, history writing and history culture in Scandinavia.

Preface

This volume presents the series of papers given at a two-day conference entitled 'Social Brain, Distributed Mind', held at the British Academy in September 2008 as part of the series of seminars and workshops organized by the British Academy's Centenary Research Project 'Lucy to Language' (the 'Lucy Project'). We would like to express our gratitude to the British Academy for their continued support in funding the Lucy Project, and for providing a conference grant that made this meeting possible, as well as for hosting the meeting at the Academy's premises. We would especially like to thank Viscount Runciman (University of Cambridge), Professor Wendy James (University of Oxford) and Professor Leslie Aiello (Wenner-Gren Foundation for Anthropological Research) for their support of the project. We are grateful to the British Academy Publications Committee for agreeing to publish the proceedings of the meeting, the editorial office for handling the publication process and Dr Fiona Coward for copy-editing the volume.

Robin Dunbar
Clive Gamble
John Gowlett

PART I

FRAMING THE ISSUES:
EVOLUTION OF THE SOCIAL BRAIN

1

The Social Brain and the Distributed Mind

ROBIN DUNBAR, CLIVE GAMBLE & JOHN GOWLETT

HUMAN NATURE IS THE PRODUCT of a long history that has brought us, over the course of some 6–8 million years, from our common ancestor with the chimpanzee lineage to modern humans. Understanding human nature—who we are, and what sets us apart from other primates—cannot be achieved in the absence of an understanding of that history, for herein lie the processes that have driven the hominin clade in the direction that it ultimately took. To understand who we are and why we are, we need to understand both modern humans as we find them now and the ancestral stages that brought us to this point. In major part, the core to that story has been the role of evolving cognition—and hence, the social brain—in mediating the changes in behaviour that we see in the archaeological record.

Hitherto, accounts of human origins and evolution have all too often been imaginative exercises, untested by the data, and hence justifiably open to the criticism of being mere 'Just-So Stories'. The reasons for this are twofold. On the one hand, some accounts are internally consistent, with assumptions drawn from either evolutionary theory or comparative stud-ies of human and animal behaviour, but remain largely untested—even untestable—by the archaeological and fossil record. Alternatively, other accounts have been built around the consequences of particular human characteristics—most notably bipedalism, technology, the control of fire and language—which have been cited as prime movers in the transition from hominid to hominin to human.[1] Such accounts invariably seem sim-plistic precisely because they focus on one dimension of an inevitably multi-stranded story, and at the same time present the transition from

---

[1] The term 'hominids' incorporates the great apes, hominins and humans. 'Hominins' include all human fossil ancestors and humans. Only modern *Homo sapiens* can be humans.

Proceedings of the British Academy **158**, 3–15. © The British Academy 2010.

some earlier stage to the full human as a major catastrophic event (a 'macro-mutation').

The aim of this particular volume has been to bring together two powerful approaches that deal, respectively, with explanations of the evolution of human brains and understandings of cognition as a distributed system, in order to illuminate the changes that took place during the later stages of human evolution—that period when, one might say, our lineage was becoming human. Our objective was to compare inter-disciplinary perspectives on these key issues across a range of disciplines (archaeology, psychology, philosophy, geography, history, anthropology) that span the Academy's interests, as well as some of those disciplines in the sciences (biology and palaeontology) that bear on our question. A particular focus is provided by consideration of the role that material culture plays as a scaffold for distributed cognition, and how almost 3 million years of artefact and tool use and manufacture provide the data for tracing key changes in areas such as language, technology, kinship, music, social networks and the politics of local, everyday interaction in small-world societies. All of this is set against a demographic background in which communities were both rapidly increasing in size and becoming more spatially dispersed. By bringing together these models of what made us human and how human cognition works in the world, rather than just inside the head, we believe we are well placed to test the social brain hypothesis with archaeological data. In this way we aim to re-introduce the material back into discussions of our evolutionary journey.

Our concept of society is modelled through the concept of networks based ultimately on interactions between dyads. The material and emotional resources that are involved in forming social bonds through such interactions have surely varied in complexity, quantity and substance during human evolution. Our social focus is the outcome of such interaction that results in a community composed of numbers of local groups. We therefore follow Knight (2008) in rejecting an earlier anthropological insistence on the family as the unit of evolutionary analysis, preferring instead the observations of primatologists and modern kinship studies, which suggest that great apes and humans live in communities. Human communities are distinguished by regular cooperation between non-kin and the individual's ability to extend their social presence across time and space, something that makes possible one of the features particularly characteristic of both chimpanzee and human sociality, namely fission-fusion organization, whereby the members of a community may be distributed over a wide area in subgroups of variable composition and temporal stability (Aureli et al. 2008). Such a capacity has clearly evolved, as has the human ability to aggregate and to organize settled populations through socially approved hierarchies.

To appreciate the departure we are arguing for, and to provide a framework for the chapters that follow, we briefly review some of the units of analysis that underpin the social brain model and then outline the major trends in human physical and material evolution.

THE SOCIAL BRAIN:
USING THEORY AS A RESEARCH TOOL

In the last decade, the 'social brain' hypothesis and its role as an explanation for the evolution of unusually large brain size in primates (Barton & Dunbar 1997; Dunbar 1998; Dunbar & Shultz 2007) has introduced a new cognitive dimension to the processes involved in social evolution. A number of features of primate social behaviour (such as community size, coalition size, time devoted to social interaction, social skills, tactical deception) have now been shown to be predictable from relative neocortex volume, and modern humans fit neatly into all these patterns (Dunbar 1992, 1998; Kudo & Dunbar 2001). Analyses of the size and structure of modern human social networks, and their implications for social bonding and interaction, suggest that grouping levels reflect levels of intimacy and trust (Hill & Dunbar 2003), as well as cognitive (specifically mindreading) abilities (Stiller & Dunbar 2007).

An important feature of the social brain hypothesis in the context of human evolution has been the linking of primates' social skills with the problems created by the disruptive effects of free-riders operating within dispersed social systems (Dunbar 1999, 2003). Given that social conformism exposes societies to free-riders, explaining the evolution of humans' unusual levels of cooperativeness and willingness to abide by the communal will has become perhaps the single greatest challenge for the study of human evolution.

The social brain hypothesis argues that the complexities of hominin social life were responsible for driving the evolution of the early hominin brain from its essentially apelike beginnings to its modern form. The theory offers a dynamic new perspective for exploring the evolutionary origins of fundamental social capabilities such as the formation of large, cooperating communities and the maintenance of high levels of intimacy and trust. Simultaneously, it informs on the specific cognitive abilities, such as theory of mind, that underpin these capabilities. The social brain model uses a number of proxies to address more directly the issue of this evolving social complexity. These proxies include brain size for community size; network densities (physical and material) for social complexity; spatial densities of archaeological evidence for local group sizes and proxies for density and distance in social relationships ranging from the appearance of hearths to intentionally fragmented objects circulating in chains of connection.

Armed with hypotheses generated by this kind of theory, our objective should be to develop a more reflexive inter-disciplinary approach in which the archaeological record identifies a problem, evolutionary psychology provides a hypothesis (or even several hypotheses) and the archaeology provides a basis for testing these hypotheses through the detailed analysis of material culture. Archaeology is unique among the human sciences in its focus on material culture and the time depth of its available data. It therefore has an unparalleled opportunity to address these issues. The study of temporal trends in the distribution of mind across the material world offers the possibility of remarkable insights into the evolution of human cognition and social life that will further our understanding of the relationship between mind and world. The key question is how the material record contributed to, and can be made to inform on, the process by which hominin 'brains' became recognizably human 'minds'.

THE EVOLUTIONARY AND
PALAEOANTHROPOLOGICAL FRAMING

The chapters in this volume map out much of the scope and complexity of a social brain in humans. In this effort, one thing becomes rapidly apparent: in some areas, we can reasonably easily establish continuity with the brains and behaviour of other species, and so work directly in a comparative framework. Social networks are an obvious example. But there are other areas where the power of the modern human mind, and its facility to operate at higher levels of intentionality, take us far beyond any possibility of immediate comparison with other animal species. Religion and philosophy are among these. Nonetheless, we believe it is essential to embrace these areas, or we leave out much of what it is to be human. The challenge is a tough one, but our task ultimately is to integrate these two immensely different areas, through building out from continuities wherever they can be found.

To do that effectively, we must both bring in the inherent complexity of modern humans and address the past without oversimplification tailored to the present. The issue is that, with a shortage of comparative possibilities, we can deal with the modern complexity in evolutionary terms largely by projecting it into the past, and testing for its presence or absence. Was there or was there not symbolism, etc.? The risk, however, is that we use the past simply to pave a way up to the present. Anthropocentrism becomes everything, the development of humans is largely unilineal, and we come close to making evolution teleological.

In the British Academy's Centenary Project (2003–10) 'Lucy to Language: The Archaeology of the Social Brain' (the 'Lucy Project' for short), and in the chapters in this volume, we seek to outflank those dangers in several ways. We seek above all to map things out by addressing each area—modern human capabilities, the comparative and its continuities, the nature of social groups and networks—and, wherever possible, we aim to carry out precise testing of archaeological evidence in the past. That is, after all, the major theme of the Lucy Project.

To achieve all this we have to embrace a broad evolutionary framework, which we set out here in the briefest outline. Primates (monkeys and apes) have an important place in it, because they too have social brains. Apes, in particular, have a long history, and have changed less conspicuously over time than most mammalian lineages. Their lifeways and encephalization appear to have been broadly consistent through as much as 20 million years. The comparable social and intellectual capabilities of the modern great apes provide good evidence of that, as they have had separate ancestries from our own for many millions of years (>10 million years for gorillas, >15 million years for orang utans) (Goodman et al. 1989). The ape adaptation is primarily to life in rainforests, and a diet of fruit and herbs. It operates chiefly in small communities that live in small territories. Within these social networks, the capacity for fission and fusion can be an important factor, as indeed it is in humans (Aureli et al. 2008). This 'apehood' provides the deep background to human origins.

Up until 10 to 12 million years ago, we can envisage a world of widespread rainforests, with numerous species of ape present in most parts of the Old World. From that time, there have been huge changes in climate, and consequently in vegetation and animal life. One of the most important events was the collision of the African and Eurasian tectonic plates, leading to extensive faunal interchanges both to north and south

(Golonka 2004; Janis 1993). At the same time, through the Miocene there was a global cooling of temperatures, and regional increases in aridity. Notable perhaps for the beginnings of the hominins, the Mediterranean dried up three times in the Messinian, probably indicating a much wider aridity. Alongside these events, there was the spread of grasslands (in particular, the C4 plants) down through Africa, and major evolution in the fauna that could exploit these changed environments. Developments include the rapid evolution of bovids as grazers and browsers; and the spread of equids from the north, through the tropical regions (Bernor & Lipscomb 1995; deMenocal 2004). In the primate world, this period was associated with the rise and diversification of the Old World monkeys. Hominins did not evolve on their own, but in the midst of this changing diversity.

First traces of the hominids or hominins are fragmentary, but what is now available is vastly better than anything we had available even a few years ago. Finds in central Africa and the eastern Rift Valley show that the earliest hominins already existed 5 to 7 million years ago, apparently occupying dense bush habitats that were certainly not rainforest, but equally were not the open savannas once supposed to be the cradle of human development (Haile-Selassie 2001).

Even with the very sparse evidence we have, a few points are certain:

- large areas became increasingly arid as the Miocene climate cooled;
- in their first 5 million years, hominins did not evolve larger brains, yet they achieved bipedalism and reduced canine teeth;
- their large chewing teeth (megadonty) suggest dietary stress;
- their presence as a 'bush' of species from 4 to 1 million years ago indicates a successful new adaptive radiation.

Thus many hominin adaptations were appearing, but the large human social brain was not one of these. However, lower population densities and wider-ranging patterns were certainly necessitated by the drier habitats. We stress these points, as also the numbers of species in the hominin bush, because they emphasize the great and crucial contrast between 'hominin in general' and 'human in particular', and hence the different explanations that are necessary. Such differences probably have to be approached through separate socio-ecological models.

When we come to the genus *Homo* in the last 2.5 million years, the larger brain can be seen as a defining characteristic. *Homo habilis* was not large-brained in absolute terms, but the move from ca. 450 cc in apes and australopithecines to 650 cc in early *Homo* was nevertheless a major change in encephalization—a 50 per cent increase, also argued to be linked with reorganization of the brain (e.g. Tobias 2005).

Why did that change come so long after the initial hominization? Some authors would see renewed climate change as the driving force. The Quaternary (2.6 Ma to present)[2] heralds further climate change, with strong temperature fluctuations, and the onset of northern latitude glaciations. These increased in intensity about 1 million years ago, when the 100,000 year glacial-interglacial cycle became predominant (Imbrie et al. 1993).

Again, in this context of climatic extremes there are certainly faunal responses. Hominins—unusually for a primate—were able to spread around most of the Old World, although the causes for that new success are far from clear. At first, hominins still existed as several species, with robust australopithecines surviving alongside *Homo* for some time. Recent developments such as the discovery of *Homo flore-siensis* and the mapping of the Neanderthal genome emphasize that *Homo* too evolved into several distinct species (e.g. Brown et al. 2004; Green et al. 2006).

Until 2.5 Ma, the probability is that hominins were restricted to Africa. It is now plain that the second phase of increased encephalization in *Homo* happened *after* the first dispersal through the Old World. The evidence suggests that this new increase in brain size was gradual and occurred over the middle part of the Pleistocene, involving the common ancestors of both Neanderthals and modern humans and continuing into the descendant species. Both species evolved large brains, but the genetics, anatomy and behavioural evidence all indicate different adaptations—different kinds of humanity.

The relevance of this background is that we are not looking at one social brain, predestined to be modern. Rather, we are looking at several series of evolutionary events in which brain enlargement was favoured a number of times over, but sometimes consistently in long-term trends. Out of all this emerged *Homo sapiens*, who evolved through the last half million years of the process, almost certainly within Africa.

---

[2] Ma = millions of years ago.

TESTING THE ARCHAEOLOGY

Advances in our understanding of Palaeolithic archaeology, combined with a much greater sophistication in our knowledge of primate behaviour, evolutionary anthropology and cognitive and neuropsychology, now provide us with an opportunity to explore the scope of these developments (including language, artistic representation and religion) with an intensity that has never previously been possible.

The integrated approach redresses the past modest contribution from archaeology towards the study of evolutionary issues. It also ties evolutionary psychology into the extensive data obtained from the past, allowing us to escape the confined timeframe of the comparatively recent human mind so as to be able to see the latter in its proper historical context.

The core to our approach in the Lucy Project has been to explore how the early hominin brain evolved from its essentially apelike beginnings among the earliest australopithecines (ca. 3–5 Ma) to the modern human potential of the 'Upper Palaeolithic Revolution' (ca. 50,000 years ago). The objective has been to focus both on the inferences we can make from primary evidence, such as stone tools, and on what we can infer about social and cognitive phenomena.

While many key questions have emerged during the course of the past five years' work on the Lucy Project, one particular focus to have emerged has been the fact that both chimpanzees and modern human hunter-gatherers live in dispersed communities in which not all members see each other every day. Even though the Neolithic (or agricultural) Revolution enabled humans to concentrate an entire community in a small, permanent settlement (something that brings its own stresses), the great bulk of our history, stretching back to the common ancestor with the chimpanzees some 6 million years ago, is constituted by these kinds of dispersed social systems. Such social systems are likely to be especially taxing cognitively because individuals have to be able to factor into their social calculations not just the interests of those with whom they happen to be living at that particular moment, but also those other members of the community who happen to be elsewhere (Aureli *et al.* 2008; Barrett *et al.* 2003). Actions or decisions that happen to suit those currently present may not suit all of those absent today but present tomorrow, or next week, or next month.

On the archaeological front, the story has developed enormously in recent years through a combination of field research and comparative and theoretical inputs (Gamble 1999, 2007; Gowlett 1996, 1997; Steele & Shennan 1996). A plethora of new sites has revealed the existence of a taxonomic 'bush' rather than linear speciation (thereby highlighting ecological competition), abundant early technology that is as refined at 2.6 Ma as it is at 1.8 Ma, and raw material transport at distances far beyond those expected. There have been new hominid finds further defining *Homo erectus*, with evidence for dispersal into Eurasia as early as 1.7 Ma. Stable isotope studies have suggested an eventual high dependence on meat-eating (corroborated by studies of butchery sites), and there has been growing evidence for a technological world beyond stone (wooden artefacts in Germany, Israel and Africa, and the probable development of shaped bone technologies from at least 100,000 years ago in Africa: Clark 2001; Goren-Inbar et al. 2002; Klein 2000; Thieme 1999).

Many of these findings are so new that their implications for the social and cognitive aspects of hominid evolution have yet to be fully assessed. In principle, the emergence of distinctively human behaviour could have occurred any time after 2 million years ago (the time at which early brain enlargement can be linked with increasing use of technology). Yet, despite the importance of elucidating the motors of change, conventional approaches in archaeology and palaeontology have isolated few landmarks in this long time sequence that can be resolved through the archaeological evidence alone. Those that have received most attention (brain size, technical developments, fire use, etc.) are ripe for testing against new lines of evidence. One thing is already plain, however: the new data are multidimensional and necessitate multi-stranded approaches, thus allowing much fuller explorations of changes in human capabilities than have been possible hitherto.

Integrating the psychological, anthropological and archaeological approaches provides a unique opportunity to triangulate many aspects of human behaviour, as well as allowing us to set humans into their historical context within the primates. Importantly, we can do so in a way that can easily be applied to fossil populations so as to explore not only the social, demographic and ecological behaviour of now-extinct species, but also the social and demographic stresses that would have been present and, hence, the reasons why individual populations of these species might have gone extinct when they did. Aiello and Dunbar (1993) provided proof of principle for this approach in their analysis of the timing of the evolution of language, and it may now be possible to extend this approach to other aspects of hominin and human behaviour.

ARCHAEOLOGY, SOCIAL BRAIN
AND DISTRIBUTED MIND

We mentioned that almost 3 million years of artefact and tool manufacture and use provide data for tracing key changes. Results from various archaeological proxies have suggested an exponential growth in hominin group size and sociality through the whole period, with the greatest increase occurring from roughly 500,000 years ago. This 'early' model is in striking contrast to studies based on material culture, which seem to show a similar trajectory taking off much more recently—according to some claims, only after around 50,000 BP. How can we compare these results and explain the discrepancies in timing? Can the different lines of evidence be reconciled? Do 'early' models suggest that later developments in material culture were purely quantitative, and what forms of social life do 'late' models attribute to early hominins? What are the implications for our understanding of the social lives of hominins and humans?

While we usually address these questions from archaeology, the concept of the *distributed mind* draws from a diverse interdisciplinary base to consider cognition as embodied, embedded, situated and emergent (Anderson 2003; Bird-David 1999; Brooks 1999; Clark 1997; Hutchins 1995; Lakoff & Johnson 1999; Strathern 1988; Varela et al. 1991). Cognition is thus both physically and socially distributed beyond the individual agent (Clark 1997; Clark & Chalmers 1998; Rowlands 2003; Wilson 2005); relations between hominins/humans and the material environment can thus be seen as facilitating the cognitive process. From an evolutionary perspective, then, material culture can be seen as *integral to* the ongoing negotiation of social practices (Gamble 1999; Knappett 2005), rather than simply a passive reflection or product of such practices.

Viewed as mediating an extended, distributed cognitive system, material culture becomes a physical correlate of that system (Gell 1998) and part of the extended phenotype of the individual agents that comprise it. The notion of the distributed mind thus affords considerable potential for examining the socio-cognitive relationships structuring hominin and human societies. What are the long-term evolutionary implications of the distribution of mind, and what are its ramifications for the study of material culture and the social lives of hominins and humans?

We have aimed to provide an interdisciplinary forum for the debate of these questions. We wanted to examine critically the role of the social brain hypothesis as a potential framework for explaining the story of human evolution and how we came to be the way we are. But we also wanted to bring the notion of distributed cognition to bear on these questions, not least because the extent to which cognition is gradually extended both into the material world and into the social world informs on the nature of what it is to be human. We hope that by following through the themes of the Lucy Project and linking them with the implications of distributed cognition for hominid evolution, we have been able to provide a fresh interdisciplinary agenda for the study of our earliest history.

REFERENCES

Aiello, L. C. & Dunbar, R. I. M. (1993). Neocortex size, group size and the evolution of language. *Current Anthropology* 34: 184–193.

Anderson M. L. (2003). Embodied cognition: a field guide. *Artificial Intelligence* 149: 91–130.

Aureli, F., Schaffner, C., Boesch, C., Bearder, S., Call, J., Chapman, A. et al. (2008). Fission-fusion dynamics: new research frameworks. *Current Anthropology* 49: 627–654.

Barrett, L., Henzi, S. P. & Dunbar, R. I. M. (2003). Primate cognition: from 'what now?' to 'what if?' *Trends in Cognitive Sciences* 7: 494–497.

Barton, R. A. & Dunbar, R. I. M. (1997). Evolution of the social brain. In: A. Whiten & R. Byrne (eds) *Machiavellian Intelligence II*, pp. 240–263. Cambridge: Cambridge University Press.

Bernor, R. L. & Lipscomb, D. (1995). A consideration of Old World hipparionine horse phylogeny and global abiotic processes. In: E. S. Vrba, G. H. Denton, T. C. Partridge & L. H. Burckle (eds) *Palaeoclimate and evolution, with emphasis on human origins*, pp. 164–177. New Haven, CT and London: Yale University Press.

Bird-David, N. (1999). 'Animism' revisited: personhood, environment, and relational epistemology. *Current Anthropology* 40: 67–91.

Brooks, R. A. (1999). *Cambrian intelligence: the early history of the new*. Cambridge MA: MIT Press.

Brown, P., Sutikna, T., Morwood, M. J., Soejono, R. P., Jatmiko, Wayhu Saptomo, E. et al. (2004). A new small-bodied hominin from the Late Pleistocene of Flores, Indonesia. *Nature* 431: 1055–1061.

Clark, A. (1997). *Being there: bringing brain, body and world together again*. Cambridge, MA: MIT Press.

Clark, A. & Chalmers, D. A. (1998). The extended mind. *Analysis* 58: 7–19.

Clark, J. D. (ed.) (2001). *Kalambo Falls prehistoric site*, vol. 3. Cambridge: Cambridge University Press.

deMenocal, P. B. (2004). African climate change and faunal evolution during the Pliocene-Pleistocene. *Earth and Planetary Science Letters* 220: 3–24.

Dunbar, R. I. M. (1992). Coevolution of neocortex size, group size and language in humans. *Behavioral and Brain Sciences* 16: 681–735.

Dunbar, R. I. M. (1998). The social brain hypothesis. *Evolutionary Anthropology* 6: 178–190.

Dunbar, R. I. M. (1999). Culture, honesty and the freerider problem. In: R. I. M. Dunbar, C. Knight & C. Power (eds) *The evolution of culture*, pp. 194–213. Edinburgh: Edinburgh University Press.

Dunbar, R. I. M. (2003). The social brain: mind, language and society in evolutionary perspective. *Annual Review of Anthropology* 32: 163–181.

Dunbar, R. I. M. & Shultz, S. (2007). Understanding primate brain evolution. *Philosophical Transactions of the Royal Society, London* 362B: 649–658.

Gamble, C. (1999). *The Palaeolithic societies of Europe*. Cambridge: Cambridge University Press.

Gamble, C. (2007). *Origins and revolutions: human identity in earliest prehistory*. Cambridge: Cambridge University Press.

Gell, A. (1998). *Art and agency: towards a new anthropological theory*. Oxford: Clarendon Press.

Golonka, J. (2004). Plate tectonic evolution of the southern margin of Eurasia in the Mesozoic and Cenozoic. *Tectonophysics* 381: 235– 273.

Goodman, M., Koop, B. F., Czelusniak, J., Fitch, D. H. A., Tagle, D. A. & Slighton, J. L. (1989). Molecular phylogeny of the family of apes and humans. *Genome* 31: 316–335.

Goren-Inbar, N., Werker, E. & Feibel, C. S. (2002). *The Acheulian site of Gesher Benot Ya'aqov, Israel: the wood assemblage*, vol. 1. Oxford: Oxbow Books.

Gowlett, J. A. J. (1996). The frameworks of early hominid social systems. In: J. Steele & S. Shennan (eds) *The archaeology of human ancestry*, pp. 135–183. London: Routledge.

Gowlett, J. A. J. (1997). Why the muddle in the middle matters: the language of comparative and direct in human evolution. In: C. M. Barton & G. A. Clark (eds) *Rediscovering Darwin: evolutionary theory in archaeological explanation*, pp. 49–65. Arizona: Archaeological Papers of the American Anthropological Association No. 7.

Green, R. E., Krause, J., Ptak, S. E., Briggs, A. W., Ronan, M. T., Simons, J. F. et al. (2006). Analysis of one million base pairs of Neanderthal DNA. *Nature* 444: 330–336.

Haile-Selassie, Y. (2001). Late Miocene hominids from the Middle Awash, Ethiopia. *Nature* 412: 178–181.

Hill, R. A. & Dunbar, R. I. M. (2003). Social network size in humans. *Human Nature* 14: 53–72.

Hutchins, E. (1995). *Cognition in the wild*. Cambridge, MA: MIT Press.

Imbrie, J., Berger, A., Boyle, E. A., Clemens, S. C., Duffy, A., Howard, W. R. et al. (1993). On the structure and origin of major glaciation cycles, Part 2. The 100,000–year cycle. *Paleoceanography* 8: 699–735.

Janis, C. M. (1993). Tertiary mammal evolution in the context of changing climates, vegetation, and tectonic events. *Annual Review of Ecology and Systematics* 24: 467–500.

Klein, R.G. (2000). Archeology and the evolution of human behaviour. *Evolutionary Anthropology* 9: 17–36.

Knappett, C. (2005). *Thinking through material culture: an interdisciplinary perspective*. Pittsburgh: University of Pennsylvania Press.

Knight, C. (2008). Early human kinship was matrilineal. In: N. Allen, H. Callan, R. Dunbar & W. James (eds) *Early human kinship: from sex to social reproduction*, pp. 61–82. Oxford: Blackwell.

Kudo, H. & Dunbar, R. I. M. (2001). Neocortex size and social network size in primates. *Animal Behaviour* 62: 711–722.

Lakoff, G. & Johnson, M. (1999). *Philosopy in the flesh: the embodied mind and its challenge to Western thought*. New York: Basic Books.

Rowlands, M. (2003). *Externalism: putting mind and world back together again*. Chesham: Acumen.

Steele, J. & Shennan, S. (eds) (1996). *The archaeology of human ancestry*. London: Routledge.

Stiller, J. & Dunbar, R. I. M. (2007). Perspective-taking and social network size in humans. *Social Networks* 29: 93–104.

Strathern, M. (1988). *The gender of the gift: problems with women and problems with society in Melanesia*. Berkeley: University of California Press.

Thieme, H. (1999). Altpaläolithische Holzgeräte aus Schöningen, Lkr. Helmstadt. *Germania* 77: 451–487.

Tobias, P. V. (2005). Tools and brains: which came first? In: F. d'Errico & L. Backwell (eds) *From tools to symbols: from early hominids to modern humans*, pp. 82–102. Johannesburg: Witwatersrand University Press.

Varela, F. J., Thompson, E. & Rosch, E. (1991). *The embodied mind: cognitive science and human experience*. Cambridge MA: MIT Press.

Wilson, R. A. (2005). Collective memory, group minds, and the extended mind thesis. *Cognitive Process online*.

2

Technologies of Separation and the Evolution of Social Extension

CLIVE GAMBLE

A tendency in the West to see emotions as soft and social attachments as messy has made theoreticians turn to cognition as the preferred guide of human behaviour. We celebrate rationality. This is so despite the fact that psychological research suggests the primacy of affect; that is, that human behaviour derives above all from fast automated emotional judgments, and only secondarily from slower conscious processes. (de Waal 2006, 6)

OFFICIAL HISTORIES AND PREHISTORIES

WHEN DID HOMININ BRAINS become human minds? Until recently the question has received few answers from archaeologists, but rather more answers than to the question of how this happened. The default position has been to rely on technology, and material culture more broadly, as a proxy for the evolving mental capabilities of larger brains. However, such simple correlations, inspired by a progressive view of human evolution, now lack conviction. The reason is simple. The evidence points to a time lag of some 500,000 years between significant advances in brain size and the much later appearance of art, architecture, writing and numeracy (Mithen 1996, 11). These were the headline changes, gradually introduced, to a complex material culture, from which a wide variety of identities were fashioned in ever increasingly complicated social geographies. It is argued that once these proxies are found the human mind had arrived, albeit rather delayed (Mellars & Stringer 1989; Mellars et al. 2007). When this process started is unclear: 'after 100kyr' covers much but not all of the data. But 'where' *is* known: Africa (see Barham ch. 18 this volume; Henshilwood & Marean 2003; McBrearty 2007; McBrearty & Brooks 2000).

Proceedings of the British Academy **158**, 17–42. © The British Academy 2010.

These proxies are widely regarded as evidence for the advent of symbol-based cognition. Human society was now running according to symbolic codes enshrined in specially designed objects such as figurines,
ornaments and hunting gear, arranged in culturally determined patterns
across regions and within living areas (Gamble 1986). After 60,000 years
ago, and along with a global diaspora (Gamble 2008), there was a marked
increase in such material proxies across many parts of the Old World,
although different continental records, notably Australia and South East
Asia, show that such step-changes in frequency were not universal
(Brumm & Moore 2005).

A late appearance of the human mind fits well with what Hutchins
(1995, 356) calls the 'official' history of cognitive science. Here cognition
takes place within the individual's skull/skin and is seen as independent
from the culture and environment that lie beyond such a boundary.
Essential to an internalist model is the competence of the brain to process
symbols, and archaeologists have enshrined such a view in their discussions of a 'symbolic revolution' late in human evolution (see Barnard ch.
12 this volume; Cauvin 2000; Chase & Dibble 1987; d'Errico et al. 2003;
Henshilwood & Marean 2003; Hodder 2001; Lindly & Clark 1990;
Renfrew 2001).

Hutchins criticizes the power of the internal model by examining
Simon and Kaplan's (1989) claim that the computer was made in the
image of a human mind. Adopting an externalist perspective to the mind
he disagrees, arguing instead that the computer was made in the image of
the formal manipulations of abstract symbols, such as arithmetic and
computing (Hutchins 1995, 363). These formal systems are not metaphors
of how cognition works inside our skulls but of the socio-cultural system
that exists both inside and outside our skins and which provides the architecture of cognition. Hutchins concludes, correctly, that we 'must carefully
distinguish between the tasks that the person faces in the manipulation of
symbolic tokens and the tasks that are accomplished by the manipulation
of the symbolic tokens' (1995, 367). Without such a distinction it is all too
easy to mistake the properties of the socio-cultural system for the properties of the person. And this is precisely what archaeologists have done with
their use of material proxies. They have inferred accomplishments, such as
language and visual representation, rather than the cognitive tasks
involved in manipulating symbolic tokens and exploring the evolutionary
contexts that led to such skills.

To address this shortfall I will argue in this chapter for a different
model based on the extended or distributed mind (Clark & Chalmers

1998; Coward & Gamble 2008; Wilson 2004). Here the skull/skin boundary is porous so that not all cognition takes place in the head. Central to this formulation is the concept that the architecture of cognition (that which allows us to cognize) is also external to the individual (Rowlands 2003). As Thomas puts it, 'Mind, body and world are not ontologically different spheres: they are categories which people have created, and which often serve to lead us to misunderstand ourselves' (1998, 151). With this perspective culture ceases to be a collection of tangible and abstract things and becomes 'a human cognitive process that takes place both inside and outside the minds of people' (Hutchins 1995, 354). Such a definition, I will argue, makes the question 'When did hominin brains become human minds?' the preserve of ancestors other than *Homo sapiens*, and opens up an avenue for understanding how this occurred. I will examine the process of hominization through the lens of the social brain and, by examining technologies of separation, move the debate away from an emphasis on the accomplishments of the modern mind to the evolutionary processes involved.

INTERNALIST MODELS OF THE PREHISTORIC MIND

Claims for the recency of human origins (Proctor 2003) resonate widely in Western societies because of the historical observation that modernity is always deferred (Andy Jones pers. comm.). It matters little if the first humans were hunter-gatherers or farmers (see Coward ch. 21 this volume) but rather that they were *Homo sapiens*. Understanding how modernity arose requires antecedents that are simply not us (Thomas 2004) and the presence/absence of material proxies for symbol-based cognition has been used by archaeologists to support this central claim.

For example, two important archaeological studies of the evolution of the mind illustrate how archaeological data are used to support an internalist model of the recent human mind. In *Human evolution, language and mind* Noble and Davidson argue that mind and language are co-extensive (1996, 10). Language is the key to distinctive modern human behaviours such as self-awareness that they regard as an expression of mindedness. Language allows us to act as the perceivers of a human world where we agonize, reminisce and make plans (1996, 215). Mind accounts for the varied ways that humans 'go about their business' (1996, 10), and language makes this possible because its constituent signs are symbols that, through convention, stand for things other than themselves. Noble and

Davidson argue that the evidence points to a late appearance in human evolution of acceptable proxies for symbol processing.

In *The prehistory of the mind*, Mithen begins by considering two metaphors of the mind: a sponge and a computer (1996, 34). He prefers the latter, where the brain is the hardware and the mind its software, but asks, what programs are running? For Mithen, minds do far more than simply compute. They create novel associations. To illustrate how this occurred during human evolution he uses an architectural metaphor of cognitive spaces to describe a general intelligence and its four mental modules, which become increasingly interlinked by a process of cognitive fluidity. This associative process had selective advantages in the context of males provisioning females with food, since females bore the costs of longer periods of infant dependency that resulted from larger-brained children (1996, 209). Cognitive fluidity achieved new connections rather than new processing power, and 'consequently this mental transformation occurred with no increase in brain size . . . It was, in essence, the origins of the symbolic capacity that is unique to the human mind' (1996, 209). Cognitive fluidity therefore accounts for the temporal lag between brain size and the late appearance of symbolic proxies. It was the ultimate internal programme, possessed only by modern humans.

However, there have been dissenting voices against a late flowering of symbolism. These concern problems of inference from the evidence:

> Measurable differences in anatomy during late stages in hominid evolution . . . can tell us little about unquantifiable differences in cognitive or symbolic capacity. Similarly, quantifiable differences in artifactual style or complexity, whether in stone tools or symbolic products, can tell us little about the capacity for problem solving or symbolic thought among these different late populations. (Marshack 1990, 459)

They also caution that evidence of absence is not necessarily absence of evidence:

> The isolated evidence for symbolic behaviour by early but behaviourally modern Australians reflects a similar pattern to the isolated evidence for symbolic behaviour in the Middle Pleistocene archaeological record of the Old World. (Brumm & Moore 2005, 169)

Marshack's arguments that hominins other than *Homo sapiens* were producing symbolic artefacts failed to convince many at the time (Chase & Dibble 1987; d'Errico & Villa 1997; Noble & Davidson 1996). His attempts to demonstrate that markings on 20,000-year-old bones by modern humans were notational systems based on lunar phases (Marshack 1972)

were also challenged (d'Errico 1996), although they are now widely
accepted as externalized memory devices forming part of practices
termed 'conscious symbolic storage' (d'Errico et al. 2003, 31–33). Some
advance has also been made in linking items of a symbolic technology
with Neanderthals (d'Errico 2003; Zilhão 2007), although close proximity in time to the arrival in Europe of modern humans from Africa makes
others sceptical that the *Homo sapiens* human mind barrier has really
been breached (Mellars 2005). However, what characterizes the debate is
that all its participants are wedded to the same concept of the internal
mind that stops at the skin. Accordingly, the mind of the 'modern
human', even if it is in a Neanderthal skull, processes symbols from
within individual heads. The outcomes of these manipulations are codes
for cultural action that interface with other similarly isolated minds to
create a collective.

EXTERNAL MINDS

The alternative notion of an extended mind has been pursued by archaeologists investigating concepts of personhood (Chapman 2000; Fowler
2004; Gamble 2007) and the agency of objects (Jones 2002; Knappett
2005; Malafouris 2004; Robb 2004). Gosden (in press) has even argued
for the death of the mind, claiming that the holistic nature of human sen-
sibility in our engagement with the material world can only be appreciated by discarding the baggage of a disembodied mental space: the mind.

Externalist approaches to cognition that fall under the banners of the
extended or distributed mind are concerned with those holistic sensibili-
ties that reunite people with the world. Clark and Chalmers (1998, 9) have
termed this engagement *active externalism* in the recognition that objects,
and features external to the individual generally, are coupled with the
human organism and so play a key role in everyday lives. Cognition is
therefore embodied (Anderson 2003; Wilson 2004), as revealed by neuroimaging (Gallese 2006), and intimately connected to the varied tasks of
manipulating symbolic tokens.

Of particular interest here is how an externalist position changes the
view of culture and the processing of symbols presented by the internalist model as the achievement of the human mind. In his discussion of
vehicle externalism, extending the architecture of cognition beyond skin,
Rowlands (2003, 166) argues that greater fitness results when individuals
get the environment to do some of their cognitive tasks. One example is

illustrated by his 'barking dog' principle (why have a dog and bark yourself?). The principle applies to evolutionary situations where, while certain activities are adaptive it may be more costly to develop internal mechanisms when the alternative exists of combining pre-existing internal mechanisms with the manipulation of the external environment.

Rowlands' (ch. 16 this volume) argument for extended cognition should not, however, be confused with archaeologists' interest in external cognitive storage (d'Errico et al. 2003; Renfrew & Scarre 1998) also known as artificial memory systems (d'Errico 1998). The latter is an example of the internal model of cognition applied to material culture and its symbolic manipulation. Written texts, measurement systems and styles of making and building things are presented as cognitive dumps outside the body; reference libraries or, to update the metaphor, memory sticks that act symbolically like the mind inside the skull. Their appearance in the archaeological record is taken to indicate that symbol-based cognition has been accomplished and entry to a human mind achieved. The ideas borrow heavily from Donald's model of cognitive evolution, which argues for a separate ontology of mind and world:

> When I coined the term 'external symbolic storage', I was simply singling out the most salient and indisputable property of material culture: *it exists only in relation to interpretive codes stored inside the heads of the people who invented it*, that is, inside their 'biological' memory systems. (Donald 1998b, 184, my emphasis)

What is lacking in such characterizations is a notion of cognitive ownership, defined by Rowlands (ch. 16 this volume) as 'the appropriate sort of integration into the life—and in particular the psychological life—of a subject'.

Finally, language is an obvious and important instance of such vehicle externalism by which cognitive processes are extended into the world (Clark & Chalmers 1998, 11). However, vehicle externalism also applies to material culture. Chapman's use of fragmentation theory in archaeology has shown that the intentional breaking of pots, dismembering animal carcasses and knapping flint were activities that enchained people and objects (2000; Chapman & Gaydarska 2007). Here material culture acts as a scaffold for relationships that tie people to the world and which clearly act as part of an internal/external cognitive architecture.

In summary, the externalist model of the mind brings the senses and emotions back into the cognitive mix, much as de Waal (2006) argues in my opening quote. Cognition becomes a relational endeavour rather than simply a rational programme. Rather than dwelling on accomplishments, archaeologists can turn instead to the tasks that required the manipulation of symbolic-tokens. As a result, the externalist model does not consider the uniqueness of the mind to reside solely its ability to process symbols, and it provides a cogent explanation of why the material world, although inanimate, has always had a form of agency.

THE ENCEPHALIZATION EVENT 600,000 YEARS AGO

The challenge that faces archaeologists is to account for evolutionary developments to external cognition without using the familiar crutch of material culture proxies for symbol-based cognition. This is where the social brain hypothesis—the assertion that our social lives drove the enlargement of our brains—acts as a framework to address emotional affect and organize the archaeological data in new ways for evolutionary analysis.

Ruff et al. have shown that in the period 1.8 Ma to 600,000 years ago the various species of *Homo* then extant were about one-third less encephalized than modern populations (1997, 174). The encephalization quotient (EQ) that scales brain to body size, moreover, shows no increase during this period. This is in marked contrast to the following 500,000 years, during which the value for EQ rises to within 10 per cent of recent populations. Rightmire (2004) confirms this trend (see Figure 2.1), pointing to a marked increase in cranial capacity and EQ for *Homo heidelbergensis* after 600,000 years ago.

Such increases in brain size are not, as Rightmire and many others have commented, matched by comparable changes in technology. A tradition of stone working (Acheulean biface) that first appeared in Africa 1.4 Ma ago is found throughout much of the inhabited Old World and continues for at least a further 300,000 years after the encephalization event. Other, older, traditions of stone working (Oldowan flake/core; de la Torre 2004) are seemingly unaffected by encephalization and continue unchanged for even longer outside the Acheulean distribution in South East Asia (Dennell & Roebroeks 2005; Moore & Brumm 2007). Alternative traditions, most notably prepared core technologies (Levallois flake and Prismatic blade) are widespread after 300,000 years ago (Foley & Lahr 1997; McNabb et al. 2004; Rolland 1995). Evidence for the control of fire becomes more common after 500,000 years ago (Gowlett ch. 17 this volume) and the data on the systematic hunting of prime-aged animals at this time is now compelling (Pope & Roberts 2005; Thieme 2005). However, both these

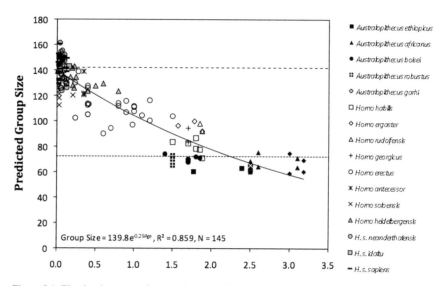

Figure 2.1. The development of group size as predicted from increases in neocortex ratios of fossil skulls. The squares plot the changing cranial volumes from which group size is interpolated (Aiello & Dunbar 1993, updated by Matt Grove). The horizontal lines indicate threshold group sizes that require 20% (lower line) and 40% (upper line) of the time budget to be devoted to integration by social grooming. The fitted line is an exponential relating group size to age.

activities—the controlled use of fire and hunting—are expected to go even further back in time to long before the encephalization event (Wrangham et al. 1999). This is not the case for changes in the organization of living spaces: traces of architecture remain elusive until after 60,000 years ago (Gamble 2007).

Encephalization and technological innovation do not therefore go brain in hand after 600,000 years ago. There is no flowering of ornament and art, although the case for burial 500,000 years ago has been strengthened by finds in the Sima de los Huesos at Atapuerca, Spain (Carbonell et al. 2003). In short, symbol-based cognition, and hence the human mind, can be as old (McBrearty 2007), or as poorly represented archaeologically (Brumm & Moore 2005), or as recent (Renfrew 2007) as you wish.

SOCIAL BRAINS AND GROUPS

The evolutionary consequences of the encephalization event 600,000 years ago are twofold. First, as Aiello and Dunbar (1993) originally proposed and Dunbar has since investigated further (2003; Dunbar & Shultz

2007), a strong relationship exists between neocortex size and group size amongst primates. Cranial capacity is one measure of brain size that does survive in fossil populations and when plotted shows predicted group sizes of 120 for *Homo heidelbergensis* 600,000 years ago, rising to 150 for anatomically modern humans (AMH) (see Figure 2.1). Second, as Aiello and Wheeler (1995) have pointed out, for metabolic reasons, such an increase in brain size had to be compensated for by a decrease in the size of another tissue: the gut. Since the brain is an energetically expensive tissue, as it expanded in size and the intestines shrank, diet quality had to be improved. This exchange was made through increased use of animal protein and cooking with fire, which compensated for the reduced processing power of the stomach (Wrangham et al. 1999).

Encephalization was therefore achieved at a considerable cost, both biological and behavioural, suggesting strong selective pressures. The best candidates for such selection pressure are the benefits that accrue to individuals as an outcome of living in larger groups. Here 'group' does not necessarily refer to an integrated group of individuals moving as a single unit, but rather to the pattern of dispersed local groups drawn from the wider community. These are the fission-fusion systems of chimpanzees and humans (Lehmann et al. 2007) where the whole community is rarely found together in one place at one time. While membership of these local foraging groups can be unstable due to local ecological conditions, it is nonetheless invariably drawn from members of the community. This dispersed form of sociality, with several grouping levels, appears to be broadly characteristic of the hominids in general, and may thus be typical of all hominins (Aureli et al. 2008).

This brief outline of the social brain model suggests at least two examples of vehicle externalism. The first is Aiello and Dunbar's (1993) proposal that larger communities inferred from brain size would have required new ways to facilitate interaction. The primate method of social grooming proves too costly in terms of time spent for group sizes above 70. Aiello and Dunbar's solution was that under this selection pressure language would provide a more efficient and rapid means of integrating the group. This adaptive solution can be evaluated in the context of the extended mind model where, as described by Clark and Chalmers, 'Language . . . is not a mirror of our inner states but a complement to them. It serves as a tool whose role is to extend cognition in ways that on-board devices cannot' (1998, 18). Language, in their terms, allows us to spread the burden of interaction between agents out into the world and was a consequence of the encephalization event.

The second example applies Rowlands' barking dog principle to a technological innovation. The consequence of larger brains is a reduced length to the intestine which results in less efficient processing of food. This is where cooking is important, as roasting in a fire breaks down the enzymes in animal protein prior to ingestion and thereby increases processing efficiency. As a result cooking has been likened to an external stomach (Aiello 1998; Wrangham et al. 1999) since it does the work of digestion that was previously an exclusively internal function. Cooking therefore became part of the cognitive architecture of hominins since it coupled an internal development (brain size) with an external manipulation of the environment (fire cooking).

TECHNOLOGIES OF SEPARATION

Here then is the relevance of the social brain hypothesis for any archaeological study of human evolution: that increases in community size due to encephalization impacted on the number of local groups and individuals that needed to be integrated. The internal mind solution, as we have seen, invokes symbol-based cognition in order to create new webs of associations between independent minds acting in groups. Evidence is then sought for artificial memory systems (AMS) (d'Errico 1998). But as we have seen, there is a chronological disconnect that is difficult to explain between the frequent appearance of symbolic proxies for AMS and the measure of social complexity indicated by encephalization. Moreover, the distributed nature of hominid sociality, seen most strongly in fission-fusion systems, suggests that extended cognition provides a better model with which to address the relation between community size and local groupings. Hominins have evolved technologies of separation using both psychotropic (Smail 2008) and material resources in response to the evolutionary pressures of larger community membership comprising more local groupings. These technologies allow cognitive ownership (Rowlands ch. 16 this volume) by integrating the psychological life of the individual within those local groups.

But how? The answer is that human societies are well wrapped and almost infinitely stretched. They are enfolded by concepts such as kinship (see Allen et al. 2008; Read ch. 10 this volume), while an individual's identity is distributed through time and across spaces they will never directly experience. Social extension would be impossible without harnessing the environment as part of our cognitive architecture. Furthermore, as the prehistory of hominin dispersal shows (Gamble 1993) three-quarters of the earth was inhabited late, beginning with the settlement of Australia some 60,000 years ago. However, people did not arrive in Australia because they first thought of symbolic sandy beaches and convinced themselves that was sufficient reason to move. They arrived because they had first accomplished the cognitive task of manipulating symbols in conjunction with the external world, which then allowed them to achieve the task of extending their social worlds and, coincidentally in this instance, their geographical extent. It would therefore be a mistake to equate a new, global distribution for *Homo sapiens* with a modern distributed mind. And the same would apply to a similar equation with the appearance of proxies such as rock art or monumental architecture. Social extension has a longer evolutionary history allied to the integration of local groups within larger communities. It needs to be understood in terms of the evolving technologies of separation that include bright ideas like boats, but equally the conceptual wrappings of active externalism.

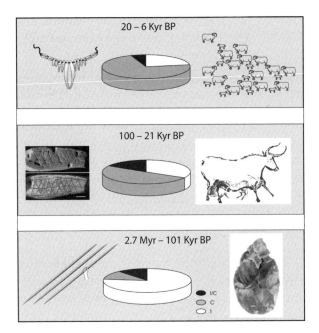

Figure 2.2. Changing popularity of instruments (I), containers (C) and hybrid forms of material culture (I/C) in three periods of human evolution. Containers enfold and include jewellery and art that wraps the body and the walls of living spaces. For a full discussion see Gamble (2007, Figure 7.1)

I have taken this last point further by examining social technologies in terms of two categories; instruments and containers (Gamble 2007). The reason for this simple division derives from the metaphorical use of material culture where one thing is experienced in terms of another. In this instance our bodies with their limbs (instruments) and trunk/head (containers) infuse material culture with its metaphorical understanding based on bodily sensation and experience.

The technologies prior to the explosion in variety after 60,000 years ago are predominantly, but never exclusively, instrument-based (Gamble 2007). It is not until much later that the world of containers, with which we are so familiar and which enfold us in a variety of sizes and forms, from socks to buildings, cars to cities, came to prominence (Figure 2.2). Indeed, the rise in popularity of containers is a key question for the archaeology of distributed cognition, since they bring with them a different metaphorical experience of ourselves as socially extended.

SOCIAL EXTENSION

To address this last question I will examine the following three aspects of social extension.

- *Ontological security*: confidence that the natural and social worlds are as they appear to be, including the basic existential parameters of self and social identity (Giddens 1984, 375);
- *Psychological continuity*: achieved by a coupling of the biological organism and external resources into an extended system so as to prevent fragmentation into occurrent states (Clark & Chalmers 1998, 18);
- *Extension of self*: how the limitations of individual 'presence' are transcended by the 'stretching' of social relations across time and space (Giddens 1984, 35).

These components of social extension were common to all hominins but varied in terms of scale and intensity as they do among extant primates.

Ontological security

Elsewhere I have introduced the concept of the childscape, or environment of development (Coward & Gamble 2008, 1972; Gamble 2007), to examine changing identities during human evolution. A childscape consists of arrays of attachment figures (Fonagy et al. 2007), material culture, sensations and emotions. In the context of the extended mind it is less the case that the child grows within this environment as it is grown by it (Gamble 2007, 227–230; Ingold 2000, 227). It is through the childscape that the child learns how the world relates to her, and she to all its myriad components. The childscape is therefore central to a person's ontological security and is another example of vehicle externalism. But what is of interest to human evolution are the components of those childscape arrays and how they contributed to change. The change in arrays from instruments to containers (Figure 2.2) implies a different set of growing experiences, just as a hominin child grown by language and music will be different from one that is not.

Likewise, if the attachment figures possessed different belief-states or intentionality, as recognized in theory of mind (ToM), then this will grow the child differently, and particularly in terms of the tasks required to accomplish social extension. Prior to the encephalization event 600,000 years ago, Dunbar has argued from brain size in primates that most early *Homo* managed level 2 intentionality and hence ToM (2003, 178; see Table 2.1). This level of ToM is reached by children over 4 years of age and is the ability to appreciate that another person holds a different view concerning your actions: that they have a different mind. This was an increase on level 1 ToM as shown by self-recognition among great apes and elephants (Plotnik et al. 2006) and, by comparison with brain size, the australopithecines. Intentionality above level 2 was certainly achievable prior to

Table 2.1. Four levels of intentionality in theory of mind (adapted from Cole 2008 with permission). In this example the use of costume, weaponry and mannerisms would all act to support Dave's intentions, and indeed without such active externalism the different belief states at level 2 could not be achieved.

Level 1	Level 2	Level 3	Level 4
Ego is self aware	Ego recognizes another person's belief-states as similar/different to theirs	Ego wants another person to recognize Ego's own belief state	Ego believes that the group understands that another person recognizes Ego's own belief states
Dave (the re-enactor) *believes* he is a Crusader	Dave *believes* that Ben (a fellow re-enactor) *thinks* he is a Crusader	Dave *desires* that Ben *believes* that Dave *thinks* he is a Crusader	Dave *knows* that the re-enactment group are *aware* that Ben *believes* that Dave *thinks* he is a Crusader

the encephalization event (Dunbar 2003, Figure 4). It involves increasingly lengthy chains of relationships predicated on assumptions and intentions about what you want others to believe about you (level 3), and the shared understandings (level 4) that sustain such cultural creations (Cole 2008). These relational chains typically include the intentions of ancestors, supernatural beings and their material manifestations. The result is a complex imaginary geography, a landscape of relationships over which social extension is laid.

Psychological continuity

The social brain model points to larger group/community sizes at the encephalization event. Since hominin societies are characterized by a fission-fusion pattern, these larger groups raise not only the issue of higher interaction costs for existing methods, such as grooming, but also pose the issue of psychological continuity; how is the identity of the self performed before different people in different social contexts? Language acted not only as an on-board means to reduce the costs of interaction, as proposed by Aiello and Dunbar, but also, as Clark and Chalmers suggest, a means of off-setting the cognitive load on individuals into the environment. It is therefore not surprising that an increase in brain size, community size and the appearance of language does not immediately transform the material worlds of these early hominins or hasten the advent of the iPhone by several hundreds of thousands of years. The explanation is that these hominins were only interested in symbols to the extent that they re-stated ontological security and provided psychological continuity in an expanded social world.

In a seminal archaeological study, Johnson (1982) showed how the fission-fusion societies of Kalahari hunters and gatherers adjust to the increasing size of local groups. When population around waterholes increased as people walked in, so the size of their camping units also changed from nuclear to extended families. In the absence of an established hierarchy to organize affairs this simple camping shift kept the number of comparable social units to be integrated at three and thereby solved some of the problems of communication stress that arise with larger aggregations. Coping with fluid membership in this manner relies on well-wrapped concepts such as kinship and can potentially be achieved without any material proxies for symbol-based cognition.

Extension of self

The final element addresses the extension of self and identity in time and space, what has been referred to as the release from proximity and which distinguishes the human from the primate community (Gamble 1998; Rodseth et al. 1991). The difficulty here is to apply the first two elements of social extension to situations outside co-presence. We extend into the world but how does the world extend back in to us? Symbols provide an answer for the internalist model and, where a mechanism such as Mithen's cognitive fluidity gives them new meaning, that results in social extension. However, an external view of cognition brings into play the senses and the emotions that suggest the following, alternative explanation.

(1) Amplifying emotions: the Acheulean gaze

The importance of emotions in human evolution has been championed by Turner (2000). He argues that natural selection worked to create more associative or positive emotions, such as happiness, sympathy and love, to build sociality and solidarity. The raw materials are the primary emotions (Table 2.2), shared with all mammals, and which ever since Darwin have been recognized as having adaptive importance.

Turner also identifies shame and guilt as two secondary emotions found only in humans (Table 2.2). These, he argues (2000, 82), depend on

Table 2.2. Turner's (2000) conception of how primary emotions vary. The levels of intensity are illustrative only and many other examples can be provided. The point is not to develop a typology of emotions but to indicate the range and nuance of human and hominin emotions that are available for constructing social ties.

Secondary emotions		Shame and guilt (about consequences to self)			Shame and guilt (at self)
High intensity	Joy	Terror		Loathing	Sorrow
Medium intensity	Cheerful	Anxiety		Displeased	Gloomy
Low intensity	Serenity	Hesitant		Irritated	Downcast
Primary emotions	**Satisfaction-happiness**	**Aversion-fear**		**Assertion-anger**	**Disappointment-sadness**

a theory of mind. As a result, they provide a moral basis for group behaviour; a situation that would be expected with advances in social complexity resulting from encephalization and the cognitive ability to infer higher levels of intentionality (Dunbar 2003). Moreover, primary and secondary emotions among humans are not limited to contexts of co-presence. And although attenuation might be expected due to time and distance between face-to-face encounters, such expectations are often contradicted by bonds of kinship and the power of objects.

Emotions form a core around which human—and by extension hominin—social lives are scaffolded. Proxies, as required by the official prehistory of the mind, will be impossible to find. However, framing the enquiry in terms of the social brain issue of community size and local group integration allows us to map the relative evolutionary position of these orders of emotion (Table 2.3) and to ask how they developed.

Humans, and by extension hominins, exhibit several unique psychotropic adaptations that amplify emotional affect. For example, Dunbar (ch. 8 this volume) proposes a solution to Deacon's dilemma (1997, 388) of why hominins have monogamous pair-bonding in terms of infatuation, commonly presented as the love-struck gaze. This human characteristic of highly focused attention between two people also applies to the world of things and ranges over everything we are enthused by, from beloved pets, shiny cars and stamp collections to national flags.

The absence of equivalent focused attention among primates is one reason for their only rudimentary manufacturing skills in wood and stone (Davidson & McGrew 2005). By contrast, the artificial symmetry achieved by hominins who made Acheulean bifaces more than a million years ago is evidence of developed attention skills (Kohn & Mithen 1999) as well as working memory and spatial competence (Wynn 1995; Wynn & Coolidge 2004). While their symmetry undoubtedly had functional advantages when butchering large animals, the affect of these objects also needs to be considered. This can be appreciated by addressing the cognitive tasks that such symmetry represented rather than dwelling exclusively on what the objects accomplished as artefacts (Gowlett 1984). The attention necessary for their manufacture and the repetition of such acts at many times and places can never be reduced to a simple emotional assessment—satisfaction and pride at aesthetic success, disgust at failure—although such responses were likely. Rather they formed elements in an external cognitive architecture by which hominins achieved social extension within local groups and a wider community. Bifaces were therefore never symbols either of cognitive processes or artificial memory systems

Table 2.3. A map of emotions, material culture and intentionality among hominins. Social crying and laughter are unique to humans and by inference any hominin that achieved a theory of mind, level 2 intentionality.

Intentionality	Hominin	Age	Community size	Emotions	Amplifying mechanisms	Material metaphors
Level 4 and greater	*Homo sapiens/neanderthalensis*	<100Ka	150	(*Memory boxes*)	Religion, myth, literature	**Containers** Instruments
Level 3	*Homo erectus/ heidelbergensis*	600Ka	120	Secondary emotions	Language, ceremony	↕
Level 2	*Early Homo habilis/ergaster*	<1.8Ma	100	(*Acheulean gaze*)	Dance, music crying, laughter, focused gaze	
Level 1	Australopithecines	2.5Ma	70	Primary emotions	Aversion, satisfaction, disappointment, assertion	**Instruments** Containers

existing only in relation to interpretive codes stored inside people's heads (Donald 1998b, 184). Instead they were necessary and highly selected elements in hominin social lives that were scaffolded around an emotional core. That core, which at its most basic contains the primary emotions shared by all social animals, was elaborated in this instance through focused attention—the Acheulean gaze, if you like. When applied to sexual partners this gaze produced novel pair-bonded arrangements (Dunbar ch. 8 this volume) and similar affection resulted in original stone objects such as symmetrical hand-axes.

But the Acheulean gaze was not the only embodied mechanism that hominins had to amplify emotional affect and so potentially impact on their ability to extend social relations in time and space. Social laughter and crying are not found in primates, but their presence in humans heightens interaction through physiological benefits. This is also the case with singing and other forms of music-making accompanied by dance (Table 2.3). These ideas are not new. Durkheim's concept of *effervescence*, identified by Allen (1998) as the emotional pleasure arising from social activity that transcends the individual participant, is enhanced by group singing, dancing and music making that bring all the senses into play.

(2) Containing emotion: memory boxes

The social brain model therefore raises the question 'Why did second-order emotions evolve in hominins?' This will not be answered by asking when symbol-based cognition arose and attempting to find material proxies for amplifying behaviours such as laughter. However, with the perspective of external rather than internal cognition we can see that the evolution of emotion, from primary to secondary orders, depended on a variety of psychotropic mechanisms that enhanced affect and changed hominin capacity for social extension. Furthermore, I would suggest that these amplifying mechanisms were instrumental in the development of higher orders of intentionality (Table 2.1).

It is in this way that the social brain issue of integrating social complexity, discussed above, can be addressed from an evolutionary perspective. Laughter, crying, music and dancing, and the affects they produce acted, as language did later (Table 2.3), to integrate members and local groups into larger communities. Consequently, there is no reason to suppose that such adaptations either came late in human evolution or were exclusive to *Homo sapiens*.

These emotional changes that extend cognition into the world also come wrapped in metaphor, experiencing something in terms of something else (Lakoff & Johnson 1980). Here containers are particularly important as material metaphors understood through the senses; houses form some of the most discussed examples (Carsten & Hugh-Jones 1995), as do pots (Gosselain 1999) and the use of containers for the production of music, whether from drums or voices (Gamble in press). Containment also forms a conceptual metaphor for systems of marriage and the reckoning of kinship in terms of generational 'boxes' that enshrine the rules of descent and recruitment (Allen et al. 2008; Gamble 2008). In Hoskins' ethnographic study containers such as bags, shrouds and drums are 'memory boxes' for the lives of others (1998, 2).

Physically and psychologically containers create technologies of separation: walls that divide and a conceptual architecture which imposes social boundaries. But as memory boxes these same containers also integrate lives through the psychology of cognitive ownership (Rowlands ch. 16 this volume). We will never know exactly what memories these boxes contained, just as the thoughts inside the heads of hominins remain unknowable. However, the fact that containers were made, multiplied and elaborated until they came to swamp human technologies, is in itself powerful evidence for the role of active externalism in the elaboration of a distributed mind.

Our well-wrapped worlds have not always been this way. In his study of chimpanzee technology, McGrew (1992) made the observation that it comprises only instruments. Even allowing for preservation and changing rules of accumulation and consumption (Gamble 2007) the history of hominin technology before 100,000 years ago is dominated by instruments, while after 20,000 years ago it is a more familiar world of containers (Figure 2.2). In other words, there was a shift in the relative frequency between these major forms of material metaphors with the result that the expression and experience of containment became prevalent. At the same time, containers offered unlimited opportunities for the exploration of sensory experiences through the elaboration of their surfaces. The result was an explosion in the variety and appearance of container styles, for example clothes, houses and pots, and the scale of the material world.

The material evidence for this shift from instruments to containers challenges the notion put forward by some evolutionary psychologists (Barkow et al. 1992) that there has been constancy in human cognition from the Pliocene savannahs to the modern Megalopolis. As Donald points out, 'we have become complex, multilayered, hybrid minds, carrying within ourselves, both as individuals and societies, the entire evolutionary heritage of the past few million years' (1998a, 16). There is still laughter, talk, dance, music and tears, and there has been for at least 600,000 years since encephalization, following the need to integrate more local groups into larger communities, and probably for much longer as we saw with the example of the Acheulean gaze.

And while these embodied mechanisms have changed during this time so too has the external cognitive architecture with which they are implicated. Material arrays in the childscape (Gamble 2007), and then the landscapes of adults, have been transformed under the selection pressure of social complexity; integrating local groupings within larger communities. Those memory boxes, be they cradles, necklaces, temples or cities are not examples of external symbolic storage, but rather the constant attempts of the self to make its way in the world of the distributed mind.

CONCLUSION: INTEGRATION AND SEPARATION

In this chapter I have sketched out a map for the evolutionary study of hominin emotions linked to a model of distributed cognition. This can now be tested with archaeological evidence as shown in several methodological studies (Chapman & Gaydarska 2007; Gamble 2007) and by examples elsewhere in this volume (see Barham ch. 18, Chapman ch. 20, Coward ch. 21, Gowlett ch. 17, Mithen ch. 22). The map I favour (Table 2.3) is drawn from the social brain hypothesis: the assertion that our social lives drove encephalization and in particular the need to cope with complexity—defined here as the integration of local groups within larger communities. Two points emerge: first, hominin evolution is characterized neither by cognitive continuity nor a moment when a hominin brain became a human mind. Second, many of the emotional mechanisms around which our social lives are built can be traced in hominins other than *Homo sapiens*. The social brain model potentially identifies the various forms of early *Homo* after 1.8 million years ago as having a theory of mind, while more complex levels of intentionality and belief states were present after the encephalization event 600,000 years ago.

Increasing brain and community size selected for mechanisms that both integrated and separated individuals in local groups. On the one hand, the cognitive load of larger numbers required psychotropic mechanisms to amplify emotions in order to promote integration in situations of face-to-face contact. And, on the other, the ecological pressures on larger communities with a wide geographical distribution in the Old World resulted in longer periods of fission and fusion among members of local groups. These two selective pressures impacted on ontological security, psychological continuity and the extension of the self to create the release from social proximity that is a hominin hallmark. And just as emotions provided the resources to amplify bonds and relationships, so selection also focused on other elements of an active externalism in the form of objects. The emotional agency of materials and things was amplified by shifting from instruments to containers (Figure 2.2) in order to develop the metaphorical opportunities that the latter presented, particularly through the elaboration of their surfaces.

None of these changes require the archaeologist to search for proxies of symbol-based cognition and the origins of the modern mind. Instead, by combining an external model of cognition with the evolutionary map drawn from the social brain it is possible to see new avenues for enquiry with archaeological data that return something of the human to all hominins.

REFERENCES

Aiello, L. C. (1998). The 'expensive tissue hypothesis' and the evolution of the human adaptive niche: a study in comparative anatomy. In: J. Bayley (ed.) *Science in archaeology: an agenda for the future*, pp. 25–36. London: English Heritage.

Aiello, L. & Dunbar, R. (1993). Neocortex size, group size and the evolution of language. *Current Anthropology* 34: 184–193.

Aiello, L. & Wheeler, P. (1995). The expensive-tissue hypothesis: the brain and the digestive system in human and primate evolution. *Current Anthropology* 36: 199–221.

Allen, N. J. (1998). Effervescence and the origins of human society. In: N. J. Allen, W. S. F. Pickering & W. Watts Miller (eds) *On Durkheim's Elementary forms of religious life*, pp. 149–161. London: Routledge.

Allen, N. J., Callan, H., Dunbar, R. & James, W. (eds) (2008). *Early human kinship: from sex to social reproduction*. Oxford: Blackwell.

Anderson, M. L. (2003). Embodied cognition: a field guide. *Artificial Intelligence* 149: 91–130.

Aureli, F., Schaffner, C. M., Boesch, C., Bearder, S. K., Call, J. Chapman, C. A. et al. (2008). Fission-fusion dynamics. *Current Anthropology* 49: 627–654.

Barkow, J. H., Cosmides, L. & Tooby, J. (eds) (1992). *The adapted mind: evolutionary psychology and the generation of culture*. New York: Oxford University Press.

Brumm, A. & Moore, M. W. (2005). Symbolic revolutions and the Australian archaeological record. *Cambridge Archaeological Journal* 15: 157–175.

Carbonell, E., Mosquera, M., Ollé, A., Rodríguez, X. P., Sala, R., Vergès, J. M. et al.
(2003). Les premiers comportments funéraires auraient-ils pris place à Atapuerca,
il y a 350,000 ans? *L'Anthropologie* 107: 1–14.

Carsten, J. & Hugh-Jones, S. (eds) (1995). *About the house: Lévi-Strauss and beyond.*
Cambridge: Cambridge University Press.

Cauvin, J. (2000). *The birth of the gods and the origins of agriculture.* Cambridge:
Cambridge University Press.

Chapman, J. (2000). *Fragmentation in archaeology: people, places and broken objects in
the prehistory of south-eastern Europe.* London: Routledge.

Chapman, J. & Gaydarska, B. (2007). *Parts and wholes: fragmentation in prehistoric
context.* Oxford: Oxbow Books.

Chase, P. & Dibble, H. L. (1987). Middle Palaeolithic symbolism: a review of current
evidence and interpretations. *Journal of Anthropological Archaeology* 6: 263–296.

Clark, A. & Chalmers, D. A. (1998). The extended mind. *Analysis* 58: 7–19.

Cole, J. N. (2008). Identity within intentionality: use of the body to relate the social
brain to the archaeological record. Conference poster presented at the 'Social
Brain and Distributed Mind' Conference, British Academy, London, September.

Coward, F. & Gamble, C. (2008). Big brains, small worlds: material culture and the
evolution of mind. *Philosophical Transactions of the Royal Society B* 363:
1969–1979.

Davidson, I. & McGrew, W. C. (2005). Stone tools and the uniqueness of human
culture. *Journal of the Royal Anthropological Institute* 11: 793–817.

d'Errico, F. (1996). Marshack's approach: poor technology, biased sciences.
Cambridge Archaeological Journal 6: 111–117.

d'Errico, F. (1998). Palaeolithic origins of artificial memory systems: an evolutionary
perspective. In: C. Renfrew & C. Scarre (eds) *Cognitive storage and material
culture: the archaeology of symbolic storage,* pp. 19–50. Cambridge: McDonald
Institute of Archaeological Research.

d'Errico, F. (2003). The invisible frontier: a multiple species model for the origin of
behavioural modernity. *Evolutionary Anthropology* 12: 188–202.

d'Errico, F. & Villa, P. (1997). Holes and grooves: the contribution of microscopy and
taphonomy to the problem of art origins. *Journal of Human Evolution* 33: 1–31.

d'Errico, F., Henshilwood, C. S., Lawson, G., Vanhaeren, M., Tillier, A.-M., Soressi,
M. et al. (2003). Archaeological evidence for the emergence of language, symbol-
ism, and music: an alternative multidisciplinary perspective. *Journal of World
Prehistory* 17: 1–70.

de la Torre, I. (2004). Omo revisited: evaluating the technological skills of Pliocene
hominids. *Current Anthropology* 45: 439–465.

de Waal, F. (2006). *Primates and philosophers: how morality evolved.* Princeton, NJ:
Princeton University Press.

Deacon, T. (1997). *The symbolic species: the co-evolution of language and the human
brain.* Harmondsworth: Penguin Books.

Dennell, R. & Roebroeks, W. (2005). An Asian perspective on early human dispersal
from Africa. *Nature* 438: 1099–1104.

Donald, M. (1998a). Hominid enculturation and cognitive evolution. In: C. Renfrew & C. Scarre (eds) *Cognitive storage and material culture: the archaeology of symbolic storage*, pp. 7–17. Cambridge: McDonald Institute of Archaeological Research.

Donald, M. (1998b). Material culture and cognition: concluding thoughts. In: C. Renfrew & C. Scarre (eds) *Cognitive storage and material culture: the archaeology of symbolic storage*, pp. 181–187. Cambridge: McDonald Institute of Archaeological Research.

Dunbar, R. I. M. (2003). The social brain: mind, language, and society in evolutionary perspective. *Annual Review of Anthropology* 32: 163–181.

Dunbar, R. & Shultz, S. (2007). Evolution in the social brain. *Science* 317: 1344–1347.

Foley, R. & Lahr, M. M. (1997). Mode 3 technologies and the evolution of modern humans. *Cambridge Archaeological Journal* 7: 3–36.

Fonagy, P., Gergely, G. & Target, M. (2007). The parent–infant dyad and the construction of the subjective self. *Journal of Child Psychology and Psychiatry* 48: 288–328.

Fowler, C. (2004). *An archaeology of personhood: an anthropological approach.* London: Routledge.

Gallese, V. (2006). Embodied simulation: from mirror neuron systems to interpersonal relations. In: G. Bock & J. Goode (eds) *Empathy and fairness*, pp. 3–19 (Novartis Foundation Symposium 278). Chichester: Wiley.

Gamble, C. S. (1986). *The Palaeolithic settlement of Europe*. Cambridge: Cambridge University Press.

Gamble, C. S. (1993). *Timewalkers: the prehistory of global colonization*. Cambridge, MA: Harvard University Press.

Gamble, C. S. (1998). Palaeolithic society and the release from proximity: a network approach to intimate relations. *World Archaeology* 29: 426–449.

Gamble, C. S. (2007). *Origins and revolutions: human identity in earliest prehistory*. New York: Cambridge University Press.

Gamble, C. S. (2008). Kinship and material culture: archaeological implications of the human global diaspora. In: N. J. Allen, H. Callan, R. Dunbar & W. James (eds) *Kinship and evolution*, pp. 27–40. Oxford: Blackwell.

Gamble, C. S. (in press). When the words dry up: music and material metaphors half a million years ago. In: N. Bannan & S. J. Mithen (eds) *Music, language and human evolution*. Oxford: Oxford University Press.

Giddens, A. (1984). *The constitution of society*. Berkeley: University of California Press.

Gosden, C. (in press). The death of the mind. In: L. Malafouris & C. Renfrew (eds) *The cognitive life of things*. Cambridge: McDonald Institute for Archaeological Research.

Gosselain, O. P. (1999). In pots we trust: the processing of clay and symbols in sub-Saharan Africa. *Journal of Material Culture* 4: 205–231.

Gowlett, J. A. J. (1984). Mental abilities of early man: a look at some hard evidence. In: R. A. Foley (ed.) *Hominid evolution and community ecology*, pp. 167–192. London: Academic Press.

Henshilwood, C. S. & Marean, C. W. (2003). The origin of modern human behaviour: critique of the models and their test implications. *Current Anthropology* 44: 627–651.

Hodder, I. (2001). Symbolism and the origins of agriculture in the Near East. *Cambridge Archaeological Journal* 11: 107–112.

Hoskins, J. (1998). *Biographical objects: how things tell the story of people's lives.* New York: Routledge.

Hutchins, E. (1995). *Cognition in the wild.* Cambridge, MA: MIT Press.

Ingold, T. (2000). *The perception of the environment: essays in livelihood, dwelling and skill.* London: Routledge.

Johnson, G. (1982). Organizational structure and scalar stress. In: C. Renfrew, M. Rowlands & B. Segraves (eds) *Theory and explanation in archaeology: the Southampton Conference*, pp. 389–422. New York: Academic Press.

Jones, A. (2002). *Archaeological theory and scientific practice.* Cambridge: Cambridge University Press.

Knappett, C. (2005). *Thinking through material culture: an interdisciplinary perspective.* Pittsburgh: University of Pennsylvania Press.

Kohn, M. & Mithen, S. (1999). Handaxes: products of sexual selection? *Antiquity* 73: 518–526.

Lakoff, G. & Johnson, M. (1980). *Metaphors we live by.* Chicago: University of Chicago Press.

Lehmann, J., Korstjens, A. H. & Dunbar, R. (2007). Group size, grooming and social cohesion in primates. *Animal Behaviour* 74: 1617–1629.

Lindly, J. & Clark, G. A. (1990). Symbolism and modern human origins. *Current Anthropology* 31: 233–240.

McBrearty, S. (2007). Down with the revolution. In: P. Mellars, O. Bar-Yosef, C. Stringer & K. V. Boyle (eds) *Rethinking the human revolution*, pp. 133–151. Cambridge: McDonald Institute of Archaeological Research.

McBrearty, S. & Brooks, A. S. (2000). The revolution that wasn't: a new interpretation of the origin of modern humans. *Journal of Human Evolution* 39: 453–563.

McGrew, W. C. (1992). *Chimpanzee material culture: implications for human evolution.* Cambridge: Cambridge University Press.

McNabb, J., Binyon, F. & Hazelwood, L. (2004). The large cutting tools from the South African Acheulean and the question of social traditions. *Current Anthropology* 45: 653–677.

Malafouris, L. (2004). The cognitive basis of material engagement: where brain, body and culture conflate. In: E. DeMarrais, C. Gosden & C. Renfrew (eds) *Rethinking materiality: the engagement of mind with the material world*, pp. 53–62. Cambridge: McDonald Institute of Archaeological Research.

Marshack, A. (1972). *The roots of civilization.* New York: McGraw-Hill.

Marshack, A. (1990). Early hominid symbol and the evolution of the human capacity. In: P. Mellars (ed.) *The emergence of modern humans: an archaeological perspective*, pp. 457–499. Edinburgh: Edinburgh University Press.

Mellars, P. (2005). The impossible coincidence: a single-species model for the origins of modern human behaviour in Europe. *Evolutionary Anthropology* 14: 12–27.

Mellars, P. A. & Stringer, C. (eds) (1989). *The human revolution: behavioural and biological perspectives on the origins of modern humans.* Edinburgh: Edinburgh University Press.

Mellars, P., Bar-Yosef, O., Stringer, C. & Boyle, K. V. (eds) (2007). *Rethinking the human revolution.* Cambridge: McDonald Institute of Archaeological Research.

Mithen, S. (1996). *The prehistory of the mind*. London: Thames & Hudson.

Moore, M. W. & Brumm, A. (2007). Stone artifacts and hominins in island Southeast Asia: new insights from Flores, eastern Indonesia. *Journal of Human Evolution* 52: 85–102.

Noble, W. & Davidson, I. (1996). *Human evolution, language and mind*. Cambridge: Cambridge University Press.

Plotnik, J. M., de Waal, F. B. & Reiss, D. (2006). Self-recognition in an Asian elephant. *Proceedings of the National Academy of Science USA* 109(45): 17053–17057.

Pope, M. & Roberts, M. (2005). Observations on the relationship between Palaeolithic individuals and artefact scatters at the Middle Pleistocene site of Boxgrove, UK. In: C. Gamble & M. Porr (eds) *The individual hominid in context: archaeological investigations of Lower and Middle Palaeolithic landscapes, locales and artefacts*, pp. 81–97. London: Routledge.

Proctor, R. N. (2003). Three roots of human recency: molecular anthropology, the refigured Acheulean, and the UNESCO response to Auschwitz. *Current Anthropology* 44: 213–239.

Renfrew, C. (2001). Symbol before concept: material engagement and the early development of society. In: I. Hodder (ed.) *Archaeological theory today*, pp. 122–140. London: Polity Press.

Renfrew, C. (2007). *Prehistory: making of the human mind*. London: Weidenfeld & Nicolson.

Renfrew, C. & Scarre, C. (eds) (1998). *Cognitive storage and material culture: the archaeology of symbolic storage*. Cambridge: McDonald Institute of Archaeological Research.

Rightmire, P. (2004). Brain size and encephalization in Early to Mid-Pleistocene *Homo*. *American Journal of Physical Anthropology* 124: 109–123.

Robb, J. (2004). The extended artefact and the monumental economy: a methodology for material agency. In: E. DeMarrais, C. Gosden & C. Renfrew (eds) *Rethinking materiality: the engagement of mind with the material world*, pp. 131–140. Cambridge: McDonald Institute of Archaeological Research.

Rodseth, L., Wrangham, R. W., Harrigan, A. & Smuts, B. B. (1991). The human community as a primate society. *Current Anthropology* 32: 221–254.

Rolland, N. (1995). Levallois technique emergence: single or multiple? A review of the Euro-African record. In: H. Dibble & O. Bar-Yosef (eds) *The definition and interpretation of Levallois technology*, pp. 333–359. Monographs in World Archaeology 23. Madison, WI: Prehistory Press.

Rowlands, M. (2003). *Externalism: putting mind and world back together again*. Chesham: Acumen.

Ruff, C. B., Trinkaus, E. & Holliday, T. W. (1997). Body mass and encephalization in Pleistocene *Homo*. *Nature* 387: 173–176.

Simon, H. A. & Kaplan, C. (1989). Foundations of cognitive science. In: M. Posner (ed.) *Foundations of cognitive science*, pp. 1–47. Cambridge, MA: MIT Press.

Smail, D. L. (2008). *On deep history and the brain*. Berkeley: University of California Press.

Thieme, H. (2005). The Lower Palaeolithic art of hunting: the case of Schöningen 13 II–4, Lower Saxony, Germany. In: C. Gamble & M. Porr (eds) *The individual hominid in context: archaeological investigations of Lower and Middle Palaeolithic landscapes, locales and artefacts*, pp. 115–132. London: Routledge.

Thomas, J. (1998). Some problems with the notion of external symbolic storage, and the case of Neolithic material culture in Britain. In: C. Renfrew & C. Scarre (eds) *Cognitive storage and material culture: the archaeology of symbolic storage*, pp. 149–56. Cambridge: McDonald Institute of Archaeological Research.

Thomas, J. (2004). *Archaeology and modernity*. London: Routledge.

Turner, J. H. (2000). *On the origins of human emotions: a sociological inquiry into the evolution of human affect*. Stanford, CA: Stanford University Press.

Wilson, R. A. (2004). *Boundaries of the mind: the individual in the fragile sciences*. New York: Cambridge University Press.

Wrangham, R. W., Jones, J. H., Laden, G., Pilbeam, D. & Conklin-Brittain, N. (1999). The raw and the stolen: cooking and the ecology of human origins. *Current Anthropology* 40: 567–594.

Wynn, T. (1995). Handaxe enigmas. *World Archaeology* 27: 10–24.

Wynn, T. & Coolidge, F. L. (2004). The skilled Neanderthal mind. *Journal of Human Evolution* 46: 467–487.

Zilhão, J. (2007). The emergence of ornaments and art: an archaeological perspective on the origins of behavioural 'modernity'. *Journal of Archaeological Research* 15: 1–54.

3

Herto Brains and Minds:
Behaviour of Early *Homo sapiens*
from the Middle Awash

YONAS BEYENE

THE FOSSIL RECORD OF HUMAN ORIGINS is most fully represented in Africa. Even within Africa Ethiopia stands out for the length of its record and richness of its finds. Very early hominids are represented in the Awash region by remains of *Ardipithecus kadabba* and *Ardipithecus ramidus* (White 2006; White et al. 1994). These are followed by the extensive finds of *Australopithecus afarensis* at Hadar and Maka (White et al. 2000), and some of the earliest known stone artefacts at 2.6 million years, at Gona (Semaw 2000). Among further Australopithecus finds (Asfaw et al. 1999), important traces of early *Homo* are reported around 2 to 1 million years ago (Asfaw et al. 2002; Gilbert & Asfaw 2008). Thereafter both hominid remains and artefacts are known from many sites along the Rift Valley, including the earliest traces of *Homo rhodesiensis* at Bodo at around 0.6 Ma (Rightmire 1996; White 1986). The finds at Herto extend this record, demonstrating important developments in behaviour and towards anatomical modernity.

Here I first describe the geographic setting and chronology of these investigations, before going on to introduce the lithic assemblages and discuss their implications for technological development in the African Pleistocene. Finally, I will provide an overview of the evidence of hominid modifications to the bone assemblages and their implications for the behaviours of these earliest anatomically modern humans.

HERTO: SETTING AND CHRONOLOGY

The Bouri peninsula juts out into the Yardi Lake, which lies just north of the Awash River in the northern part of the Ethiopian rift valley, about

120 km south of Hadar. The late J. Desmond Clark pioneered archaeological work on the peninsula, correcting the gross chronostratigraphic
errors of the initial investigators during an initial visit with J. W. K. Harris
in 1981 (Clark et al. 1984; Gilbert & Asfaw 2008).

The Herto Member unconformably overlies or is in fault contact with
the locally extensive Dakanihylo Member which has yielded *H. erectus*
remains along with abundant early Acheulean artefacts and fauna (Asfaw
et al. 2002 and references therein; Gilbert & Asfaw 2008). At the base of
the local succession is the much older Hatayae Member, which has yielded
the 2.6 Ma *Australopithecus garhi* remains along with the earliest evidence
of hominid activity involving the butchery of large mammals (Asfaw et
al. 1999; de Heinzelin et al. 1999). The Herto sediments measure between
15 and 20 meters thick and are divided into Lower and Upper Members
by an intervening temporal and stratigraphic unconformity (Clark et al.
2003).

Clark resumed work in the area during the 1990s, first focusing on
Acheulean sites east of the modern Awash River at Bodo and Hargufia,
and then probing into the then little known Bouri succession. His efforts
in the Lower Herto sediments resulted in the discovery of artefacts which
were attributed to the Upper Acheulean. In the process of this work a
capping vitric ash horizon of the Lower Herto Member was dated to 260
± 16 thousand years (Clark et al. 2003). Surface collections, excavations,
faunal analysis and refitting studies showed that the Herto Lower
Member artefacts were associated with large mammal bones bearing
modifications demonstrating extensive hominid butchery activities on the
Middle Pleistocene landscape at Bouri. However, while Clark's work—
especially at excavations at BOU-A8 and BOU-A10—demonstrated hippopotamus butchery (Schick & Clark 2000), neither he nor subsequent
work produced any hominid remains. Clark's focus on the Upper
Acheulean of the Lower Herto Member meant that the relatively thin
overlying sedimentary package went little studied until 1997.

The importance of the archaeological localities around the Herto village increased dramatically after the discovery of the first hominid there
in the autumn of 1997 (described in White 2006).

Following the discovery of the first hominids in the Upper Herto
Member sediments adjacent to the Herto village, further archaeological
work was conducted on the Upper Herto sediments, including two major
excavations at Bouri Archeological Locality 19 (B and HT). Excavations
in 2000 resulted in the discovery of additional hominid remains, a mod-
erately rich fauna, extensive zooarchaeological samples, and a complex of

localities exposed across several kilometres in the vicinity (Clark et al. 2003; White et al. 2003).

The Lower and Upper Herto Member archaeological occurrences are widely distributed across an area that stretches for approximately 5 km along the Bouri peninsula. The Lower Herto Member occurrences are located primarily to the north and immediate south of the modern Bouri village. The Upper Herto Member sediments are located further south around the Herto village. The superimposition of these geological packages is best seen in the areas immediately south of Bouri and immediately east of Herto village.

The Upper Herto Member sediments are widely exposed east of the modern Yardi Lake. These sediments are characterized by sandstones, volcanic ash, silt, silty clay and sand deposited in a lake margin environment: the archaeological occurrences and hominids of the Upper Herto Member derive from the sand layers dated to between 160,000 and 154,000 years ago (Clark et al. 2003).

THE ARCHAEOLOGY OF HERTO

Palaeontological and archaeological collection localities were established following Middle Awash project protocols (Gilbert and Asfaw 2008): the major localities are clustered east and south of Herto village, at BOU-A19, BOU-A26 and BOU-A29, and were delineated based on local contiguous outcrop and surface content. Controlled surface collection of archaeological lithic assemblages was undertaken within defined areas inside these localities (designated by letters suffixed to the archaeology localities). Three sites were excavated: (1) BOU-A19-B (the hippo cranium locus); (2) BOU-A19-HT (the complete hominid cranium locus) and (3) BOU-A26C (the *in situ* pick locus). Additional test pits were excavated at four locations to define the stratigraphy and determine the spatial distribution of archaeological materials. These test pits produced much more limited archaeological materials.

All of the Upper Herto Member archaeological assemblages derive from a single lithostratigraphic horizon comprising cross-bedded pumaceous sands positioned unconformably above the underlying dated vitric tuff that caps the Lower Herto Member. They are therefore effectively contemporaneous with each other. Surface finds on these beds, including two of the three hominid crania, are clearly from this stratigraphic unit, as attested to by (in two cases) adhering matrix, the *in situ* provenance of the more intact adult and the absence of overlying deposits which could have contaminated the original sediments.

The archaeology of the Upper Herto Member includes artefact forms characteristic of both Acheulean and Middle Stone Age technologies of Africa as traditionally defined. The total number of artefacts collected and analysed from the three localities identified above is 640. Surface-collected and excavated artefacts consist of ordinary flakes (66.1%), biface trimming flakes (2.18%), retouched tools on flakes (9.37%), Levalloisian techniques (7.5%), hand-axes (4.37%), cores (8.28%), picks (0.47%), blades (0.63%), hammer stones (0.78%), an anvil (0.15%), a point (0.15%) and a retouched hippopotamus canine fragment.

The raw material comprising the combined lithic assemblage is mostly fine-grained basalt. Obsidian and chert were also used, the former more commonly (although thick hydration rinds and spalling suggest that post-depositional dissolution of small obsidian *débitage* may have shifted the raw material abundance counts). Obsidian was obviously a heavily used raw material, and the point and blades were made on obsidian by prefer-ence. Although not abundant, chert of varied colours was also used for scrapers. The basalt is usually fine-grained and good quality. Basalt does not outcrop in the vicinity of the archaeological localities, and the pro-curement outcrop is not easily identified; it was at least several kilometers away from the depositional locus, probably one of the outcrops to the east of the modern Awash River at Bunketo. All the Acheulean bifaces, almost all cores, almost 90 per cent of artefacts with Levalloisian tech-niques and 90 percent of the retouched tools on flakes (end and side scrapers) were made on basalt.

The rarity of hand-axe preparation flakes, along with the absence of large cores such as those documented from Bodo (Clark & Schick 2000), suggest that these tools were made elsewhere and imported to the occu-pation loci. The absence of cortical flakes suggests that basalt was quar-ried from the flow outcrop rather than collected from river conglomerate cobbles. The rarity of retouched tools and diagnostic tool types on obsid-ian could be due to rapid degradation of this volcanic glass. Obsidian sourcing studies of these tools are currently under way.

The chert is usually of good quality. Although it is rare when com-pared with other raw material types (4.2%), it represents 15 per cent of the total retouched tool category, suggestive of preference for fine-grained exotic materials whenever available.

Levalloisian techniques are well represented in the lithic assemblage. Out of the 63 tools on flakes, 9 were made on Levallois flakes. In addition to that, 46 Levallois flakes and a unifacial hand-axe made on a Levallois flake were collected and analysed. The 56 artefacts showing Levalloisian technique show that preparation was usually radial centripetal. The flakes are mostly elliptical with a flat section, and their platforms almost always facetted convex. They are typologically '*chapeaux de gendarme*' and '*en aile d'oiseau*' with a platform angle always between 90 and 95 degrees. The technological sophistication attained in the various '*modes opératoire*' is confirmed by the presence of 16 Levallois cores. Of the 53 cores collected and analysed, 28 are examples of discoid cores. Experimentation conducted in this '*châine opératoire*' suggests that the discoid cores could be result of exhaustive exploitation of the Levallois cores.

The flake tools comprise 60 artefacts. Simple side scrapers with convex edges are the most represented tool types (22 out of 25 retouched pieces). The rest are convergent side scrapers and double side scrapers with biconvex edges. Most specimens show direct retouch. The denticulates are less represented (8.3%). They are mostly made by adjacent notches.

A group of 15 end scrapers/rabots are present. They are made on thick flakes which sometimes conserve cortical surface. The working edges are usually convex and regular, made with lamellar retouch. Most of these tools are on the same piece as side scrapers.

Four blades made on obsidian are also present. One blade, from BOU-A19-B, is *in situ* while the other three are surface-collected from BOU-A26-C. Two of the points are unifacial, whereas one is bifacially made. A transverse burin on an angle and a backed knife (made on basalt) are also present.

All hand-axes (there are 28) are made on fine-grained basalt. The hand-axe group is represented by ovates and elongate ovates, a triangular biface, cleaver/bifaces (which are ovate elongate in plan form), unifaces, a cleaver, a knife, a pick, a biface scraper, a biface nucleus, and two broken hand-axes.

A total of 61 per cent of the hand-axes show ovate and elongate ovate plan forms. With the exception of a pick made on a cobble, all the hand-axes are made on flakes. The platforms of the ovates and elongate ovates bear inverse flake scars. The dorsal face shows exhaustive flaking scars, except on rare occasions when the mesial dorsal face is left unworked. These hand-axes show shallow flake scars and their edges are regular and show secondary edge regularization retouches attesting to use of mostly soft hammer techniques. They have mostly biconvex and sometimes plano-convex cross-sections. The hand-axe subassemblage of the Upper

Herto could be viewed as a stage whereby evolved forms of the Acheulean technologies merged with the Levalloisian techniques of the Middle Stone Age.

Based on the above analysis, the Herto assemblages could be techno-logically divided into three major groups. The first group is the bifacially worked group that includes ovates, ovate elongates, cleavers, triangular bifaces, knives, biface scraper, and picks. The second group is character-ized by the high representation of the Levalloisian technology which shows a technological control in the various '*modes opératoire*' of this technology. The third group is represented by retouched tools made on flakes. These are composed of side scrapers, denticulates and points that are typical of the African Middle Stone Age. Rabots/end scrapers made on thick flakes are reminiscent of more ancient technologies. A few burins and backed knives complete the assemblage series.

The presence of such a large biface component in a strongly Levalloisian assemblage blurs the distinction between the Acheulean and the Middle Stone Age, and one explanation could be that the assemblage is mixed. However, the local geological circumstances of recovery, the abundance of hand-axes, the same preservational characteristics of the Levallois-based flakes and cores, and the presence of hand-axes found *in situ* during natural exposure and excavation of the Upper Herto Member sands show that these markers of the Acheulean persisted alongside more derived tools here at Herto.

A BROADER PERSPECTIVE

Earlier research done on the Horn of Africa region shows that some com-parable industries were present, specifically at Garba III in the Melka Kunture site, Ethiopia (Chavaillon et al. 1979; Hours 1976). As in Herto, the Garba III archaeological materials show the presence of hand-axes of terminal Acheulean type, typical Levalloisian techniques, and a good number of retouched tools made on flakes (side and end scrapers, backed knives, burins, unifacial and bifacial points). Hours (1976) considers this a transitional stage between the Acheulean and the Middle Stone Age traditions.

Recent work conducted in the Gaddemota and Kapthurin areas of Ethiopia and Kenya, respectively, shows that the notion of a simple tran-sition from the Acheulean to the Middle Stone Age in Africa is no longer tenable. The former site shows typical Middle Stone Age technologies at ca. 300 Ka (Morgan & Renne 2008; Wendorf & Schild 1974), without Acheulean, whereas the latter shows very early Levalloisian and blade technologies (Tryon & McBrearty 2002).

The complex nature of the transition from what has traditionally been described as Acheulean in Africa to assemblages typically called Middle Stone Age was appreciated by Clark 20 years ago when he stated that, although the beginning of the Middle Stone Age is identified by the changes in technology and artefact types, the transition from the Acheulean to the Middle Stone Age is not easy to define clearly (Clark 1988). In the Lower Herto, Late Acheulean assemblages recovered during his last work in Africa, Clark found that the refined, symmetric and soft hammer retouched bifaces made on finer raw materials were indicative of regular access to and butchery of whole carcasses of large animals such as hippopotami. Furthermore, without knowledge of the Upper Herto assemblage, he had predicted that Upper Herto would provide artefacts characteristic of the Middle Stone Age technologies (Schick & Clark 2000).

It is ironic that adjacent to the Lower Herto Member assemblages that were recovered and insightfully analysed by Clark and Schick, the Middle Awash team has been able to further this research and confirm Clark's prognostications regarding the complexity of the transition from what has been called 'Acheulean' to what has been called 'Middle Stone Age'. Most researchers agree that the transition from Acheulean to Middle Stone Age, as traditionally viewed, is marked by the appearance of new knapping techniques (Levallois and blade), the appearance of smaller and new hand-axe types, and high proportions of retouched flake tools. All of these are present in the Herto assemblage, accompanied by the late persistence of Acheulean bifaces.

If we accept that the Middle Stone Age had its roots in the Acheulean and is distinguished as a distinct technology through the abandonment of the biface component and the adoption of new forms of knapping techniques, we can infer that, as Chavaillon et al. (1979) and Tryon and McBrearty (2002) have suggested, there was no clear and simple gradual process of transition. The nature of the technological shift from assemblages traditionally labelled Acheulean to those traditionally described as Middle Stone Age is clearly being cast in a different light by discoveries across Africa. The well-calibrated Middle Awash succession of Ethiopia confirms that the shift was complex and patterned by various topographic, ecological and perhaps local cultural factors that are only beginning to be understood. We are far from understanding this transition even locally, let alone on a continental scale, and more research of this type is clearly called for now that we have escaped the nomenclatural bounds of earlier pan-continental models.

The extensive surface collections and excavation probes into the Upper Herto Member sands have revealed important aspects of the behaviour of these early humans and of the environment they occupied. The presence of aquatic animals such as hippotamus, crocodiles and fish, indicate nearby rich aquatic environments along the shore of a shallow lake whose modern analogue is the current Yardi Lake just west of the Bouri horst.

The co-occurrence of abundant lithic remains and well-preserved fauna offers some insights into the diet of the human inhabitants. Zooarchaeological analyses are still under way, but it is already evident that the Pleistocene occupants of the Bouri region engaged in the acquisition and processing of large mammals for millions of years. There is evidence of marrow processing and defleshing from Hata times (2.5 Ma) onward, often involving large mammals (de Heinzelin et al. 1999). The Upper Herto Member excavations provide the most important evidence for later involvement with large mammal carcasses. In our team's two large excavations at BOU-A19, the association between fresh stone tools and processed remains of large mammals is clear cut. There is abundant evidence of cutmarks to the bones of hippopotamus as well as rhinoceros, large bovids (presumably *Pelorovis*) and medium-sized bovids. This evidence for repeated hippopotamus butchery builds on that presented elsewhere (Clark et al. 2003), in which the processing of very young animals was evident. The presence of multiple cut-marked and intentionally percussion-fractured bones of large and small hippopotami is indicative of access to these territorial and aggressive animals that are not easy to hunt. That they were repeatedly acquired and butchered is not open to doubt given the zooarchaeological and associational evidence. However, whether the carcasses were obtained by scavenging or hunting is not yet possible to determine given the limited samples, and this remains a key research question to be addressed in further work on these unique open-air occurrences.

The Upper Herto Member early humans had mastered both the Acheulean and Levallois techno-complexes at ca. 160 Ka, and were using these tools to butcher and exploit carcasses of the largest mammals in the landscape. There is no associated evidence of fire, but this absence of evidence does not necessarily preclude its control and use.

MODERN HUMANS AND SYMBOLISM

There is an ongoing debate about the degree to which these earliest African *Homo sapiens* of the late Middle Pleistocene had begun to express themselves symbolically. Opposing schools of thought are exemplified by the work of McBrearty and Brooks (2000), who see the very early acquisition of novel behaviours in Africa prior to 100,000 years ago, and Klein (2000) who interprets the archaeological record as favouring the emergence of more advanced symbolic behaviours at a later date. The Upper Herto Member archaeological occurrences, and additional evidence from earlier, typical Acheulean-bearing deposits in the same study area (at Bodo) contribute to this debate.

Despite intensive collection and modest excavation of the Upper Herto Member, there is so far no evidence for items of personal adornment. There is no red ochre, no geometrically incised stone or bone, and no evidence of intentionally patterned stone or bone. The Upper Herto Member lithic technology shows an advance over the Lower Herto assemblages also associated with animal tissue procurement. However, neither assemblage shows evidence of the kinds of artefacts that, in somewhat later Middle Stone Age contexts, are interpreted to represent symbolic behaviour (McBrearty & Brooks 2000). The best evidence for non-subsistence behaviour, therefore, comes from the hominid remains themselves.

Evidence for very early, ca. 500,000-year-old mortuary practices was found on the Bodo cranium (White 1986). This evidence was confined to a single individual and was difficult to interpret, particularly given its poor archaeological context. In contrast, the three Herto hominid crania show a clear pattern of early mortuary practice involving intensive modification over protracted periods by skilful manipulators.

At Herto, hundreds of lithic artefacts and faunal remains were found in association with the three hominid crania within very close proximity and a limited stratigraphic interval. It is particularly significant that of these three individuals, only cranial remains were found. The more intact cranium was found *in situ* in the sand deposit emplaced immediately above the occupation horizon excavated at BOU-A19-HT. It showed isolated cutmarks. At the other excavated locality but from the same stratigraphic horizon BOU-A19-B, the surface find of parts of a second adult (also presumed male) shows both functional defleshing cutmarks and more 'decorative' repeated scratching around the vault perimeter. Unfortunately, the specimen demonstrated considerable weathering, preventing a more detailed account of its overall modification.

Finally, the presence of very fine cutmarks (presumably made by chert or obsidian flake edges) on the basicranium of a 7-year-old child in the same stratigraphic horizon demonstrates that all three hominid skulls recovered show evidence of peri-mortem bone modification. The absence of any other associated body parts of any of these individuals is particularly provocative, as is the polish on the infant's cranial vault. It is evident that some form of mortuary practice involving the transport and curation of the cranium after death was occurring at Herto ca. 160–154 Ka. The details of these practices will only be illuminated by additional discoveries.

CONCLUSIONS

The emergence of fully anatomically modern humans post-dated the Upper Herto Member *Homo sapiens idaltu* population at Bouri. Evidence of these modern humans has been recovered in the Middle Awash at Halibee (unpublished; ca. 100,000 years ago) in a purely Middle Stone Age archaeological context. Later hominids and more derived Middle Stone Age occurrences have been documented at the nearby site of Aduma (Yellen et al. 2005).

The Middle Awash discoveries, combined with those from other Ethiopian sites, have confirmed that the technological changes accompanying the evolution of anatomical modernity in this part of Africa were more complex than once thought. They have also shown that important cognitive changes were happening in this part of Africa just before the emergence of modern people and their spread across the Old World. The brains of these people were fully modern in size, but the organization of these brains is only accessible indirectly, through an archaeological record that is growing rapidly and promises to reveal more about the lives and even thoughts of these ancestors.

Note. Work in the Middle Awash research area was conducted through the financial support of the National Science Foundation (US), the Institute of Geophysics and Planetary Physics (University of California at Los Alamos National Laboratory) and the Japan Society for the Promotion of Science. Additional financial contributions were made by the Hampton Fund for International Initiatives, Miami University. The ARCCH (Authority for Research and Conservation of Cultural Heritages, Ethiopian Ministry of Culture and Tourism) has provided field permits, administrative facilitation and laboratory facilities. The Afar Regional Government and the Afar people living in the research area (Bouri and Herto in Bouri-Modaito) have supported the field research. I thank the hundreds of Middle Awash research group members who have all contributed to the research in the Bouri and Herto areas. The late J. D. Clark pioneered this research and his contributions are paramount. I would like to thank Tim White for his valuable comments and editorial of this chapter.

REFERENCES

Asfaw, B., White, T. D., Lovejoy, C. O., Latimer, B., Simpson, S. & Suwa, G. (1999). *Australopithecus garhi*: a new species of early hominid from Ethiopia. *Science* 284: 629–635.

Asfaw, B., Gilbert, W. H., Beyene, Y., Hart, W. K., Renne, P. R., WoldeGabriel, G. et al. (2002). Remains of *Homo erectus* from Bouri, Middle Awash, Ethiopia. *Nature* 416: 317–320.

Chavaillon, J., Chavaillon, N., Hours, F. & Piperno, M. (1979). From the Oldowan to the Middle Stone Age at Melka-Kunture (Ethiopia): understanding cultural changes. *Quaterneria* 21: 87–114.

Clark, J. D. (1988). The Middle Stone Age in East Africa and the beginnings of regional identity. *Journal of World Prehistory* 2: 235–308.

Clark, J. D. & Schick, K. (2000). Acheulean archaeology of the eastern Middle Awash. In: J. de Heinzelin, J. D. Clark, K. D. Schick & W. H. Gilbert (eds) *The Acheulean and the Plio-Pleistocene deposits of the Middle Awash Valley Ethiopia*, pp. 51–121. Royal Museum of Central Africa (Belgium): Annales Sciences Géologiques 104.

Clark, J. D., Asfaw, B., Harris, J. W. K., Walter, R. C., White, T. D. & Williams, M. A. J. (1984). Paleoanthropological discoveries in the Middle Awash Valley, Ethiopia. *Nature* 307: 423–428.

Clark, J. D., Beyene, Y., WoldeGabriel, G., Hart, W. K., Renne, P. R., Gilbert, H. et al. (2003). Stratigraphic, chronological and behavioural contexts of Pleistocene *Homo sapiens* from Middle Awash, Ethiopia. *Nature* 423: 747–752.

de Heinzelin, J., Clark, J. D., White, T. D., Hart, W., Renne, P., WoldeGabriel, G. et al. (1999). Environment and behavior of 2.5-million-year-old Bouri hominids. *Science* 284: 625–629.

Gilbert, H. & Asfaw, B. (2008). *Homo erectus: Pleistocene evidence from the Middle Awash, Ethiopia*. Berkeley: University of California Press.

Hours, F. (1976) Le Stone Age de Melka Kontouré. In: B. Abebe, J. Chavaillon & J. E. G. Sutton (eds.), *Proceedings of the Seventh Panafrican Congress of Prehistory and Quaternary Studies, 1971*, pp. 99–104. Addis Ababa: Ministry of Culture.

Klein, R.G. (2000). Archaeology and the evolution of human behavior. *Evolutionary Anthropology* 9: 17–36.

McBrearty, S. & Brooks, A.S. (2000). The revolution that wasn't: a new interpretation of the origin of modern human behavior. *Journal of Human Evolution* 39: 453–563.

Morgan, L. & Renne, P. (2008). Diachronous dawn of Africa's Middle Stone Age: new 40Ar/39Ar ages from the Ethiopian Rift. *Geology* 36(12): 967–970.

Rightmire, G. P. (1996). The human cranium from Bodo, Ethiopia: evidence for speciation in the Middle Pleistocene? *Journal of Human Evolution* 31: 21–39.

Schick, K. & Clark, J.D. (2000). Acheulean archaeology of the western Middle Awash. In: J. de Heinzelin, J. D. Clark, K. D. Schick & W. H. Gilbert (eds) *The Acheulean and the Plio-Pleistocene deposits of the Middle Awash Valley Ethiopia*, pp. 125–181. Royal Museum of Central Africa (Belgium): Annales Sciences Géologiques 104.

Semaw, S. (2000). The world's oldest stone artifacts from Gona, Ethiopia: their implications for understanding stone technology and patterns of human evolution between 2.6–2.5 million years ago. *Journal of Archaeological Science* 27: 1197–1214.

Tryon, C. A. & McBrearty, S. (2002). Tephrostratigraphy and the Acheulean to Middle Stone Age transition in the Kapthurin Formation, Kenya. *Journal of Human Evolution* 42: 211–235.

Wendorf, F. & Schild, R. (1974). *A Middle Stone Age sequence from the Central Rift Valley, Ethiopia*. Warsaw: Ossolineum.

White, T. D. (1986) Cutmarks on the Bodo cranium: a case of prehistoric defleshing. *American Journal of Physical Anthropology* 69: 503–509.

White, T. D. (2006). Human evolution: the evidence. In: J. Brockman (ed.) *Intelligent thought: science versus the intelligent design movement*, pp. 65–81. New York: Vintage.

White, T. D., Suwa, G. & Asfaw, B. (1994). *Australopithecus ramidus*, a new species of early hominid from Aramis, Ethiopia. *Nature* 371: 306–312.

White, T. D., Suwa, G., Simpson, S. & Asfaw, B. (2000). Jaws and teeth of *Astralopithecus afarensis* from Maka, Middle Awash, Ethiopia. *American Journal of Physical Anthropology* 111: 45–68.

White, T. D., Asfaw, B., DeGusta, D., Gilbert, H., Richards, G. D., Suwa, G. et al. (2003). Pleistocene *Homo sapiens* from Middle Awash, Ethiopia. *Nature* 423: 742–747.

Yellen, J., Brooks, A., Helgren, D., Tappen, M., Ambrose, S., Bonnefille, R. et al. (2005). The archaeology of Aduma Middle Stone Age sites in the Awash Valley, Ethiopia. *PaleoAnthropology* 10: 25–100.

PART II

THE NATURE OF THE NETWORK: THE BONDS OF SOCIALITY

4

Social Networks and Social Complexity in Female-bonded Primates

JULIA LEHMANN, KATHERINE ANDREWS
& ROBIN DUNBAR

Most primates live in closely bonded social groups in which they have differentiated social relationships (Cheney & Seyfarth 1990; Silk 2007). This, together with the ability of some primates to recognize not only their own position within a social group but also to understand third party relationships (e.g. Cheney & Seyfarth 1980), has led to the hypothesis that primates may have evolved what has been termed a 'social brain' (Dunbar 1998; Jolly 1966). In relation to body size, primates have the largest brains in the animal kingdom (Jerison 1973) and it is especially the neocortex that is enlarged in comparison to other taxa (Finlay & Darlington 1995). The neocortex has long been recognized as the part of the brain responsible for higher cognitive functions, enabling more complex behaviours and learning (Campbell & Reece 2005). It has been suggested that the unusually large neocortex in primates has evolved under selection to manage and maintain complex social relationships (Byrne & Whiten 1988; Dunbar & Shultz 2007a, 2007b). In support of this, it has been found that in primates neocortex size correlates positively with the typical size of the social groups across species (Dunbar 1992a, 1998; Dunbar & Shultz 2007b). Furthermore, individuals of species with larger neocortices have also been found to have larger grooming networks (Kudo & Dunbar 2001), adding further support to the suggestion that the neocortex has evolved to manage social relationships.

However, while most of the studies supporting the social brain hypothesis have used group size as a proxy for social complexity, there is very limited evidence as to how group size really relates to social complexity. Worse still, there is no agreed definition for what exactly it is that makes one social system more complex than another. Although group size and neocortex size correlate positively (Dunbar 1992a; Lehmann et al.

Proceedings of the British Academy **158**, 57–82. © The British Academy 2010.

2007), it is unlikely that the neocortex has evolved simply to process a larger number of social relationships (as would be the case in larger groups). Indeed, the social brain hypothesis is based on the relationship between social complexity (e.g. managing a more complex network of relationships) and brain size, not simply on the quantitative relationship between group size and brain size (Dunbar 1998; Dunbar & Shultz 2007a). In addition, more recent analyses suggest that this quantitative relationship between brain size and group size only exists in anthropoid primates; in most other higher vertebrates, the relationship seems rather to be a function of social system in that pair-bonded species have the largest brains (Pérez-Barbería et al. 2007; Shultz & Dunbar 2007).

Only a few studies have attempted to use parameters other than group size to analyse the relationship between brain size and aspects of social complexity: these variables have included social play (Lewis 2000), tactical deception (Byrne & Corp 2004), mating tactics (Pawlowski et al. 1998) and cooperation (Dunbar & Shultz 2007b). All of these studies suggest that species with larger neocortices/brains may use cognitively more demanding behavioural strategies (assuming that deception and cooperation are indeed cognitively demanding), so that individuals with a 'social brain' may have available a larger number of behavioural elements/ manipulations to reach their goals and so ultimately to increase their fitness (see Silk 2007). However, there is no intrinsic reason why complexity should be indexed by large numbers of relationships, irrespective of whether these are direct or indirect. Indeed, there is clear evidence, for Old World monkeys at least, that even though grooming time may increase with group size, grooming network size may actually decrease (gelada; Dunbar 1984), probably in order to enable core alliances to be invested in more heavily (Dunbar in press).

In this study, we do not seek to test the social brain hypothesis (that has been well established by a long series of analyses over many years; for a recent review, see Dunbar & Shultz 2007b). Rather, we aim to explore the nature of social complexity by asking (1) whether social network properties vary between species depending on neocortex size and (2) whether we can use these properties to give us more insight into what social complexity might be in primates. To do so, we use social network analysis, which has previously been used successfully to describe social groups across a variety of animal species (see e.g. Krause et al. 2007; Wey et al. 2008). Here, social relationships between individuals of a group are used to derive a network of relationships from which formal descriptors (definitions and measures) for characterizing social groups can be derived. In addition, social network analysis also allows the testing of statistical models about relationships and structure (see Wey et al. 2008). Being able to pinpoint which network properties vary with brain size will help us to understand what exactly it is that makes a social network more complex (as postulated by the social brain hypothesis). This type of analysis moves away from asking what individuals can or cannot understand about social relationships to look at the effects of social intelligence on the group structure *per se*: in other words, do network parameters vary systematically with brain size in such a way that species with larger brains exhibit significantly different group structures?

This largely exploratory study represents a first step towards such a definition, using social network analysis to compare the properties of female primate grooming networks across a variety of Old World monkeys. We are interested in the relationship that grooming network structure has to both group size and brain size. Because it has previously been suggested that being divided into smaller subgroups while simultaneously maintaining a higher-order grouping level is cognitively more demanding than spreading social effort evenly across the group (Aureli et al. 2008), we are particularly interested in how relationships are distributed across the network, the extent of subgrouping that occurs and whether these patterns might give us insight into the nature of social complexity.

METHODS

Data collection

Data on Old World monkey grooming (in the form of individual grooming matrices) were compiled from the literature for as many populations and species as possible by scanning relevant journals using the internet search engine 'Web of Science' (including all available years and scientific information indices) and relevant key-words. We also supplemented our dataset with data from colleagues who kindly provided grooming matrices from their study populations. Only species in which females are philopatric and form female-bonded matrilines were included to allow us to compare network parameters across similar social systems. By concentrating on female–female social relationships in species in which females remain within their natal communities throughout their lives, we avoided the complicating issues of male–female relationships and different dispersal patterns which would have been hard to control for. Because we are interested in the possible limiting effects of brain size, species were only included in our analysis if we were able to derive a species-specific neo-cortex ratio: this yielded a sample of 11 species in total (see Table 4.1). Whenever possible, we calculated neocortex ratios (volume of the neo-cortex/volume of the rest of the brain) based on actual brain tissue vol-umes as given by Stephan et al. (1981). For the six species for which no published data on neocortex volumes were available, we estimated neo-cortex ratio from brain weight or brain volume using the equations given by Kudo and Dunbar (2001).

In addition to data on grooming effort, we also collated data on group size. Group size creates a potential problem because the various network indices were not designed for comparative analysis and hence do not always take network size into account. Consequently, as James et al. (2009) point out, inter-species comparisons of network metrics may be confounded by group size effects if network metrics scale with group size: in such cases, a significant correlation between the network metric in question and group size would simply be a mathematical by-product of the way the measures are defined. Unfortunately, at the present time it is unclear whether such effects are real (i.e. network dynamics do change predictably depending on group size) or are mere mathematical by-products. Nonetheless, in order to address this problem we did a two-step analysis: first, we assessed the independent effects of group size and brain size on network parameters, and then in a second step we statistically con-trolled for the confounding variable in each case by including it simulta-neously into the analysis. This should allow us to partial out effects that are purely due to group size.

Whenever data were available we collated networks for more than one population per species, thereby avoiding the pitfall of the representative-ness of single networks (see James et al. 2009). Whenever grooming matri-ces were available from more than one study/population per species, we used average values across those studies for all between-species compar-isons (see Table 4.1). The dataset includes data from both wild and captive populations and we originally treated these as two different datasets. However, as there were no significant differences between the two datasets (Andrews 2007), they were combined for all the analyses reported here.

Network parameters

For all grooming matrices, we calculated the percentage of total individual grooming effort directed towards a particular partner. These percentages

Table 4.1. Data included in the analysis

Species	No. of troops	Mean no. females	Mean clan size	% clan membership	NCr ratio	Source
Chlorocebus aethiops	3	7.7	7.7	1.00	2.17	Seyfarth 1980
Cercopithecus mitis	1	17	12.4	.73	2.46	Rowell et al. 1991
Erythrocebus patas	1	18	7.9	.42	2.96	Kaplan and Zucker 1980
Miopithecus talapoin	1	5	5.0	100	2.33	Wolfheim 1977
Macaca radiata	5	12.8	9.4	81	2.28	Sugiyama 1971; Silk, pers. comm.
Macaca fuscata	3	10	5.2	56	2.60	Oi 1988
Macaca fascicularis	2	8	7.3	89	2.24	Butovskaya et al. 1995
Macaca sylvanus	2	12.5	8.1	77	2.37	Deag 1972; Bellingham 2002
Papio papio	1	8	5.0	63	2.76	Anthoney 1975
Papio anubis	1	16	9.0	56	2.76	Frank, pers. comm.
Theropithecus	16	5.4	3.5	72	2.55	Dunbar and Sharman 1984; Dunbar, pers. comm.

NCr ratio = Neocortex ratio

represent the distribution of individual grooming effort across same-sex group members. Using these matrices we calculated network density by dividing the number of existing grooming relationships by the total number of possible relationships ($N^2 - N$ in the case of directed relationships; Wasserman & Faust 1994). This measure of network density therefore

allowed us to assess what proportion of the existing dyads actually inter-
acted. We are further interested in the size, number and composition of
grooming networks. In order to analyse these we had first to make the
matrices symmetric and then dichotomize the matrix, both of which were
done using UCInet (6.170, Analytic Technologies, Lexington, USA).

Matrices were made symmetrical using the maximum effort rules, i.e.
any particular dyad was given its maximum value (irrespective of whether
this was grooming given or grooming received, i.e. assuming that a social
bond exists irrespective of the direction of the behaviour exchanged). In
addition, dichotomized matrices were filtered to include only significant
grooming relationships in the analyses. To determine an appropriate cut-
off value, graphs were plotted for each population with the mean number
of grooming partners set against a range of discriminant values (DV) (see
Appendix). The DV at which there was a steep drop-off in the number of
grooming partners per individual was chosen as the cut-off value. Across
populations, the mean and the modal DV value was 0.1; this was therefore applied to all populations. Thus, only those relationships in which
one of the partners invested more than 10 per cent of their total grooming effort was considered a real relation (link) and included in the network
analysis. This edge filtering technique allows us to concentrate our analysis on relatively strong relationships, thereby reducing the problem of the
possible distorting effects that casual relationships might have on network
metrics and that can be easily overlooked in shorter-term studies (for
details see James et al. 2009).

The transformed symmetric binary matrices were then used to analyse
subgrouping patterns. Network analysis provides a multitude of different
algorithms to analyse subgrouping patterns. In this study, we used an
algorithm to identify all subgroups in which each individual is connected
to each other individual by a maximum distance of two links (n-clans in
UCInet). Thus, in Figure 4.1 (inset) all black circles are members of the
same clan while the white circle is not part of the black-circle clan as it is
not connected to all other circles by a maximum of two links (three
links are needed to connect white to the black circle in the upper left
corner). In line with network terminology we termed these subgroups
in our dataset grooming clans. The use of 2-clans, a common network
algorithm, allows the discovery of subgroups in a larger network, and we
do not consider larger distances to be meaningful for these animals since
very few Old World monkeys have grooming clusters that contain more
than three individuals (Kudo & Dunbar 2001). We determined the overall number of existing clans within each network, average clan size, the

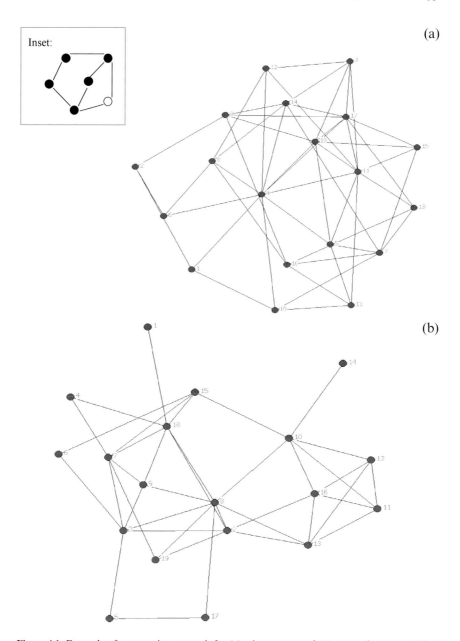

Figure 4.1. Example of a grooming network for (a) a large group of *Macaca sylvanus* and (b) a similar sized group of *Erythrocebus patas*. Numbered circles represent individual females, while lines represent non-directional grooming relationships (more than 10% of total individual grooming effort). Inset figure (not part of the grooming network in (a)): example for a 2-clan (black circles) and an individual not belonging to the clan (white circle). Each black dot is connected to every other black dot by a minimum of two steps (thus forming a 2-clan), but the white dot needs three steps to connect to some black dots (and so is excluded).

total number of clans a particular female belonged to and the percentage of all clans in that group that a female belonged to. In addition, we also calculated individual connectivity (i.e. the number of links that need to be deleted so that there is no longer a connection between a given dyad) as an indicator of network cohesiveness (a cohesive network is assumed to be less vulnerable to the removal of any one individual). Individual values were averaged within populations.

Finally, in order to determine how important individual females are for the average network connectivity, we removed the statistically most and the least central female (see below for definition) respectively from the network and recalculated average connectivity. A statistically significant decrease in overall connectivity following the removal of the most but not the least central individual indicates that the overall network structure is dominated by a few very central individuals. (Note that this analysis is not affected by changes in group size because comparisons are done within species and hence between groups of virtually identical size: N versus N − 1 after the removal). Centrality was measured using Freeman's betweenness index: a highly central female is an individual that links otherwise unconnected individuals; such an individual would have a high betweenness value (Wasserman & Faust 1994). Such individuals are often referred to as 'brokers' (Lusseau & Newman 2004) and it has been hypothesized that socially more complex species rely more on weak links (Kudo & Dunbar 2001), which are functionally brokers.

Statistical analysis

Although a number of recent studies have shown that phylogenetic relationships do not affect the outcome of these kinds of socio-cognitive comparisons (Deaner et al. 2007; Pérez-Barbería et al. 2007; Shultz & Dunbar 2007), we nonetheless controlled for the possible non-independence problem arising in cross-species comparisons by using the method of independent contrasts. Phylogeny was based on Purvis (1995) and we used standardized branch lengths to calculate independent contrasts. Thus, all analyses and graphs are based on independent contrast data (with the exception of the connectivity analysis, where most comparisons are made within species).

First, we used Pearson correlation analysis to identify the relationships between network parameters and group size or neocortex ratio, respectively. We included this analysis because we are interested in the effects of group size on network parameters. However, since it has been suggested that network parameters could scale with group size and, in addition, it has previously been shown that neocortex ratio and group size are interrelated (Dunbar 1992a; Lehmann et al. 2007), we subsequently re-analysed the data using mixed models with the respective network parameters as independent variables and both neocortex size and number of adult females simultaneously as covariates. This procedure allows us to determine the influence of neocortex ratio on grooming networks while controlling for the effect of group size (and vice versa). All models originally also included an interaction term (neocortex ratio $\times$ group size) which was subsequently dropped as it was never significant. Data on connectivity following the removal of the most and least central females were compared to average connectivity of the group before the removal, using paired-sample t-tests.

RESULTS

Effects of group size on network structure

Figure 4.1 represents an example of a grooming network for two groups of primates. As can be seen in Table 4.2, group size is positively correlated with clan size and absolute clan membership, indicating that primates living in larger groups are generally members of larger grooming clans and that each individual female is a member of absolutely more clans. In addition, we found a negative correlation between group size and relative clan membership (percentage of all existing clans), indicating that females in larger groups are members of relatively fewer grooming clans compared to those available to them within their social group. Finally, there was a near-significant negative correlation between density and group size, indicating that larger grooming networks are less dense: i.e. the number of grooming relations in relation to the total number of possible relationships decreases. This is in line with the suggestion that, in large groups, individual females tend to concentrate their grooming effort on a few key individuals rather than aiming to maintain close grooming relationships with all group members (Dunbar 2003; Dunbar & Sharman 1984). A similar negative relationship between network size and network density has also been found in human social networks (Carter & Feld 2004; Hislop 2005). Finally, the total number of grooming clans increased positively with group size.

While some of these effects could be due to the increased availability of social partners in larger groups (e.g. large clans can only be formed in

Table 4.2. Results of Pearson correlations and mixed model analyses

Pearson corr.		Density	Connectivity	Clan size	Clan mem.	%clan_mem	#clans
	n	10	10	10	10	10	10
Group size	r	*–0.591*	0.38	**0.798**	**0.927**	**–0.715**	**0.713**
	p	*0.072*	0.28	**0.006**	**<0.001**	**0.020**	**0.021**
NCr	r	**–0.917**	–0.34	0.032	**0.68**	**–0.912**	*0.552*
	p	**<0.001**	0.336	0.929	**0.031**	**<0.001**	*0.098*
Mixed model							
grpsz(NCr)	F	0.19	**9.6**	**88.3**	**26.34**	2.890	3.48
	ß	–0.77	**0.686**	**0.87**	**0.943**	–0.17	1.16
	p	0.675	**0.017**	**<0.001**	**0.001**	0.133	0.104
NCr(grpsz)	F	**22.4**	**9.07**	**27.6**	1.8	**21.8**	0.41
	ß	**–4.31**	**–3.45**	**–2.53**	1.26	**–2.38**	2.06
	p	**0.002**	**0.02**	**0.001**	0.227	**0.002**	0.54

Corr. = correlation; n = sample size; r = Pearson correlation coefficient; clan mem. = number of clans a female belongs to; %clan_mem = percentage of clan membership; #clans = total number of clans detected; NCr = neocortex ratio; grpsz = group size; bold values indicate significant results; values in italic indicate tendencies to significance ($0.05 < p < 0.1$).

large groups, and large groups allow a larger number of clans to be formed), other effects, such as the decrease in network density and in the percentage of clan membership in larger groups, are more likely to be genuine emergent properties of primate grooming networks when groups get larger, because density as well as percentage of clan membership are network indices that are independent of group size.

Effects of neocortex ratio on grooming networks

The results of the correlation analyses for neocortex size are summarized in Table 4.2. We found that neocortex ratio was significantly negatively correlated with network density and per cent clan membership, indicating that species with larger neocortices form networks that are less dense and in which individual females are members of relatively fewer subgroups. In addition, there was a positive correlation between neocortex ratio and clan membership.

Social complexity and cognitive constraints

In order to establish the relationship between social complexity and brain size, we controlled for the effects of group size by using a mixed model. Neocortex ratio was found to be negatively related to most of the network parameters (see Table 4.2). When group size was controlled for, species with larger neocortices form smaller clans and were members of relatively fewer grooming clans (Figure 4.2). In addition, after controlling for group size the networks of larger-brained species were found to be significantly less dense and had a lower connectivity (Figure 4.2). However, there was no longer any effect on absolute clan membership (Table 4.2). These results suggest that grooming networks in species with larger brains are more fragmented: in other words, in these cases individual females are involved in relatively few direct relationships, with a large number of indirect relationships. By indirect relationships, we mean relationships in which a female is not directly involved via grooming with another individual, but which can nonetheless be reached via a series of direct grooming links through other females.

On the other hand, when neocortex ratio is held constant, group size was found to be positively related to most network metrics: females in larger groups form larger clans and are members of more clans, while grooming networks of larger groups have higher connectivity (Figure 4.3). Density, the number of clans and relative clan membership were not affected by group size (after controlling for brain size).

Key players in female social networks

Average connectivity between female primates dropped significantly when the individual with the highest betweenness centrality was removed from the analysis (Figure 4.4: paired samples t-test: $t = 12.1$, $df = 10$, $p<0.0001$), indicating that one (or at most a few) central female might be responsible for much of the overall group connectivity. In contrast, there was no change in overall connectivity when we removed the individual with the lowest betweenness value (Figure 4.4: paired samples t-test: $t = -0.9$, $df = 10$, $p = 0.38$).

DISCUSSION

Our analysis shows that, in female-bonded primate species, social network parameters are affected by both group size and neocortex size, with both variables having independent effects on social networks. While the effects of group size are similar to those found in other studies (Carter & Feld 2004; Hislop 2005), we demonstrate for the first time an effect of brain size on social network structure.

(a)

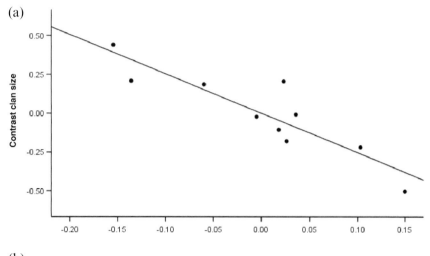

(b)

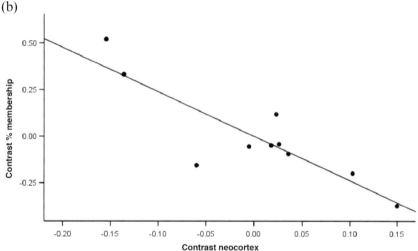

Figure 4.2. Relationship between neocortex ratio and (a) mean clan size, (b) percent clan membership.

Effects of group size

Although comparisons between networks of different sizes are not always easy to interpret, we believe that at least some of the effects reported here are a consequence of group size rather than simply being a scaling problem (cf. James et al. 2009). For example, it has previously been shown in human social networks that density is negatively correlated to the size of the network (Carter & Feld 2004; Hislop 2005). This effect is not surpris-

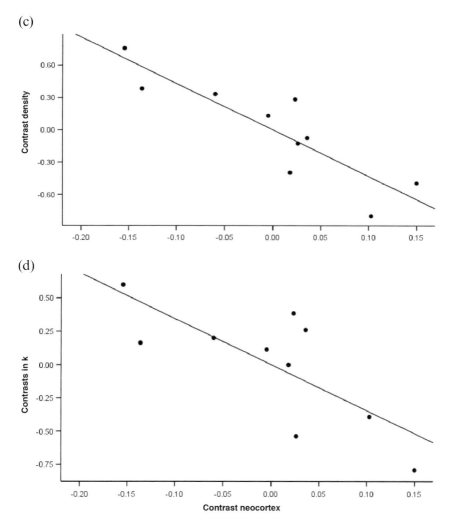

Figure 4.2 continued. (c) network density and (d) connectivity (k). Graphs represent partial plots, controlling for group size; calculations are based on independent contrasts. For statistical values see Table 4.2.

ing, given that the number of possible links in a network increases rapidly with network size. However, given that the number of individual ties is constrained by the time available for grooming as well as by neocortex size (presumably reflecting cognitive constraints), we might also expect that, in larger groups, the number of actual ties decreases relative to the number of possible ties.

(a)

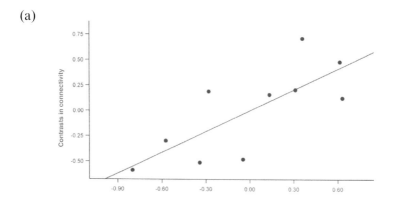

(b)

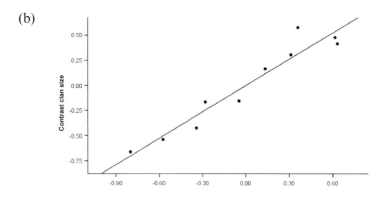

(c)

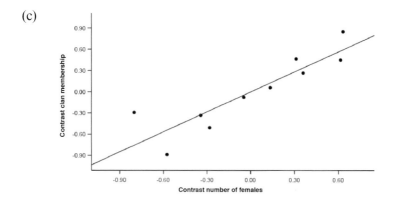

Figure 4.3. Relationship between group size and (a) connectivity, (b) mean clan size and (c) absolute clan membership. Graphs represent partial plots, controlling for neocortex ratio; calculations are based on independent contrasts. For statistical values see Table 4.2.

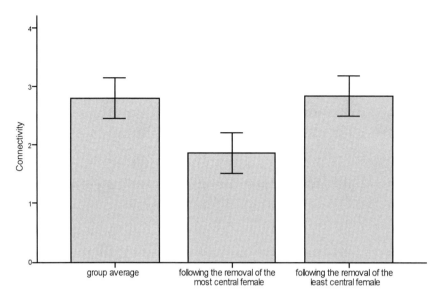

Figure 4.4. Effect of the removal of the most or the least central individual on overall group connectivity; only one female was removed in each of the removal conditions. Plotted values are means ($\pm$ 1 SE) across species.

We further found that clan size and clan membership show a positive correlation with group size, while relative clan membership (as a percentage of available clans) is negatively related to group size. While the latter effect disappeared when controlling for neocortex ratio, we believe that the first two effects are indeed due to a scaling effect (i.e. larger groups inevitably allow the formation of more and larger clans compared to smaller groups). Finally, group size was found to be positively correlated to overall connectivity (when controlling for neocortex ratio) and this relationship remained significant even after the removal of the most central female in the group. This suggests that females in large groups are better connected and less affected by the removal of a central individual. If this is indeed the case, it further suggests a dissociation between the effects of group size and those of social cognition (as measured by neocortex size), indicating that using group size may not always be a reliable proxy for social complexity.

Social complexity

The finding that neocortex size was negatively correlated with clan size and relative clan membership (i.e. that in species with larger brains,

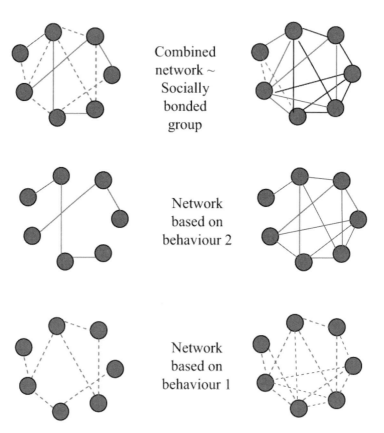

Figure 4.5. Illustration of social complexity measured by social networks based on different behaviours. We suggest that (i) a bonded social group emerges by overlaying networks based on different behaviours and (ii) that in socially highly complex species more behaviours are needed because networks are more differentiated than in socially less complex species. Circles represent individuals and lines represent relationships between individuals (dotted grey lines for behaviour 1, full grey lines for behaviour 2, black lines for links present in both networks). Under the low social complexity condition networks based on different behaviours are very similar and dense, while under the high social complexity condition networks are fragmented and dissimilar. See discussion for more details.

females form smaller grooming clans and each female is a member of fewer clans) was unexpected. This finding appears to contradict a previous study, which found that in primates grooming network size is positively correlated with brain size (Kudo & Dunbar 2001). However, there are a number of fundamental differences between our study and that by Kudo and Dunbar (2001). First, we only used female-bonded species and analysed only female social networks, while Kudo and Dunbar used a larger range of Old World monkey and ape species and did not differentiate between males and females. We expect that using social networks involving both sexes will mask the effects reported here because males and females are expected to use different social strategies as they pursue different social goals. Furthermore, relationships between the sexes are driven by different motivations and presumably differ in quality, making comparisons between networks of different species/groups difficult to interpret. To fully understand social complexity, however, it would be interesting to compare networks of groups with variable sex ratios, as all social relationships (within and between sexes) will ultimately add to time and cognitive constraints. Second, in our study we controlled for the effects of group size on social networks, whereas Kudo and Dunbar did not. Third, and perhaps most importantly, Kudo and Dunbar calculated egocentric networks, in which each individual group member is the centre of its own network; in contrast, our study focused on overall network structure, looking at the social group as a unit (thereby allowing us to investigate the influence of individual strategies on the group structure as a whole). While Kudo and Dunbar were interested in individual females' direct grooming networks, we were interested in how the group as a unit is structured as a result of individuals' social interactions (i.e. what it is that makes a system more or less complex). The grooming networks used in the Kudo and Dunbar (2001) study are therefore not comparable to the concept of grooming clans used in our study, and any comparison needs to be undertaken with caution.

Our results (i.e. negative relationships between neocortex size and network density, clan size, percentage clan membership and connectivity) suggest that increased brain size enables individuals to focus their direct social efforts on a few key individuals: 'friends' or 'allies' (Silk 2007; Silk et al. 2003). This leads to a number of relatively distinct clans and results in low levels of overall network density and connectivity. At the same time, however, each individual member has to manage a larger number of indirect social relationships (i.e. relationships in which they are not directly involved through grooming), because in a socially bonded group each group member has to maintain some level of social knowledge of every other group member. Previous studies have shown that such knowledge can be very fine-grained (e.g. Bergman et al. 2003; Cheney et al. 1995), a trait that distinguishes the primate groups in our analysis from simple aggregations. Thus, we suggest that maintaining a highly fragmented network in which members of the same social group are organized into smaller clans with relatively little overlap, while at the same time maintaining a higher-level grouping structure (as a bonded social group), is socially more complex.

It may be this capacity to concentrate social efforts on a few key individuals without losing group cohesion that ultimately allows group members to avoid such problems as time-budgeting conflicts (grooming every individual would be too time-consuming to do in a large group) and ecological competition (e.g. by having a few but reliable allies) among group members that would otherwise make living in large, densely packed groups very difficult. Additionally, it could be hypothesized that the existing relationships in such complex networks are more 'intense', involving either more fine-grained information or are more time-consuming (as compared to those in less complex networks) and may hence impose higher cognitive demands on individuals ('quality instead of quantity').

In this study, we only analysed one behavioural component, namely grooming, and we assumed the existence of a higher social structure (namely, the group as a whole) as all species in this analysis live in bonded social groups. This is an important restriction to our analysis. Ideally, these analyses should be based on several behavioural components simultaneously, as it is likely that primates use several modes of interaction to form social relationships (see also Hinde 1976). Similar analyses should also be undertaken for species that live in non-bonded groups (i.e. aggregations). The fact that we used socially bonded groups (i.e. groups in which members of the group cooperate to exclude non-members trying to join) only allows us to analyse one facet of social complexity. In human social network analysis, social complexity has been described as a multi-level phenomenon in which the macro-levels emerge from the micro-levels (Goldspink & Kay 2004). Based on our analysis, we hypothesize that the same may apply to primates: the macro-level (i.e. the socially bonded group) emerges from micro-level behavioural interactions (cf. Hinde 1976). We also hypothesize that the more complex the network, the more behavioural components will be needed to describe the macro-level because of the increasing levels of fragmentation in more complex networks (see Figure 4.5). In other words, we would predict that, in a complex social system, individuals might need to use a variety of different behavioural processes to manage and maintain group cohesion, such as proximity, coalition formation, mutual tolerance, etc., in addition to grooming.

Social networks could be analysed for all these behaviours, and we predict that, in larger-brained species, there will be an increasing dissociation between these parameters such that grooming networks are increasingly dissimilar to association networks. If this is so, then overlaying networks based on different behaviours will be necessary to provide a full description of socially bonded groups. Support for this comes from chimpanzee social networks, where it has been found that association networks are very stable over time, whereas grooming networks are much more fluid (Lehmann & Boesch 2009). However, taken together, the two networks produce a socially coherent group in terms of network metrics (Lehmann & Boesch 2009). In less complex networks, on the other hand, different behavioural measures would show a much stronger overlap, so that few behavioural parameters may be needed to describe the macro-level. Simpler networks of this kind should be predominantly found in species with smaller neocortices, which are predicted to live in less complex social systems. We further predict that these characteristics also distinguish socially bonded groups from simple random aggregations, in which no higher-order grouping level emerges, no matter how many behavioural parameters are used. Unfortunately, although more data on animal social networks are becoming available (Manno 2008; Miller et al. 2008; Ryder et al. 2008) there is a complete dearth of data suitable to test these predictions. However, the few studies using primate social networks in this context support our claim (cf. Lehmann & Boesch 2009; Maryanski 1987).

The importance of 'brokers'

It has previously been suggested that weak ties become increasingly important in socially more complex systems because they often link several otherwise unlinked subgroups (Maryanski 1987). In the present study, we tested this hypothesis by analysing the effects of removing individual females ('brokers') from the analysis on overall network connectivity. This method is more robust than actually identifying each weak tie within the network because it is less sensitive to potential oversights of such links (James et al. 2009).

Flack et al. (2006) demonstrated in a real removal experiment that it is often males that act as brokers in large bonded primate groups (a result first demonstrated in a cross-species analysis by Kudo and Dunbar [2001]). However, even though removal experiments (Flack et al. 2006) or the analysis of changes in networks after the death of a group member (Dunbar 1979; Engh et al. 2006) may help to elucidate the importance of key players in a social network, it remains questionable whether we will be able to fully understand the importance of individual members in animal social networks in this way. The definition of a broker is usually an individual who links two subgroups which, following their removal, will no longer be connected, resulting in two unconnected networks (Lusseau & Newman 2004). However, in socially complex species, we should expect a high degree of social flexibility and hence individual group members should be able to adjust their networks relatively quickly to the new conditions (Flack et al. 2006), thereby maintaining overall group cohesion. Thus, actual removal experiments may be of limited value for this particular question. A more theoretical analysis (i.e. the virtual removal of individuals out of a network), on the other hand, indicates that socially more complex networks are intrinsically more diverse in that a few key individuals contribute a lot to overall connectivity, such that when this individual is removed, connectivity decreases significantly.

Social complexity in human evolution

Our results suggest that increased brain power and cognition enables primates to maintain large closely bonded social groups despite concentrating social effort on only a few key group members. As brain size and group size increased during human evolution (e.g. Aiello & Dunbar 1993), we would thus expect that social network structure changed accordingly: social networks would have become increasingly fragmented as social investment became concentrated on a few key individuals within the group (presumably relatives and family members) with whom individuals would spend a lot of time. In support of this, Coward (ch. 21 this volume) found that even large-scale human networks of the Epipalaeolithic and early Neolithic became increasingly fragmented: this can be interpreted as suggesting increasing social complexity in human networks achieved by enlarging networks through focusing on 'brokers' between tightly bonded smaller units.

However, if higher-order grouping levels need to be maintained (e.g. for territory defence), individuals also need to keep track of all other group members and their relationships, even though time constraints would not allow intense social interactions. Primates need to gain direct visual or at the very least auditory information about changes in social relationships, and so need to encounter all other group members individually on a regular basis in order to do this. This need to manage what we have termed indirect (i.e. third party) social relationships will ultimately limit group size in primates.

In contrast to primates, humans have evolved a unique way to overcome this problem of information exchange: the evolution of language allows individuals to exchange information about social changes in increasingly fragmented networks without the need of direct social interactions between all group members (Dunbar 1992b, 1996). Social information can be exchanged through gossiping, making direct social contact unnecessary to track social developments within the group. This important step may have allowed humans to increase their group sizes even further (for comparative data on primate and human group sizes, see Layton & O'Hara ch. 5 this volume) and to establish complex relationships with other groups (such as trading relationships), embedding human social groups into a much larger social network across space and even time (see e.g. Layton & O'Hara ch. 5 this volume).

CONCLUSION

Our study is the first to demonstrate how social network analysis can be used to characterize social complexity across a variety of species. We show that social network structure changes as neocortex size changes. Our data suggest that, with increasing brain size, networks become increasingly fragmented: they are less dense, less well connected and consist of more clans with relatively fewer members. This might function as an operational definition of social complexity and suggests that the evolution of a large brain enables individuals to maintain a higher-order group structure while at the same time concentrating social effort on only a few key individuals. As a consequence, individuals will have to manage either an increasingly large number of indirect social relationships (i.e. those in which they are not actively involved but which need monitoring) or, alternatively, they have to manage an increasing number of different social networks which—as a whole—reflect the higher-order social level (i.e. the bonded group).

While primates need to be in visual (or at least auditory) contact to obtain information about social relationships between other group members (such as rank reversals), humans may have used language to exchange

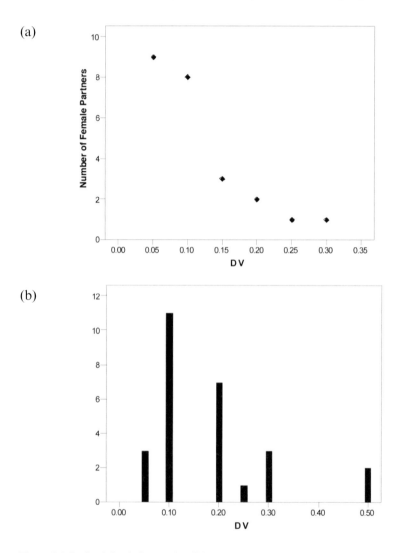

Figure 4.6. Optimal discriminant value (DV) to use in dichotomizing grooming matrices. (a) The plotted value is the number of female grooming partners obtained for a given discriminant value for one example species. (b) Distribution of optimal discriminant values in individual groups for the full sample of species.

relevant information (gossip) without the need to encounter all group members on a regular basis. This would have made the maintenance of indirect relationships much more manageable in human social groups, allowing humans to be part of a relatively large group while at the same time concentrating their social relationships on a few key individuals.

Although further analysis is needed to fully test the framework proposed here, what data are available so far support this proposal. In the meantime, this provides us with a promising and testable operational definition for one aspect of social complexity and social bonds in animals and humans.

Note.   JL and KA were funded by the British Academy Centenary Research Project. RD was supported by a British Academy Research Professorship. We would also like to thank several colleagues who generously shared their unpublished data with us and Susanne Shultz for discussions during data analyses.

APPENDIX

In order to identify an appropriate discriminant value (DV) to differentiate core from casual social partners, we analysed each grooming matrix separately to determine the number of female grooming partners that would result from using a range of values for the proportion of total grooming effort devoted to individual females. A plot of these values typically reveals a striking phase shift in the number of grooming partners at one particular DV (Figure 4.6a). With too small a DV, almost every female in the group was included as a grooming partner; a larger DV constrains the range of grooming partners to an identifiable core. The distribution of these values is highly skewed (Figure 4.6b), with a median value of DV = 0.1 (10% of grooming effort devoted to one individual) (see also Dunbar 1984; Kudo & Dunbar 2001). Although individual cases had higher values, we used this value in all analyses.

REFERENCES

Aiello, L. & Dunbar, R. I. M. (1993). Neocortex size, group size and the evolution of language. *Current Anthropology* 34: 184–93.
Andrews, K. (2007). *Social cohesion in primate societies*. Unpublished MPhil. thesis, University of Liverpool.
Anthoney, T. R. (1975). *Evolution of social structure in baboons (Papio spp.): detailed analysis of social structure in a captive group of guinea baboons (P. papio) and a comparative review and analysis of social structure in all species of the genus.* Unpublished PhD thesis, University of Chicago.

Aureli, F., Bearder, S., Call, J., Connor, R., Holekamp, K. E., Lehmann, J. et al. (2008). Fission-fusion dynamics: new research frameworks. *Current Anthropology* 49: 627–654.

Bellingham, L. (2002). *Principles of social attraction in female Barbary macaques, macaca sylvanus.* Unpublished PhD thesis, University of Liverpool.

Bergman, T. J., Beehner, J. C., Cheney, D. L. & Seyfarth, R. M. (2003). Hierarchical classification by rank and kinship in baboons. *Science* 302: 1234–1236.

Butovskaya, M. L., Kotzintsev A. G. & Welker, C. (1995). Grooming and social rank by birth: the case of *Macaca fascicularis. Folia Primatologica* 65: 30–33.

Byrne, R. W. & Corp, N. (2004). Neocortex size predicts deception rate in primates. *Proceedings of the Royal Society of London Series B-Biological Sciences* 271: 1693–1699.

Byrne, R. W. & Whiten, A. (eds) (1988). *Machiavellian intelligence.* Oxford: Oxford University Press.

Campbell, N. A. & Reece, J. B. (2005). *Biology.* San Francisco: Pearson Benjamin Cummings.

Carter, W. C. & Feld, S. L. (2004). Principles relating social regard to size and density of personal networks, with applications to stigma. *Social Networks* 26: 323–329.

Cheney, D. L. & Seyfarth, R. M. (1980). Vocal recognition in free-ranging vervet monkeys. *Animal Behaviour* 28: 362–367.

Cheney, D. L. & Seyfarth, R. M. (1990). *How monkeys see the world.* Chicago: University of Chicago Press.

Cheney, D. L., Seyfarth, R. M. & Silk, J. B. (1995). The role of grunts in reconciling opponents and facilitating interactions among adult female baboons. *Animal Behaviour* 50: 249–257.

Deag, J. (1972). *Social behaviour in Barbary macaques.* Unpublished PhD thesis, University of Bristol.

Deaner, R. O., Isler, K., Burkart, J. & van Schaik, C. (2007). Overall brain size, and not encephalization quotient, best predicts cognitive ability across non-human primates. *Brain Behavior and Evolution* 70: 115–124.

Dunbar, R. I. M. (1979) Structure of gelada baboon reproductive units I: stability of social relationships. *Behaviour* 69: 72–87.

Dunbar, R. I. M. (1984) *Reproductive decisions: an economic analysis of gelada baboon social strategies.* Princeton, NJ: Princeton University Press.

Dunbar, R. I. M. (1992a). Neocortex size as a constraint on group size in primates. *Journal of Human Evolution* 20: 469–493.

Dunbar, R. I. M. (1992b). Coevolution of neocortex size, group size and language in humans. *Behavioral and Brain Sciences* 16: 681–735.

Dunbar, R. I. M. (1996). *Grooming, gossip and the evolution of language.* London: Faber & Faber.

Dunbar, R. I. M. (1998). The social brain hypothesis. *Evolutionary Anthropology* 6: 178–190.

Dunbar, R. I. M. (2003) Evolution of the social brain. *Science* 302: 1160–1161

Dunbar, R. I. M. (in press). Brain and behaviour in primate evolution. In: P. H. Kappeler & J. Silk (eds) *Mind the gap: tracing the origins of human universals.* Cambridge, MA: MIT Press.

Dunbar, R. I. M. & Sharman, M. (1984). Is social grooming altruistic? *Zeitschrift Fur Tierpsychologie—Journal of Comparative Ethology* 64: 163–173.

Dunbar, R. I. M. & Shultz, S. (2007a). Evolution in the social brain. *Science* 317: 1344–1347.

Dunbar, R. I. M. & Shultz, S. (2007b). Understanding primate brain evolution. *Philosophical Transactions of the Royal Society of London Series B-Biological Sciences* 362: 649–658.

Engh, A. L., Beehner, J. C., Bergman, T. J., Whitten, P. L., Hoffmeier, R. R., Seyfarth, R. M. et al. (2006). Behavioural and hormonal responses to predation in female chacma baboons (*Papio hamadryas ursinus*). *Proceedings of the Royal Society of London Series B-Biological Sciences* 273: 707–712.

Finlay, B. L. & Darlington, R. B. (1995). Linked regularities in the development and evolution of mammalian brains. *Science* 268: 1578–1584.

Flack, J. C., Girvan, M., de Waal, F. B. M. & Krakauer, D.C. (2006). Policing stabilizes construction of social niches in primates. *Nature* 439: 426–430.

Goldspink, C. & Kay, R. (2004) Bridging the micro-macro divide: a new basis for social science. *Human Relations* 57: 597–618.

Hinde, R. A. (1976). Interactions, relationships and social structure. *Man* 11: 1–17

Hislop, D. (2005). The effect of network size on intra-network knowledge processes. *Knowledge Management Research & Practice* 3: 244–259.

James, R., Croft, D. P. & Krause, J. (2009). Potential banana skins in animal social network analysis. *Behavioural Ecology and Sociobiology* 63(7): 989–997.

Jerison, H. J. (1973). Evolution of the brain and intelligence. London: Academic Press.

Jolly, A. (1966). Lemur social behavior and primate intelligence—step from prosimian to monkey intelligence probably took place in a social context. *Science* 153: 501–508.

Kaplan, J. R. & Zucker, E. (1980). Social organization in a group of free-ranging patas monkeys. *Folia Primatologica* 34: 196–213.

Krause, J., Croft, D. P. & James, R. (2007). Social network theory in the behavioural sciences: potential applications. *Behavioral Ecology and Sociobiology* 62: 15–27.

Kudo, H. & Dunbar, R. I. M. (2001). Neocortex size and social network size in primates. *Animal Behaviour* 62: 711–722.

Lehmann, J. & Boesch, C. (2009). Sociality of the dispersing sex: the nature of social bonds in West African female chimpanzees (*Pan troglodytes*). *Animal Behaviour* 77: 377–387.

Lehmann, J., Korstjens, A. H. & Dunbar, R. I. M. (2007). Group size, grooming and social cohesion in primates. *Animal Behaviour* 74: 1617–1629.

Lewis, K. P. (2000). A comparative study of primate play behaviour: implications for the study of cognition. *Folia Primatologica* 71: 417–421.

Lusseau, D. & Newman, M. E. J. (2004). Identifying the role that animals play in their social networks. *Proceedings of the Royal Society B-Biological Sciences* 271: S477–S481.

Manno, T. G. (2008). Social networking in the Columbian ground squirrel, *Spermophilus columbianus*. *Animal Behaviour* 75: 1221–1228.

Maryanski, A. R. (1987). African ape social structure: is there strength in weak ties? *Social Networks* 9: 191–215.

Miller, J. L., King, A. P. & West, M. J. (2008). Female social networks influence male vocal development in brown-headed cowbirds, *Molothrus ater*. *Animal Behaviour* 76: 931–941.

Oi, T. (1988). Sociological study on the troop fission of wild Japanese monkeys (*Macaca fuscata yakui*) on Yakushima Island. *Primates* 29: 1–19.

Pawlowski, B., Lowen, C. B. & Dunbar, R. I. M. (1998). Neocortex size, social skills and mating success in primates. *Behaviour* 135: 357–368.

Pérez-Barbería, J., Shultz, S. & Dunbar, R. I. M. (2007). Evidence for intense co-evolution of sociality and brain size in three orders of mammals. *Evolution* 61: 2811–2821.

Purvis, A. (1995). A composite estimate of primate phylogeny. *Philosophical Transactions of the Royal Society of London Series B-Biological Sciences* 348: 405–421.

Rowell, T. E., Wilson, C. & Cords, M. (1991). Reciprocity and partner preference in grooming of female blue monkeys. *International Journal of Primatology* 12: 319–336.

Ryder, T. B., Mcdonald, D. B., Blake, J. G., Parker, P. G. & Loiselle, B. A. (2008) Social networks in the lek-mating wire-tailed manakin (*Pipra filicauda*). *Proceedings of the Royal Society B-Biological Sciences*. 275: 1367–1374.

Seyfarth, R. M. (1980). The distribution of grooming and related behaviors among adult female vervet monkeys. *Animal Behaviour* 28: 798–813.

Shultz, S. & Dunbar, R. I. M. (2007). The evolution of the social brain: anthropoid primates contrast with other vertebrates. *Proceedings of the Royal Society of London Series B-Biological Sciences* 274: 2429–2436.

Silk, J. B. (2007). Social components of fitness in primate groups. *Science* 317: 1347–1351.

Silk, J. B., Alberts, S. C. & Altmann, J. (2003). Social bonds of female baboons enhance infant survival. *Science* 302: 1231–1234.

Stephan, H., Frahm, H. & Baron, G. (1981). New and revised data on volumes in brain structures in insectivores and primates. *Folia Primatologica* 35: 1–29.

Sugiyama, Y. (1971). Characteristics of the social life of Bonnet macaques (*Macaca radiata*). *Primates* 12: 247–266.

Wasserman, S. & Faust, K. (1994) *Social network analysis: methods and applications*. Cambridge: Cambridge University Press.

Wey, T., Blumstein, D. T., Shen, W. & Jordan, F. (2008). Social network analysis of animal behaviour: a promising tool for the study of sociality. *Animal Behaviour* 75: 333–344.

Wolfheim, J. H. (1977). A quantitative analysis of the organization of a group of captive talapoin monkeys (*Miopithecus talapoin*). *Folia Primatologica* 27: 1–27.

5

Human Social Evolution: A Comparison of Hunter-gatherer and Chimpanzee Social Organization

ROBERT LAYTON & SEAN O'HARA

WE COMPARE THE SOCIAL BEHAVIOUR of human hunter-gatherers with that of the better-studied of the two chimpanzee species, *Pan troglodytes*, in an attempt to pinpoint the unique features of human social evolution. Chimpanzees have presumably followed their own evolutionary trajectory, and we do not assume they represent the social behaviour of any common ancestral species. Humans and chimpanzees nonetheless share a fission-fusion type of social dynamic, although such systems are unusual in primates (Aureli et al. 2008).[1] In both species small temporary, task-specific parties of variable membership form within the residential community that later rejoin other parties, again of variable membership. This shared pattern in spatial distribution within the community can help define the role of the community for both humans and chimpanzees, and that of human bands, which appear absent in chimpanzees. Our primary data for chimpanzees come from six study sites: Budongo, Ngogo and Kanyawara in Uganda; Gombe and Mahale in Tanzania; and Taï, Côte d'Ivoire. Our primary data on hunter-gatherers are taken from ethnographic studies of 26 hunter-gatherer peoples, ranging from those who occupy the same environment as chimpanzees (Mbuti, Aka) and those occupying similar environments on other continents, to those occupying very different environments such as tropical and arctic deserts (because data on some are incomplete, our samples vary in size). In order to compare like for like, we confine our analysis to the observable behaviour of both species. It is, however, difficult completely to disregard intentions.

---

[1] Found in only eight species of non-human primate: South American spider monkeys (two species) and muriquis; Asian apes: orangutans, African apes: chimpanzees and bonobos; African cercopithicines: gelada and hamadryas baboons.

Proceedings of the British Academy **158**, 83–113. © The British Academy 2010.

Male hunter-gatherers set off with the deliberate intention of hunting, whereas chimpanzee hunts can be more opportunistic; males may be foraging, resting or undertaking a border patrol when a troop of monkeys approach and stimulate the start of a hunt, and chimpanzee hunting party size may thus be determined by patrol size.

The behaviour of both hunter-gatherers and chimpanzees today is affected by the presence of more powerful human neighbours. Neither represents the 'original condition' of the species. Because hunter-gatherers survived longest in environments unsuitable for farming, our sample is also biased by its lack of data on hunter-gatherers living in resource-rich environments. Our case studies are in the 'ethnographic present' of the time they were recorded. The Mbuti have since been caught up in the civil wars on the Rwandan-Congo border, while the government of Botswana is currently (2008) denying G/wi access to bore water in the Kalahari Game Reserve. Disease had reduced many populations by the time they were first studied by anthropologists, although some have since recovered (Cree—Rogers 1972, 94; Northwest Coast— Rohner & Rohner 1970, 84; G/wi—Silberbauer 1972, 303; Gugadja— Cane 1990, 150). Furthermore, most hunter-gatherers today rely to some extent on cultivated or purchased foods and this may affect not only the size, but even the shape, of foraging ranges. Mbuti territories, for example, consist of long, narrow strips extending from a farming village to the deep forest (Ichikawa 1978, cited in Bahuchet 1992). However, through a comparison of those human communities whose subsistence strategies are closest to those of chimpanzees, we identify consistencies in behaviour that throw light on the species' characteristic social strategies, and variability that indicates how such strategies have been adapted to specific ecological constraints.

Although the total size of a typical hunter-gatherer community is greater than that of a chimpanzee community, the size of the action sets that forage together is similar. Male chimpanzees move in parties of up to 4–5, while human hunters frequently hunt singly or in pairs. Cooperative drives similar to those claimed for male chimpanzees take place in larger parties of 10–30. Female chimpanzees move in parties of up to seven (O'Hara unpublished data), foraging women in parties of up to ten (see Table 5.1). The size of the group within which day-to-day interaction occurs—the community among chimpanzees and the band among humans—is comparable, ranging from 40 to 150 among chimpanzees and 35 to 80 among hunter-gatherers. However, while the hunter-gatherer band has frequently been treated as the human equivalent of the chimpanzee community, we argue that this is incorrect. The chimpanzee community should be compared with the human community, and the band treated as a more enduring fusion phase within a wider pattern of fission and fusion sustained by inter-band movement. We consider the functional benefits of band membership, and of membership in a wider community.

BAND OR COMMUNITY?

Social anthropologists have long equated hunter-gatherer society with the band (Radcliffe-Brown 1930; Steward 1936). Men were supposed to remain in the same band all their lives, while women transferred from one band to another at marriage. When it was discovered that the male chimpanzee has to spend his entire life living in the community into which he was born while female chimpanzees typically change community at adolescence, the chimpanzee community was equated with the hunter-gatherer band (e.g. Foley & Lee 1989 and commentators on Hawkes et al. 1997). The band, however, is a much more fluid and permeable grouping than Radcliffe-Brown and Steward appreciated. Human adults of both sexes often freely change band membership, whereas the chimpanzee community appears to be a closed reproductive unit (Wrangham 2000).

Among chimpanzees, the males of the community defend the boundary of their territory and attack individuals from neighbouring communities that they discover in the border zone (Wilson et al. 2004). Men may range more widely than women within the human band territory, but this is probably due to prey distribution rather than boundary defence (Aka—Bahuchet 1992, 222; Cree—Rogers 1972, 106, 109, 127; G/wi—Silberbauer 1972, 287, 290; Nukak—Politis 2007, Table 6.2; Numamiut—Binford 1976, 169).

Neighbouring hunter-gatherer bands often acknowledge mutual rights of access over each others' territories. Richard Lee writes that camp composition among the Ju/'hoansi changes monthly and even daily, due mainly to inter-camp visiting (1979, 54). Colin Turnbull wrote of the Mbuti (sympatric with chimpanzees), that 'individuals or whole families sometimes wander . . . until they are several territories distant from their home territory' (1965, 96). Visiting between Hadza camps was continuous and it was 'not uncommon' for individuals or single families to change camp (Hawkes et al. 1997, 553). Winter band composition among the Cree varies from year to year (Rogers 1972, 121).

Table 5.1. Foraging party size, band size, community size and population density in a range of groups and habitat types

	Foraging party size (a) male	(b) female	Band size range	mean	Community size	Pop. density/km²
Tropical forest						
Ache (Paraguay)			15–70	50	<500	0.03
Aka (Central African Republic)			c. 24–28		500	0.031 (Bagandu [1]) 0.28 (Bagandu [2]) 0.017 (N'Delé)
Batek De (Malaysia)	1–2	2–3	'20 families'	c. 80?	200	0.11
Cholanaickan (India)			5–28	20	250	0.6
Mbuti (Zaire)	1–5	2–3	37–62			0.17–0.2
Nukak (Colombia)	1–3	2–11 (mixed parties)	12–63	20–30	125	0.034
Tropical coast						
Gidjingali (Australia)	1–3	2–7	14–80	34	300	0.46
Gunwinggu (Australia)			18–44		175	0.05
Tiwi (Australia)	1–3; 15	2–3	40–50		1000	0.4
Yolngu (Australia)				32.7	>500	0.34
Savanna						
Hadza (Tanzania)	1	2–10	35–60		750	0.34
Yolngu (Australia)						0.06
Semi-desert						
G/wi (Kalahari)	1–2; 12		21–85	57	2000	0.07
Ju/'hoansi (Kalahari)	1–2	2–4	9–75 (<141)*	42	460	0.017
Warlpiri (Australia)			25–30		>200	0.01
Western Desert (Aus)			6–30	13.6	250–600	0.01–0.02
Temperate coast						
Kwakiutl (Canada)			50–60		280	0.24 [1] 0.57 [2]
Nootka (Canada)	1 to 'several'					0.4 [1] 0.66–0.77 [2]
Tlingit (Canada)	1–2; 20–60		<50			

Boreal forest					
Cree (Canada)			15–50	450 [1] 250–1000 [2]	0.004
Khanti (Siberia)			1–6 households / c. 14?	800	0.005
Arctic coast					
Central Canadian Inuit			Winter 50–150 / Summer 15–30	500	0.012–0.005
Hudson Bay	1–8			500–700 (Itivimiut) / 150 (Qiqiqtamiut)	0.016
Netsilik (Canada)	2–3	20–30 (mixed)	Winter 50–100 / Summer 20–30	260	0.005
Taremiut (Alaska)	2; 35		30–100 [1] 12–75	336 [1] av 450 [2]	0.05–0.15 [1] 0.07 [2]
Arctic interior					
Nunamiut (Alaska)			Winter 50–150 (Gubser) / Summer 18–36 (Binford)		0.02

*Population at /Xai/xai is exceptionally large (141); the next largest waterhole group size is 75. Where two sets of figures are given for male parties, the larger figure refers to collective hunting (e.g. fire drives, seals, caribou).

Sources

Ache—Hill & Hurtado 1996, 41–49, 61, 81; **Aka**—Bahuchet 1992, 219 [1]; Hewlett et al. 1982, 425 [2]; Bahuchet 1988 cited in Kelly 1995; **Batek Dé**—Endicott 1979, 11; 1988, 110; **Cholanaickan**—Bhanu 1992, 48; Kelly 1995, Table 6.4 cites similar densities for Hill Pandaran and Paliyan; **Mbuti**—Bahuchet 1992, 212; Turnbull 1965, 167; Harako 1981, 506–507; **Nukak**—Politis 2007, 25, 36, 77–78, 164; **Gidjingali**—Jones 1980, 137; Meehan 1982, 13, 15, 90–105; Peterson & Long 1986, 40–42; White et al. 1990, 177; **Gunwinggu**—Altman 1987, 15, 22, 23; **Tiwi**—Hart & Pilling 1960, 33–37; Goodale 1986, 199; **Yolngu**—Peterson & Long 1986, 135; Williams 1986, 131; **Hadza**—Woodburn 1972, 193–194, Hawkes et al. 1997, 552–555; **G/wi**—Silberbauer 1972, 273, 295; **Ju/'hoansi**—Lee 1979, 53 and pers. comm., 351; **Warlpiri**—Meggitt 1962, 47; Peterson & Long 1986, 38, 69; **Western Desert**—Gould 1969, 64; Layton 1986, 43; Peterson & Long 1986, 135; Tonkinson 1991, 71; **Kwakiutl**—Codere 1950, 50–52 [data for 1853], [1]; Hunn 1994, 2]; Kelly 1995, Table 6.4 citing Mitchell & Donald, and Shalk; **Nootka**—Drucker 1965, 17, 19, 150, [1] estimated from map; Drucker 1965, 3, [2]; Kelly 1995, Table 6.4 citing Mitchell and Donald; **Tlingit**—Emmons 1991, 105–132; **Cree**—Scott 1988, 38, [1]; Rogers 1972, 91, [2]; Feit 1983, 417; **Khanti**—Jordan 2003, 40–42, 73–74, 85, 251–260; Kelly 1995, Table 6.4 cites same density for Yukaghir; **Central Canadian Inuit**—Damas 1969, 45, 51, 113; 1984 cited Kelly 1995, Table 6.4; **Hudson Bay Itivimiut**—Smith 1991, 112; Hunn 1994; **Qiqiqtamiut**—Guemple 1988, 131; **Netsilik**—Balikci 1970, xxiii, 56; Kelly 1995, Table 6.4; **Taremiut [1]**—Andrews 1989, 21, 93–94, [2; community figure for 1880]; Burch 1988, 96–97; **Nunamiut**—Binford 1976, 204–205, 231, 236; Gubser 1965, 167; Kelly 1995, Table 6.4 citing Hall.

To increase sample size in the box plots we have added secondary data from Kelly on band size and population density for the Bihor, Hill Pandaram, Paliyan, Semang and Andaman Islanders, and population density for the Great Basin (USA), Bella Coola, Haida, Tsimshian, Chipewan, Tutchone, Gilyak, Round Lake Ojibwa, Ojibwa, Yaghan and Yukaghir. We have not used Kelly's data on band sizes for these high latitude societies as these appear to be based on winter aggregations (see discussion in text).

It is harder for hunter-gatherers to move between regional communities (Kalahari—Wiessner 1982; Nukak—Politis 2007, 164) and the hunter-gatherer community sometimes acts collectively to defend subsistence resources (Alaskan Inuit—Andrews 1989, 30; Burch 1988, 98; Gubser 1965, 166–167: Gidjingali—White et al. 1990, 177). On the Northwest Coast of North America, the winter village community contained several lineages that came together for mutual defence (Boas 1966, 35–36; Drucker 1965, 47; Hunn 1986, 33–34).

The human community is most frequently characterized as an endogamous breeding unit. The Alaskan Inuit community was 80 per cent endogamous (Burch 1988, 96) and there was a high rate of endogamy among the Nukak *munu* (Politis 2007, 164). Wobst's pioneering paper predicted, on the basis of computer simulations, that a demographically stable hunter-gatherer breeding population would require a minimum of 175–475 individuals (Wobst 1974, 169). Data in Table 5.1 support this prediction.

Thus the human *community* seems the best parallel with the chimpanzee community. Central to our argument is the hypothesis that bands are better seen as intermediate groups which have crystallized during human social evolution, emerging as social bonds of cooperation and reciprocal exchange between individuals became stronger during the evolution of modern hunter-gatherer strategies. Equating the regional community, rather than the band, with the chimpanzee community is more consistent with Dunbar's (1993) prediction of group size from brain evolution, although Barton (2006) has recently argued that specific aspects of social complexity, including the tracking of relationships with absent individuals, provides a better explanation for human brain evolution. The capacity to move between bands, according to this hypothesis, would persist from the earlier pattern of fission-fusion within the wider community, but enhanced by specifically human traits such as language, and gift exchange with members of other bands.

In the great majority of societies included in this survey, band recruitment is flexible. The greatest degree of fluidity appears to exist among the Batek De, where, according to Endicott (1979, 10–11), there are no lineages, bands or other corporate groups larger than the conjugal family. In most cases, the core of the band consists of a few bilaterally related families, to which other families attach themselves for a greater or lesser period (Ache—Hill & Hurtado 1996, 66; Aka—Bahuchet 1992, 219; Cholanaickan—Bhanu 1992, 48; Hadza—Hawkes et al. 1997, 553; Ju/'hoansi—Lee 1976, 77, 1979, 58, 65, 338; Yellen 1976, 60; G/wi—

Silberbauer 1972, 308; Cree—Rogers 1972, 106, 119, 121; Hudson Bay Inuit—Smith 1991, 110). In Australia's Western Desert, individuals began life with potential rights in the father's and mother's bands, and also to the place where they were born, but only become 'kin to the country' by looking after it (Layton 1995). Myers (1986: 183) argues that while individuals must affiliate themselves to a residential group, rights to land in the Western Desert are best seen as the outcome of individual claims and assertions rather than descent.

SOCIAL FUNCTIONS OF FISSION AND FUSION AMONG HUNTER-GATHERERS

To investigate the adaptive value of the distinctive patterns of fission-fusion behaviour among hunter-gatherers, we look at the activities that take place during both fission and fusion phases.

Meat consumption

One of the most striking differences between hunter-gatherers and chimpanzees is that humans consume much more meat. Stiner (2002) concludes that systematic hunting of large ungulates by humans began about a quarter of a million years ago. Humans living in tropical forest consume up to ten times more meat than chimpanzees (see Table 5.2) and this has consequences both for population density and the social organization of hunting. Hayden (1981) and Marlowe (2001) found that male hunting contributes from between 20–25 per cent to 100 per cent of the human hunter-gatherer diet. Hunting contributes most to the diet in high latitudes, both because there is less plant food for women to gather and because more of the diet is derived from fishing. While information on weight of meat consumed per person is relatively hard to locate, the difference between chimpanzees and central African hunter-gatherers is striking.

As a consequence of our species' greater reliance on predation, hunter-gatherers occupying the same environment as chimpanzees live at considerably lower densities (Table 5.3; Figure 5.1; see also Grove ch. 19 this volume). In less rich environments humans are even more dispersed (Figure 5.1: $p < 0.001$). Hunter-gatherer population densities are thus very responsive to habitat type.

Because the human community is considerably more dispersed than the chimpanzee community, the coherence of the community cannot be

Table 5.2. Meat consumption

	Kg/individual/day	% meat in diet	Source
	Chimpanzee		
Gombe (male)	0.055	equivalent to 2–6%	Boesch & Boesch-Achermann
(female)	0.007	of total	2000, 165
		Kcalories/day	
Taï (male)	0.186		
(female)	0.025		
	Human hunter-gatherer		
Tropical forest			
Mbuti	0.5	30%	Ichikawa 2005, 159
	0.45		Hart 1978 in Kelly 1995, 103
	1.06		Tanno 1976 in Kelly 1995
Ache	1.78	87%	Hill et al. 1985, cited Kelly 1995, 103; Hill & Hurtado 1996, 65
Nukak (dry season)	0.237	10%	Politis 2007, 75
Nukak (wet season)	0.306		
Huaoroni	0.200+		Rival 2002, 75
Batek	0.2	67%	Endicott 1981 in Kelly 1995; Endicott 1988
Tropical coast			
Gunwinggu	0.621	50%+	Altman 1987, 36
Savannah			
Hadza	<1.00	50%	O'Connell et al. 2002, 858
Semi-desert			
Ju/'hoansi	0.256	30%	Lee 1979, 265 based on 28 days obs.
G/wi (October)	0.03		Silberbauer 1972, 285
G/wi (January and June)	0.22	30%	
Western Desert	0.56	15–30%	Gould 1980 in Kelly 1995, 103

Notes: Figures are for meat rather than protein and are taken from data in Hayden 1981, Table 10.3 (where hunting is distinguished from fishing), except Gunwinggu (Altman 1987, 42, 44), Nukak, based on raw weights of fruit and meat (quoted in Politis 2007), and Hadza, for whom O'Connell et al. (2002, 836) give figure of 50% 'for full-time foragers' (Hayden quotes a figure of 20% meat in Hadza diet). 87% of Gunwinggu bush protein derived from men's hunting and fishing (Altman 1987, 41), yielding 0.621 kg meat/person/day. Figure for Ache from Hill and Kaplan 1988 in Betzig, Borgerhoff-Mulder and Turke, via Hewlett 1991. Ichikawa's (2005) figure for the Mbuti is based on his report that a medium-sized duiker contains enough meat for 9 adult-days. Silberbauer (1972, 286) calculates that a duiker yields 10 lbs of meat (Lee 1979, 214 gives the meat yield from a duiker as 9.3 kg). Hayden (1981, 353) questions the validity of some data. He points out, for example, that while Gould estimates that Western Desert Aborigines consumed 0.5 kg meat per day, the returns on the hunting trips he observed were much lower. Silberbauer (1981, 486) notes that his data on yields are sometimes estimates.

Table 5.3. Body weight, population densities and foraging ranges, central Africa

	Male	Female
	Body weight in kg (Smith & Jungers 1997)	
Chimpanzee	42.7–59.7	33.7–45.8
Pygmies	47.9	42.2
	Population densities per km^2	
Chimpanzee	2.5	Wrangham et al. 1993
Aka	0.31	Hewlett et al. 1982 (*Man*)
	0.28 in Bagandou	Bahuchet 1988, cited in Kelly 1995
	0.17 in N'Delé	Hewlett et al. 1982
Mbuti	0.17 to 0.2	Turnbull 1962; Ichikawa 2005
	Home range size in km^2	
Chimpanzee (Gombe)	9.0–12.0 (male)	
	5.8–11.0 (female; smallest recorded range)	
Chimpanzee (Ngogo)	35 (largest recorded range)	
Mbuti	260	Turnbull 1968, 134, cited in Abruzzi 1980, 22
Aka	490	Hewlett et al. 1982, 422, 424

guaranteed by daily interaction and humans have evolved cultural mechanisms such as gift exchange and classificatory kinship to sustain relationships with individuals beyond the band whom they may meet only infrequently. Why, then, has the human community persisted, despite the greater difficulty of maintaining it? We also consider various functional benefits of retaining the ability to move between bands in the community.

THE FISSION PHASE (FORAGING PARTIES)

Although the size of the 'action sets' that forage together is of the same order among human hunter-gatherers and chimpanzees, human parties last for several hours while chimpanzee parties are of much shorter maximum duration, ranging from 69 minutes at Gombe (Halperin 1979) to 19 minutes in Budongo (Reynolds 2005). Unlike chimpanzee females, hunter-gatherer women very rarely forage alone. Hawkes et al. (1997, 558) write that Hadza women usually forage as a group. Warner (1958, 129) writes that the women in a Yolngu band frequently forage together as men claim to have practised sorcery on women encountered alone, while Hart and Pilling write that the young wives of Tiwi men are rarely allowed to

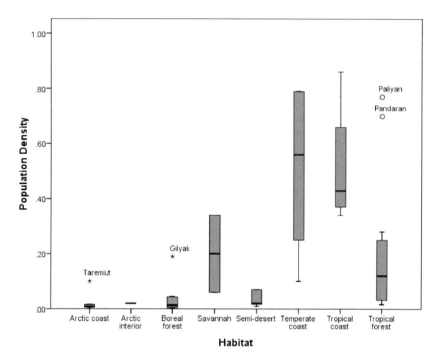

Figure 5.1. Hunter-gatherer population density as individuals per km² by habitat type

forage without a chaperone (1960, 36–37). According to Tonkinson (1991, 45), Mardu women usually forage in groups because it allows them to be sociable and share child-minding.

Hunting techniques

Male chimpanzees hunt animals smaller than themselves, typically monkeys. The most commonly hunted species across sites is the red colobus (Newton-Fisher et al. 2002) although, in the absence of red colobus at Budongo, chimpanzees there hunt black and white colobus and blue duiker. Chimpanzees hunt singly or in the company of others. In group hunts, a single prey is separated from a group and cornered. West African Taï chimpanzees are reported to collaborate, taking on the roles of 'drivers' and 'blockers' in hunts (Boesch & Boesch 1989). Once killed, any chimpanzee (male or female) present at the place will attempt to gain some of the meat. Active or passive sharing occurs (Newton-Fisher 2007).

(a)

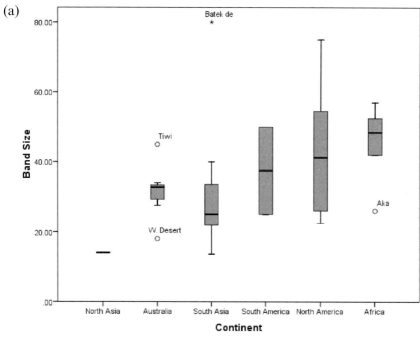

(b)

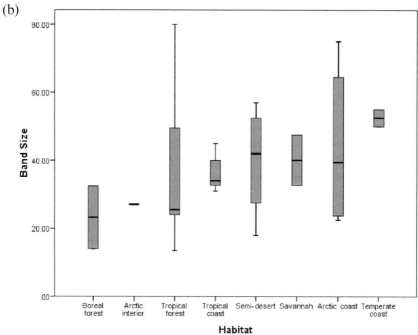

Figure 5.2. Band size by continent and habitat type

Some human hunting strategies appear similar, although using sophisticated technology and communication. In Mbuti net-hunting, for example, several families cooperate, joining their nets together. Men drive small game toward the net, while women and children kill any animal that is trapped (Harako 1981, 519; Turnbull 1965, 154). Aka bands on the same trail periodically form a single camp to enable more effective net-hunting (Bahuchet 1992, 226). Meat is always taken back to camp to be divided. Even those who were not present (such as elderly people and children) can expect a share. Fire drives among the Tiwi involve 10–15 men, with women and children acting as beaters (Hart & Pilling 1960, 33–37, 42). Finlayson (1935, 44) describes a similar fire drive in the Australian Western Desert. Inuit men cooperate to catch seals: each seal keeps several breathing holes open in the ice, and one man must stand by each hole to corner the seal.

Humans also have a different hunting strategy, hunting by stealth, where men go out from camp singly or in twos, to hunt larger prey. They creep up on the animal until it can be speared or shot with an arrow. Again, the meat is taken back to camp to share. Human hunting techniques are thus determined by both hunting technology and the behaviour of the prey species. Nunamiut congregate at the spring and autumn caribou hunting sites, located to intercept the migrating herd, but scatter in summer to hunt dispersed game (Binford 1976, 204, 235, 277, etc., cf. Damas 1969). Men in the Cree winter camp combine to hunt caribou, but moose/elk are solitary and are usually hunted by pairs of men (Rogers 1972, 111) or single hunters among the Khanti (Jordan 2003, 250).

A second key variable in human hunting strategies is the predictability of herd locations. Herd movements are more predictable in the arctic and boreal forest than in savannah and semi-deserts. Where the location of game is unpredictable, hunters of the band can reduce the risk of failure by dispersing. Hadza men routinely hunt independently, reducing but not eliminating the risk of failure (O'Connell et al. 2002, 836). Even though they target herd animals, G/wi hunters generally operate in pairs (Silberbauer 1981, 474). Each pair leaves camp in a different direction. Smith attributes the large winter aggregations of the Inuit to the wish to reduce risk in seal hunting through the winter ice by including more than one hunting team in the same camp (Smith 1991, 330). The success of this strategy depends crucially on hunters' willingness to bring meat back to camp and distribute it beyond the hunting party (Smith 1991, 330; cf. Damas 1969, 51).

FUSION PHASE 1: THE BAND

The overnight camp is a defining feature of human hunter-gatherer adaptation. A band is a group whose members meet up at the end of the day, assembling at a camp site which has been pre-arranged and may be used for a number of days at a time. Sharing of resources, such as the meat from game animals, takes place at this base camp. Chimpanzees do not assemble in this way; there are no set base camps and individuals build a new nest site wherever they find themselves at nightfall. The mean number of bands per community in our sample is approximately 17–18, ranging from 5 among the Kwakiutl to 30 in the Western Desert (Australia) and the G/wi, and up to 67 among the Khanti (see Table 5.1). The frequency with which the band moves camp location is variable. The Nukak band moves 70–80 times in a year, the mean distance between camps 3.85 km in the wet season and 7.65 km in the dry season (Politis 2007, 100, 166–167). Cholanaickan bands move weekly (Bhanu 1992, 48). Aka and Mbuti bands move camp on average six times a year; successive sites are usually one hour's walk apart, about 6 km (Bahuchet 1992, 212, 222).

Binford (1980) distinguished between 'logistic organization' and 'foraging', arguing that the Nunamiut were logistically organized while the San were foragers. Logistic organization is adapted to a highly seasonal environment, where the location of key food resources differs in a predictable way from season to season. Under such conditions, hunter-gatherers can cache seasonally used equipment at the appropriate site and move camp to another resource as it becomes available. Living in fine-grained environments with low seasonal variation, foragers exploit diverse resources and seek to locate their camps at places that will minimize travel distance to *all* resources. However Yellen (1976) argued that the Ju/'hoansi also strive for logistic organization, but are mapping onto a different resource distribution. Foragers in semi-desert environments must camp near scarce water supplies. The Ju/'hoansi occupy small, widely scattered and short-lived camps in the rainy season, and more permanent ones near secure water sources in the dry season. In the Western Desert of Australia, each band territory contains a permanent or semi-permanent water source that forms the base camp during drought (Layton 1986, 39–41). Hawkes et al. (1997) record that one Hadza band predicated its camp locations on the local abundance of plant foods, moving to fresh plant foods as they ripened.

Functional benefits of the band

Among non-human primates, party size is explained as a trade-off between reducing the increased predation risk experienced by small parties, and the increased competition for food experienced by large parties (Sterck et al. 1997; van Schaik 1989). Not only does human band size show no significant variation between Africa, where there is a high predation risk, and other continents (Figure 5.2a: p = 0.201), nor does it vary significantly between habitat type (Figure 5.2b: p = 0.505). Given the sensitivity of forager population densities to ecology, this is remarkable.

We therefore hypothesize that band size is the outcome of trade-offs between social costs and benefits. The flexibility of band composition is consistent with individuals' need to balance or 'trade off' competing benefits of joining different bands, in particular the husband's and wife's parents' bands. We identify four advantages of living in a band: child-minding, prior rights to resources, food sharing and information exchange. The primary cost of band life is competition for food resources within a day's range from camp.

Child-minding

Hawkes et al. (1997) found that Hadza mothers reduce the time they spend foraging at the birth of a new child. Older, weaned children too young to support themselves will therefore suffer. This is where the grandmother steps in: grandmothers spend most time foraging when their infant grandchild is youngest and their weaned grandchildren are receiving least from the mother. Thus a young mother will benefit from living with her parents' band. While Gurven and Hill (1997, 566) point out that only two of the eight older women tracked in the study were mother's mothers, five out of the eight were matrilateral relatives, and there is therefore evidence for the adaptive value of adult daughters living with maternal relatives. The specific value of the maternal grandmother's role has since been supported by Sear et al.'s (2000) study of infant survival among subsistence cultivators in the Gambia, and Gibson and Mace (2005) in Ethiopia. Leaving children in camp was a common practice (Ache—Hill & Hurtado 1996, 66; Cholanaickan—Bhanu 1992, 40; Ju/'hoansi—Lee 1979, 310, but in the context of Lee's seminal work on the relationship between carrying children when gathering and birth-spacing).

The ability of women to gather into old age is an important aspect of hunter-gatherer behaviour, but does not necessarily lead to young women remaining permanently in their mother's band. Newly married couples typically live with the bride's parents for a few years before returning to the husband's band (Aka—Bahuchet 1992, 219; Nukak—Politis 2007, 82; Cree—Rogers 1972, 106; G/wi—Silberbauer 1972, 303). Our data show that only one-third to a quarter of women live matrilocally. Despite the flexibility of recruitment to bands, which may be due in part to the marginal environments in which most recent hunter-gatherers live, there is widespread evidence for a patrilineal bias. Terashima (1985, quoted in Bahuchet 1992) reported that about three-quarters of men in a Mbuti band live with their paternal kin, one-fifth with maternal kin and one-fifth with their wife's kin. Bahuchet (1992, 219) also found two-thirds of Aka families living with the husband's band, one-third with the wife's. In the Uluru region of the Western Desert, 70 per cent of people joined their father's band, 20 per cent their mother's and 10 per cent the band of a more distant relative (Layton 1983, 25). The *numayms* (totemic clans) of the Kwakiutl, on the Northwest Coast of North America were recruited bilaterally, but with a slight patrilineal bias (Drucker & Heizer 1967, 10), although elsewhere on the Northwest Coast recruitment was ambilineal or matrilineal (Richardson 1986). There are evidently conflicting advantages of patrilocal and matrilocal residence that individuals must resolve when deciding which band to join.

Prior rights to resources

In two cases among the societies sampled (Batek De—Endicott 1979, 10; Hadza—Woodburn 1972, 193) there are no band prerogatives over foraging in any area. In a few instances the community, rather than the constituent band, is the land-holding unit (see above). Generally, however, the band holds prerogatives, but not exclusive rights, over resources in its territory (Cholanaickan—Bhanu 1992, 39; Ju/'hoansi—Lee 1979, 70; Mbuti—Turnbull 1965, 93, 174, 222–223; Nukak—Politis 2007, 163; Nunamiut—Gubser 1965, 165–167). Peterson and Long argue that even in the rich tropical woodland of Arnhem Land, an Aboriginal band of 40 occupying a territory of 400 km^2 would have had to defend a boundary of 70 km, equivalent to 2 km/man. Boundary defence is therefore not practised anywhere in Australia (Peterson & Long 1986: 29). Greeting rituals, where visitors wait for permission to enter a camp, are widespread in Australia (Peterson & Long 1986: 27–28). Peterson (1975) coined the term 'social boundary defence' to describe the strategy of controlling access to the group that asserts prior rights to the band territory or, in

Stanner's (1965) term, 'estate'.[2] However, some cases in which the band defends its territory are known (Ache—Hill & Hurtado 1996, 70, 72; Northwest Coast lineages in summer—Boas 1966, 35–36; Drucker 1965; 47; Hunn 1986: 33–34).

Information exchange

Among the G/wi, all information about game is relayed to hunters when the band camps together (Silberbauer 1981, 474). Information about caribou herd movements is exchanged in the Nunamiut village (Binford 1976, 178). Marshall (1976, 351) wrote that talking maintains good, open communication among band members, releases emotion, sanctions behaviour, and exchanges information about events, plans and movement of people. Men retell hunting exploits, women recall good gatherers.

Food distribution

Meat sharing is probably the best known, and most debated, aspect of band behaviour. Ichikawa (2005) points out that hunting success is uneven, but a large antelope in the Kalahari contains enough meat for 90–135 adult consumption days. Non-human carnivores cope with daily fluctuations through gluttony, whereas primates have a herbivore feeding rhythm. Ichikawa argues humans have inherited the latter pattern, despite their greater dependence on meat, and fluctuating supplies are dealt with by sharing. Sharing is most simply explained as an example of reciprocal altruism, a practice identified by Trivers (1971). Trivers argues that where there is a risk of death, e.g. from starvation, and where no-one knows who will be successful on any one occasion, yet those who are successful in obtaining food get more than their immediate need, it will pay to share, because when the once-successful individual is unsuccessful on another occasion, the debt can be repaid. Both partners will therefore survive whereas, on their own, both would have died. It has been shown that such reciprocity is only reliable where two other conditions hold good (Winterhalder 1990, 1996): individuals must have long-term social relationships, to allow for the balancing of give and take between partners, and it must be possible to detect, and pun-

---

[2] Australian anthropologists usually distinguish between band and clan, where the co-residential group is the band, the territorial group the clan (Stanner 1965). The distinction makes most sense where individuals have a presumptive right to a parent's territory from birth, and least sense where rights are only established through residence. Practice generally lies between these extremes, with clans most clearly existing in northern Australia and effectively absent in the Western Desert.

ish, 'cheaters', who try to avoid sharing when they do well, but take when they do badly. Band organization allows these conditions to be satisfied. The practice of sharing meat and honey within the Ache band increased nutritional status by 60 per cent (Kaplan & Hill 1985b, 233). Among the Nukak, even water and firewood are shared (Politis 2007, 79, 125). Sharing meat helps to keep stress and hostility over food at a low intensity, and fear of hunger is mitigated by knowledge that the receiver will share when he later has food (Ju/'hoansi—Marshall 1976, 357).

Convincing evidence in favour of the risk-reduction hypothesis lies in the nature of the foods that are most widely distributed, primarily large game (Gunwinggu—Altman & Peterson 1988, 78–79; Ju/'hoansi—Marshall 1976, 357). Among the Ache all meat is subject to the same sharing rules but the distribution of gathered foods is less extensive than of meat and honey (Hawkes 1990, 155ff; Kaplan et al. 1990, 114, 124). An Ache hunter, though he will fail on most days to feed a family, would bring in a larger amount than a family could possibly consume often more than once a week (Hawkes 1990, 151; Kaplan et al. 1990, 114).

The care taken to diffuse possible disputes during meat sharing is well known (Aka—Bahuchet 1992, 229–231; Ache—Kaplan et al. 1990, 129; Cholanaickan—Bhanu 1992, 42; Gunwinggu—Altman & Peterson 1988, 80; Mbuti—Ichikawa 2005; Nunamiut—Binford 1976, 235). Among the Netsilik, where successful winter seal hunting depends on the cooperation of a number of hunters, hunting partners were *not* close kin, but were chosen by the hunter's mother at birth or during the hunter's childhood, creating complex interlocking sets of relationships in the winter camp (Balikci 1970, 133–135).

Against the risk-reduction hypothesis

Two principal arguments claim the risk-reduction hypothesis is inadequate: first, some hunters are better than others, and therefore always give more meat than they receive and, second, hunters often receive little or nothing from their own kills (Hawkes & Bliege Bird 2002; O'Connell et al. 2002; cf. Bahuchet 1992, 229–231). The striking differences in hunting success documented by Lee are well known: of 127 men in Lee's Ju/'hoansi sample, 37 had never killed a kudu, whereas 43 had killed 10 or more (Lee 1979, 243). This may, however, be exceptional. Differential success in hunting affects the Mbuti to a lesser degree: of 10 net-hunters in an Mbuti camp, the most successful obtained 140 kg meat in four weeks, whereas the least successful got 24 kg (Ichikawa 2005). We argue that, just as the grandmothering hypothesis placed women's foraging activities in a lifetime perspective, the costly signalling hypothesis for hunting effort (see below) must be placed in a man's lifetime perspective, to resolve the apparent contradiction identified by O'Connell et al. (2002).

Married men

Lee reports that, among the Ju/'hoansi:

> Many good hunters did no hunting at all for weeks or months at a time, while their wives and children waited patiently and ate the meat distributed by other hunters . . . A period of hunting inactivity allows the hunter to enjoy the benefits of some of the reciprocal obligations he has built up. (Lee 1979, 248–249)

Above-average foragers may be willing to give more than their share to avoid the risk of long stretches without food if they suffer injury (Kaplan & Hill 1985b, 237). Kaplan and Hill argue that high producers can expect to be well treated to prevent them joining another band. Wiessner, moreover, has shown that good hunters among the Ju/'hoansi fathered twice as many children as poor hunters, and also had more surviving children (2002, 419; cf. Ache—Kaplan & Hill 1985a).

Single men

Single men among the Ache are the biggest losers because they hunt frequently but most of their game is distributed to other members of the band (Kaplan & Hill 1985b, 233; Kaplan et al. 1990, 127; cf. Gunwinggu—Altman 1987, 134, 139; Altman & Peterson 1988, 80). This requires further explanation. Hawkes and Bliege Bird (2002, 60–61) conclude that hunting is a form of costly signalling, by which meat distribution becomes a medium of communication through which the hunter transmits information to potential mates, allies and competitors. We propose that male foraging strategies must be interpreted within a lifetime perspective. Women can gather effectively into old age, but successful hunting demands good eyesight. Among the Ju/'hoansi age is an important factor in hunting success, although not the only one (Lee 1979, 243–244). Ju/'hoansi men continue to hunt into their fifties, but 'the camp core of older people want to encourage the sons-in-law to stay with the group permanently, as more hunters mean more meat' (Lee 1979, 242). Hawkes et al. (1997, 555) write that among the Hadza, older women spend significantly more time foraging than females in any other category, whereas the male pattern is quite different, '*the peak for males comes before marriage*' (italics added). Among Aka, hunting nets are frequently owned by adult men, *but it is young men who do the hunting* (Ichikawa 2005). As Nicholas Peterson long ago pointed out (pers. comm. to RL), a young man's best asset is his hunting ability, whereas one of the best assets an older man has is a marriageable daughter (cf. Lee 1979, 240). It is when a hunter's eyesight is failing that his daughter is ready for marriage, and he must entice young men to hunt for him. Among the Tiwi of northern Australia, where women are betrothed at birth, a man might bestow his infant daughter on someone he wanted as an ally, or he might bestow her on a younger man as 'old-age insurance', in which case he would look for a younger man in his late twenties or thirties who showed signs of being a good hunter and fighting man (Hart & Pilling 1960, 34; Hart et al. 1988, 19). We conclude that while hunting success may be a form of costly signalling for the young, unmarried hunter, surrendering the kill is a long-term investment that will eventually guarantee him meat in old age.

FUSION PHASE 2: THE COMMUNITY

Defining the community

Many hunter-gatherer communities number between 250 and 500 individuals (Table 5.1). Where hunter-gatherers live in the same or similar environments to chimpanzees, the community is up to five times larger than the chimpanzee community. A few hunter-gatherer communities are apparently even larger (1,000–3,000), or even 10,000 (Nootka—Drucker 1965, 144), but the literature does not state whether individuals could move between bands throughout this larger population. Drucker describes the Northwest Coast winter village as an alliance of local groups whose territories were contiguous, and calls village communities 'tribes' (1965, 70). Boas wrote specifically of the Kwakiutl: 'The people speaking the *Kwa'g·ul* dialect inhabit many villages, each of which is considered as a separate unit, a tribe' (1966, 37). On the Northwest Coast of North America, it seems safer to treat the aggregate of bands/lineages that formed a single winter village as the community. The Yolngu of northern Australia, another apparently very large community of 2,500–3,000, are actually an aggregate of speakers of up to six related dialects; clans speaking the same dialect belong to the same *mala*.

Although clans on the border between two *mala* claimed dual affiliation, the *mala* seems better to correspond to our 'community' (Keen 1982, 632; Warner 1958, 35–36; Williams 1986, 64–65). Among the Inuit there was regular movement between winter villages and here we have taken the named community (-miut = people of a named area) as the community. In the literature on the Cree, the term 'band' is applied to the community rather than the band as we have defined it above.

In some of our case studies, the total population comprises a single community (e.g. Batek De, Hadza and Cholanaickan). Like the smaller Nukak communities, these may be isolated remnants whose size may have been reduced by disease or loss of territory (see Bhanu 1992, 31).

Population density

Although there is little difference in weight between central African hunter-gatherers and chimpanzees, human communities occupy much larger territories, both because humans live at lower population densities (Table 5.3), and because their communities are bigger (Table 5.1). We concluded above that this is due to the greater contribution meat makes to the human diet (Table 5.2). The lower population densities of hunter-gatherers, and the larger size of the community, pose serious problems for the coherence of the community. In many cases, unlike the situation in most chimpanzee communities, no individual will know all other members. Such dispersal renders the expensive tissue hypothesis (Aiello & Wheeler 1995) paradoxical. If a higher quality, meat-rich diet was an adaptation associated with increase in brain size, then increased carnivory posed its own cognitive problems for tracking social relationships.

Why do hunter-gatherers sustain inter-band links in the community?

(a) Inter-access between territories
The band territory rarely enables self-sufficiency in subsistence resources. 'Aborigines, and most other hunter-gatherers, live in environments subject to great fluctuations in the weather and in the abundance of game and plant resources' (Peterson & Long 1986, 143). When water fails at one waterhole, during drought, people can join relatives or exchange-partners at other waterholes. Rain falls unevenly in the deserts of Australia and southern Africa, and after rain everyone converges on the fortunate area, to exploit its plant foods (see Layton 1986, 26, 34–35; Western Desert— Myers 1986, 183). In the Kalahari, drought occurs two out of five years

and is severe in one year out of four, but rainfall can vary by a factor of ten over a few miles (Lee 1979, 352). Mutual insurance against local drought was one of the main reasons for maintaining inter-band links among the G/wi (Silberbauer 1981, 459). A well-rounded set of partners is better than a few promising ones; the variety of resources in Ju/'hoansi *hxaro* partners' areas is more important than distance (Wiessner 1982, 74, 76). Even in the monsoon zone of northern Australia, Tiwi bands invite others to share local concentrations of resources (Goodale 1986, 201). Among the Inuit and Northwest Coast Native Americans, there was a seasonal fluctuation between dispersed bands in summer and community aggregations in winter. The Cree practised the opposite pattern, with summer aggregation, traditionally at good fishing locations, and winter dispersal into separate bands for hunting.

In more fine-grained environments such as equatorial forest (Bahuchet 1992, 207–210) the function of the community is less clear. Through kinship, an Aka has access to the territories of ten different lineages, and Aka travel furthest to visit relatives (Hewlett et al. 1982, 427), but it is not clear what benefits these kin networks provide. The Mbuti describe a lack of relatives in other bands as '"walking emptily" thus emphasizing the necessity to have friends elsewhere for travelling to' (Bahuchet 1992, 217, quoting Turnbull 1965).

(b) Dispute avoidance
Woodburn (1982) argued that the desire to avoid disputes and overbearing would-be leaders was the main reason for movement between bands among the Hadza. Turnbull and Abruzzi reach the same conclusion with regard to movement between Mbuti bands (Abruzzi 1980; Turnbull 1965, 106, 223). Equalizing band size may be an underlying consideration. A newly married Mbuti couple's residence is usually based on the relative size of the spouses' home bands (Turnbull 1965, 219).

How often will any two members of the community meet?

The entire community can generally assemble, if at all, only during times and at places where resources are exceptionally dense. *If* the Northwest Coast winter village can be equated with the community (see above), this is a rare example among recent hunter-gatherers of the whole community assembling in one place, relying in this case on stored food. The Cree form summer aggregations of several hundred, but these are probably facilitated by White Canadian stores (Feit 1983, 417; Rogers 1972, 91). Before the fur trade, summer aggregations met at favourable fishing spots for weddings and feasts (Rogers 1972, 107, 123). The winter aggregations of coastal Inuit are undoubtedly traditional, and dictated by seal hunting on sea ice (see above), but aggregations of 50 to 200 were drawn from a community of c. 500 (Damas 1969, 52).

Among the Ache, up to half the community (i.e. up to 250 people) might assemble in one place once every two to three years for ritualized club fights. After six weeks the assembly dispersed, with many changing band membership and new sexual relations established (Hill & Hurtado 1996, 73). A similar ritual is performed by all bands within the Nukak *munu* (Politis 2007, 82), but this is a smaller group of c. 125 people. The Aka are divided into clusters of bands which live on the same hunting trail. Camps on the same trail meet for several days at a time to perform a ceremony and enable more efficient net-hunting (Bahuchet 1992, 215, 226, 230).

In harsher environments, assemblies are infrequent and short-lived. In good summers, two G/wi bands can combine for a couple of weeks to socialize, exchange news and commodities, and play games. A maximum of 150 people can camp together for short periods (Silberbauer 1981, 459). In the Western Desert, groups of 200 assembled for ceremonies, but could only do so in years of good rainfall and restricted to a period of about two weeks (Layton 1986, 35–37).

How are inter-band links sustained?

(a) Reciprocal gift-giving

Mauss (1954 [1925]) argued that gift exchange was fundamental to human social organization and it may indeed be that exchange enabled the human communities to persist even as their members dispersed over far larger areas than are occupied by chimpanzee communities. In many hunter-gatherer societies, people constantly give each other gifts. Given the impossibility, among most hunter-gatherer communities, of all assembling in one place, the hunter-gatherer community is generally sustained by overlapping networks of kinship and friendship among members (e.g. Aka—Bahuchet 1992, 232; G/wi—Silberbauer 1972, 305; 1981, 463; Lehmann et al. ch. 4 this volume). Among the Netsilik, namesakes exchanged gifts that had to be identical, such as a knife for a knife; the exchanges were not carried out for material benefit but 'to give expression to . . . enduring friendliness' (Balikci 1970, 139). Among the Pintupi (central Australia), gifts are tokens of friendship providing a moral basis for continued and on-going co-residence and cooperation (Myers 1988; cf.

Tonkinson 1991, 53). The Ju/'hoansi (Kalahari) exchange system called *hxaro*, which maintains friendships between people in different bands, is well known. Wiessner (1982, 66) described *hxaro* partnership as 'a bond of friendship accompanied by mutual reciprocity and access to resources' (cf. Marshall 1976, 367). Women play the main part in maintaining these partnerships, going on long journeys to visit *hxaro* partners and giving them ostrich-shell necklaces, water carriers, etc. (Marshall 1976, 363).

(b) Marriage

The combination of band exogamy and community endogamy also underpins inter-band movement. Among the Ndelé Aka, men range almost twice as widely as women; the most wide-ranging are young Aka bachelors who leave their camp as individuals (Hewlett et al. 1982, 425; cf. Bahuchet 1992, 222, 233). 'The main purpose of interband visits' among the Mbuti 'is the extension of the social horizon, particularly necessary in view of the preferred [band] territorial exogamy' (Turnbull 1965, 96–97). Lee (1976, 72) writes that the single Ju/'hoansi male travels more widely and more frequently than the single female, in search of casual liaisons and marriages. In the Western Desert, young men were taken on long expeditions to visit distant bands by their future fathers-in-law (Layton 1995).

(c) Classificatory kinship

Among the Yankunytjatjara, members of neighbouring bands were addressed as brother and sister, and they frequently foraged together. Marriage was expected to take place between members of more distant bands separated by at least 70 km, who were addressed as brother- and sister-in-law and who provided refuge during local drought (Layton 1995). Relationships modelled on kinship are extended among the Ju/'hoansi and Netsilik through the use of namesakes, where two individuals with the same personal name treat each other as siblings (Barnard 1992, 265–281; Balikci 1970). In Australia, 'section systems' assign everyone at birth to a category that determines their 'kin' relationship to all other members of the community (see e.g. Layton 1999; Read ch. 10 this volume).

(d) Language

The human community sometimes corresponds to the group speaking a distinctive dialect or language, as is the case among the G/wi, and !Ko of the Kalahari (Cashdan 1983, 54; Silberbauer 1972, 273). Community and language or dialect commonly coincide in Australia (Dixon 1997). This probably arises from the greater intensity of social interaction within the community, although in some cases the correspondence may arise because the community is isolated from other hunter-gatherers by surrounding farmers or herders, e.g. the Hadza. Elsewhere, the language group is larger than the community. This may be because the region has been colonized by its current hunter-gatherer population relatively recently (e.g. Inuit, Australian Western Desert: McConvell & Evans 1997) while in extreme cases separate dialects may emerge at the band level (Sutton 2001). Mellars (1998) argued that language embodying tense and the subjunctive would be necessary to talk about social relationships with people displaced in time and space characteristic of hunter-gatherers ('Should this drought continue I may visit Y, whom we allowed to camp with us three years ago'). Terms universal to modern human language include words equivalent to 'now', 'before', 'after', 'here' and 'far', 'the same', 'other/else' and 'because' (Wierzbicka 1996). Language was probably essential to enable the distinctively human form of fission-fusion society we have outlined.

CONCLUSIONS

Our analysis began with the observation that humans and chimpanzees share a form of social organization that is unusual among primates, but we continued by identifying a number of differences between the distinctive patterns of fission and fusion in chimpanzees and human hunter-gatherers. The hunter-gatherer community is larger than the chimpanzee community, yet human population densities are lower. Parties formed during fission phases last longer among humans, and the bands characteristic of hunter-gatherer society are far more durable than the fusion phases of chimpanzee social behaviour. We found that the greater contribution of hunting to the human diet had a number of important consequences. The predatory nature of human subsistence compels a lower population density than chimpanzees can sustain, while the larger size, and frequently unpredictable occurrence of large game, is efficiently exploited by sharing at band camps. Band residence confers a number of other advantages (child-care, territorial prerogatives, information exchange), but these may conflict. Male and female strategies must be assessed within a lifetime perspective.

The persistence of the larger community can be explained by the need to keep membership options in a number of bands open. The persistence of the community is facilitated by a number of distinctively human traits: gift-giving, inter-band marriage, classificatory kinship and language. The idea that hunting was crucial to human evolution gained a bad press as a result of the exaggerated claims made by early writers (Ardrey 1967; Dart 1959). We argue that increased carnivory during the course of human evolution may indeed be responsible for some of the most striking differences between human and chimpanzee social behaviour: not aggression and territoriality, but rather sharing, cooperation and exchange.

Note. The stimulus for this chapter arose from two events: the Wenner-Gren funded workshop on fission-fusion societies organized by Filippo Aureli following the 2004 meeting of the International Primatological Society (see Aureli et al. 2008) and a 2006 workshop organized by Robin Dunbar under the auspices of the British Academy Centenary 'Lucy to Language' Research Project. We thank Russell Hill for substantial help with creating the box plots, also Filippo Aureli, Catherine O'Hara, Jamie Tehrani and Jeremy Kendall for comments on draft versions, and Peter Sutton for references to language boundaries.

REFERENCES

Abruzzi, W. S. (1980). Flux among the Mbuti Pygmies of the Ituri Forest. In: E. B. Ross (ed.) *Beyond the myths of culture*, pp. 3–31. New York: Academic Press.

Aiello, L. & Wheeler, P. (1995). The expensive-tissue hypothesis: the brain and digestive system in human and primate evolution. *Current Anthropology* 36: 199–221.

Altman, J. (1987). *Hunter-gatherers today.* Canberra: Aboriginal Studies Press.

Altman, J. & Peterson, N. (1988). Rights to game and rights to cash among contemporary Australian hunter-gatherers. In: T. Ingold, D. Riches & J. Woodburn (eds) *Hunters and gatherers: property, power and ideology*, pp. 75–94. Oxford: Berg.

Andrews, E. (1989). *The Akulmiut: territorial dimensions of a Yup'ik Eskimo society.* PhD thesis, University of Alaska Fairbanks.

Ardrey, R. (1967). *The territorial imperative: a personal enquiry into the animal origins of property and nations.* London: Collins.

Aureli, F., Schaffner, C., Boesch, C., Bearder, S., Call, J., Chapman, C. et al. (2008). Fission-fusion dynamics: new research frameworks. *Current Anthropology* 49: 627–654.

Bahuchet, S. (1992). Spatial mobility and access to resources among African pygmies. In: M. Casimir & A. Rao (eds) *Mobility and territoriality: social and spatial boundaries among foragers, fishers, pastoralists and peripatetics*, pp. 205–257. New York: Berg.

Balikci, A. (1970). *The Netsilik Eskimo.* Garden City, NY: Natural History Press.

Barnard, A. (1992). *Hunters and herders of Southern Africa: a comparative survey.* Cambridge: Cambridge University Press.

Barton, R. (2006). Primate brain evolution: integrating comparative, neurophysiological and ethological data. *Evolutionary Anthropology* 15: 224–236.

Bhanu, A. (1992). Boundaries, obligations and reciprocity: levels of territoriality among the Cholanaickan of South India. In: M. Casimir & A. Rao (eds) *Mobility and territoriality: social and spatial boundaries among foragers, fishers, pastoralists and peripatetics*, pp. 29–54. New York: Berg.

Binford, L. (1976). *Nunamiut ethnoarchaeology*. New York: Academic Press.

Binford, L. (1980). Willow smoke and dogs' tails: hunter-gatherer settlement systems and archaeological site formation. *American Antiquity* 45: 4–20.

Boas, F. (ed. H. Codere) (1966). *Kwakiutl ethnography*. Chicago: University of Chicago Press.

Boesch, C. & Boesch, H. (1989). The hunting behaviour of wild chimpanzees in the Taï National Park. *American Journal of Physical Anthropology* 78: 547–573.

Boesch, C. & Boesch-Achermann, H. (2000). *The chimpanzees of the Taï forest*. Oxford: Oxford University Press.

Burch, E. (1988). Modes of exchange in north-west Alaska. In: T. Ingold, D. Riches & J. Woodburn (eds) *Hunters and gatherers: property, power and ideology*, pp. 95–109. Oxford: Berg.

Cane, S. (1990). Gugadja of Great Sandy Desert, NW Western Australia. In: B. Meehan & N. White (eds) *Hunter-gatherer demography past and present* (Oceania Monograph 39), pp. 149–159. Sydney: University of Sydney Press.

Cashdan, E. (1983). Territoriality among human foragers: ecological models and an application to four bushman groups. *Current Anthropology* 24: 47–66.

Codere, H. (1950). *Fighting with property.* New York: Augustin.

Damas, D. (1969). Environment, history, and central Eskimo society. *Contributions to anthropology: ecological essays. Proceedings of conference on cultural ecology.* Ottawa: National Museum of Canada Bulletin 230.

Dart, R. (1959). *Adventures with the missing link*. London: Hamilton.

Dixon, R. (1997). *The languages of Australia.* Ann Arbor: University of Michigan Press.

Drucker, P. (1965). *Cultures of the North Pacific coast.* San Francisco: Chandler.

Drucker, P. & Heizer, R. (1967). *To make my name good.* Berkeley: University of California Press.

Dunbar, R. (1993). Co-evolution of neocortical size, group size and language in humans. *Behavioural and Brain Sciences Evolution* 16: 681–735.

Emmons, G. (1991). *The Tlingit Indians*, ed. F. de Laguna. Seattle: University of Washington Press.

Endicott, K. M. (1979). *Batek Negrito religion: the world-view and rituals of a hunting and gathering people*. Oxford: Clarendon Press.

Endicott, K. M. (1988). Property, power and conflict among the Batek of Malaysia. In: T. Ingold, D. Riches & J. Woodburn (eds) *Hunters and gatherers: property, power and ideology*, pp. 110–127. Oxford: Berg.

Feit, H. (1983). Negotiating recognition of Aboriginal rights. In: N. Peterson & M. Langton (eds) *Aborigines, land and land rights*, pp. 416–438. Canberra: Aboriginal Studies Press.

Finlayson, H. (1935). *The red centre*. Sydney: Angus & Robertson.

Foley, R. & Lee, P. (1989). Finite social space, evolutionary pathways, and reconstructing hominid behaviour. *Science* 243: 901–906.

Gibson, M. & Mace, R. (2005). Helpful grandmothers in rural Ethiopia. *Evolution and Human Behaviour* 26: 469–482.

Goodale, J. (1986). Production and reproduction of key resources among the Tiwi. In: N. Williams & E. Hunn (eds) *Resource managers: North American and Australian hunter-gatherers*, pp. 197–210. Canberra: Aboriginal Studies Press.

Gould, R. (1969). *Yiwarra: foragers of the Australian desert*. London: Collins.

Gubser, N. (1965). *The Nunamiut Eskimos, hunters of caribou*. New Haven, CT: Yale University Press.

Guemple, L. (1988). Teaching social relations to Inuit children. In: T. Ingold, D. Riches and J. Woodburn (eds) *Hunters and gatherers: property, power and ideology*, pp. 131–149. Oxford: Berg.

Gurven, M. & Hill, K. (1997). Comment on Hawkes et al. 1997. *Current Anthropology* 38: 566–567.

Halperin, S. (1979). Temporary association patterns in free ranging chimpanzees: an assessment of individual grouping preferences. In: D. A. Hamburg & E. M. McCown (eds) *The great apes*, pp. 491–499. Menlo Park, CA: Benjamin/Cummings.

Harako, R. (1981). The cultural ecology of hunting behaviour among Mbuti pygmies. In: R. V. O. Harding & G. Teleki (eds) *Omnivorous primates*, pp. 499–555. New York: Columbia University Press.

Hart, C. & Pilling, A. (1960). *The Tiwi of north Australia*. New York: Holt, Rinehart & Winston.

Hart, C., Pilling, A. & Goodale, J. (1988). *The Tiwi of North Australia*, 3rd edn. New York: Holt, Rinehart & Winston.

Hawkes, K. (1990). Why do men hunt? Benefits from risky choices. In: E. Cashdan (ed.) *Risk and uncertainty in tribal and peasant economies*, pp. 145–166. Boulder, CO: Westview Press.

Hawkes, K. & Bliege Bird, R. (2002). Showing off, handicap signaling and the evolution of men's work. *Evolutionary Anthropology* 11: 58–67.

Hawkes, K., O'Connell, J. F. & Blurton Jones, N. G. (1997). Hadza women's time allocation. *Current Anthropology* 38: 551–577.

Hayden, B. (1981). Subsistence and ecological adaptations of modern hunter/gatherers. In: R. Harding & G. Teleki (eds) *Omnivorous primates: gathering and hunting in human evolution*, pp. 344–421. New York: Columbia University Press.

Hewlett, B. (1991). Demography and childcare in pre-industrial societies. *Journal of Anthropological Research* 47: 1–37.

Hewlett, B., van der Koppel, J. & Cavalli-Sforza, L. (1982). Exploration ranges of Aka pygmies of the Central African Republic. *Man* (n.s.) 17: 418–430.

Hill, K. & Hurtado, M. (1996). *Ache life history: the ecology and demography of a foraging people*. Hawthorne, NY: Aldine de Gruyter.

Hunn, E. (1986). Mobility as a factor limiting resource use in the Columbia Plateau of North America. In: N. Williams & E. Hunn (eds) *Resource managers: North American and Australian hunter-gatherers*, pp. 17–43. Canberra: Aboriginal Studies Press.

Hunn, E. (1994). Place-names, population density and the magic number 500. *Current Anthropology* 35: 81–85.

Ichikawa, M. (2005). Food sharing and ownership among central African hunter-gatherers: an evolutionary perspective. In: T. Widlok & W. G. Tadesse (eds) *Property and equality*, vol. 1: *Ritualisation, sharing, egalitarianism*, pp. 151–164. Oxford: Berg.

Jones, R. (1980). Hunters in the Australian coastal savanna. In: D. Harris (ed.) *Human ecology in savanna environments*, pp. 107–146. London: Academic Press.

Jordan, P. (2003). *Material culture and sacred landscape: the anthropology of the Siberian Khanty*. Walnut Creek, CA: AltaMira.

Kaplan, H. & Hill, K. (1985a). Hunting ability and reproductive success among male Ache foragers. *Current Anthropology* 26: 131–133.

Kaplan, H. & Hill, K. (1985b). Food sharing among Ache foragers: tests of explanatory hypotheses. *Current Anthropology* 26: 223–246.

Kaplan, H., Hill, K. & Hurtado, M. (1990). Risk, foraging and food sharing among the Ache. In: E. Cashdan (ed.) *Risk and uncertainty in tribal and peasant economies*, pp. 107–143. Boulder, CO: Westview Press.

Keen, I. (1982). How some Murngin men marry ten wives. *Man* (n.s.) 17: 620–642.

Kelly, R. (1995). *The foraging spectrum*. Washington, DC: Smithsonian Institution Press.

Layton, R. (1983). Ambilineal descent and Pitjantjatjara rights to land. In: N. Peterson & M. Langton (eds) *Aborigines, land and land rights*, pp. 15–32. Canberra: Aboriginal Studies Press.

Layton, R. (1986). *Uluru, an Aboriginal history of Ayers Rock*. Canberra: Aboriginal Studies Press.

Layton, R. (1995). Relating to the country in the Western Desert. In: E. Hirsch & M. O'Hanlon (eds) *The anthropology of landscape: perspectives on place and space*, pp. 210–231. Oxford: Clarendon Press.

Layton, R. (1999). The Alawa totemic landscape: economy, religion and politics. In: P. Ucko & R. Layton (eds) *The archaeology and anthropology of landscape*, pp. 219–239. London: Routledge.

Lee, R. B. (1976). !Kung spatial organisation: an ecological and historical perspective. In: R. B. Lee & I. DeVore (eds) *Kalahari hunter-gatherers: studies of the !Kung San and their neighbours*, pp. 74–97. Cambridge, MA: Harvard University Press.

Lee, R. B. (1979). *The !Kung San: men, women and work in a foraging society.* Cambridge: Cambridge University Press.

McConvell, P. & N. Evans (eds) (1997). *Archaeology and linguistics*. Melbourne: Oxford University Press.

Marlowe, F. (2001). Male contribution to diet and female reproductive success among foragers. *Current Anthropology* 42: 755–760.

Marshall, L. (1976). Sharing, talking and giving. In: R. Lee & I. DeVore (eds) *Kalahari hunter-gatherers*, pp. 350–371. Cambridge, MA: Harvard University Press.

Mauss, M. (1954 [1925]). *The gift*. London: Cohen & West.

Meehan, B. (1982). *Shell bed to shell midden*. Canberra: Aboriginal Studies Press.

Meggitt, M. (1962). *Desert people*. Sydney: Angus & Robertson.

Mellars, P. (1998). Neanderthals, modern humans and the archaeological evidence for language. In: N. G. Jablonski & L. Aiello (eds) *The origin and diversification of language*, pp. 89–115. San Francisco: Memoirs of the California Academy of Science.

Myers, F. (1986). Always ask: resource use and land ownership among Pintupi Aborigines. In: N. Williams & E. Hunn (eds) *Resource managers: North American and Australian hunter-gatherers*, pp. 173–195. Canberra: Aboriginal Studies Press.

Myers, F. (1988). Burning the truck and holding the country. In: T. Ingold, D. Riches & J. Woodburn (eds) *Hunters and gatherers: property, power and ideology*, pp. 52–74. Oxford: Berg.

Newton-Fisher, N. (2007). Chimpanzee hunting behaviour. In: W. Henke & I. Tattersall (eds) *Handbook of paleoanthropology*, pp. 1295–1320. New York: Springer.

Newton-Fisher, N. E., Notman, H. & Reynolds, V. (2002). Hunting of mammalian prey by Budongo Forest chimpanzees. *Folia Primatologica* 73(5): 281–283.

O'Connell, J. F., Hawkes, K., Lupo, K. D. & Blurton Jones, N. G. (2002). Male strategies and Plio-Pleistocene archaeology. *Journal of Human Evolution* 43: 831–872.

Peterson, N. (1975). Hunter-gatherer territoriality: the perspective from Australia. *American Anthropologist* 77: 53–68.

Peterson, N. & Long, J. (1986). *Australian territorial organisation* (Oceania monograph 30). Sydney: University of Sydney Press.

Politis, G. (2007). *Nukak: ethnoarchaeology of an Amazonian people*. Walnut Creek, CA: Left Coast Press.

Radcliffe-Brown, A. R. (1930). The social organisation of Australian tribes. *Oceania* 1: 34–63.

Reynolds, V. (2005). *The chimpanzees of the Budongo Forest*. Oxford: Oxford University Press.

Richardson, A. (1986). The control of productive resources on the Northwest Coast of North America. In: N. Williams & E. Hunn (eds) *Resource managers: North American and Australian hunter-gatherers*, pp. 93–112. Canberra: Aboriginal Studies Press.

Rival, L. (2002). *Trekking through history*. New York: Columbia University Press.

Rogers, E. S. (1972). The Mistassini Cree. In: M. G. Bicchieri (ed.) *Hunters and gatherers today*, pp. 90–137. New York: Holt, Rinehart & Winston.

Rohner, R. & Rohner, E. (1970). *The Kwakiutl: Indians of British Columbia*. New York: Holt, Rinehart & Winston.

Sear, R., Mace, R. & McGregor, I. A. (2000). Maternal grandmothers improve nutritional status and survival among children in rural Gambia. *Proceedings of the Royal Society B* 267: 1641–1647.

Scott, C. (1988). Property, practice and Aboriginal rights among Quebec Cree hunters. In: T. Ingold, D. Riches & J. Woodburn (eds) *Hunters and gatherers: property, power and ideology*, pp. 35–51. Oxford: Berg.

Silberbauer, G. (1972). The G/wi bushmen. In: M. G. Bicchieri (ed.) *Hunters and gatherers today*, pp. 271–326. New York: Holt, Rinehart & Winston.

Silberbauer, G. (1981). Hunter/gatherers of the central Kalahari. In: R. S. O. Harding & G. Teleki (eds) *Omnivorous primates*, pp. 455–498. New York: Columbia University Press.

Smith, E. A. (1991). *Inujjuamiut foraging strategies*. New York: Aldine de Gruyter.

Smith, R. & Jungers, W. (1997). Body mass in comparative primatology. *Journal of Human Evolution* 32: 523–559.

Stanner, W. (1965). Aboriginal territorial organisation. *Oceania* 36: 1–26.

Sterck, E. H. M., Watts, D. P. & van Schaik, C. P. (1997). The evolution of female social relationships in nonhuman primates. *Behavioural Ecology and Sociobiology* 41: 291–309.

Steward, J. (1936). The economic and social basis of primitive bands. In: R. H. Lowie (ed.) *Essays on anthropology in honour of Alfred Louis Kroeber*, pp. 311–350. Berkeley: University of California Press.

Stiner, M. (2002). Carnivory, coevolution and the geographic spread of the genus *Homo*. *Journal of Archaeological Research* 10: 1–63.

Sutton, P. (2001). Talking language. In: J. Simpson, D. Nash, M. Laughren, P. Austin & B. Alpher (eds) *Forty years on: Ken Hale and Australian languages*, pp. 453–464. Canberra: Australian National University Pacific Linguistics.

Tonkinson, R. (1991). *The Mardu Aborigines*. New York: Holt, Rinehart & Winston.

Trivers, R. (1971). The evolution of reciprocal altruism. *Quarterly Review of Biology* 46: 35–57.

Turnbull, C. (1962). *The forest people*. New York: Simon & Schuster.

Turnbull, C. (1965). *Wayward servants: the two worlds of the African pygmies*. Westport, CT: Greenwood Press.

van Schaik, C. P. (1989). The ecology of social relationships among female primates. In: V. Standen & R. A. Foley (eds) *The behavioural ecology of humans and other mammals*, pp. 195–218. Blackwell: Oxford.

Warner, W. (1958). *A black civilisation*. New York: Harper.

White, W., Meehan, B., Hiatt, L. & Jones, R. (1990). Demography of contemporary hunter gatherers: lessons from Central Arnhem Land. In: B. Meehan & N. White (eds) *Hunter-gatherer demography past and present* (Oceania Monograph 39), pp. 171–185. Sydney: University of Sydney Press.

Wierzbicka, A. (1996). *Semantics: primes and universals*. Oxford: Oxford University Press.

Wiessner, P. (1982). Risk, reciprocity and social influences on !Kung San economics. In: E. Leacock & R. Lee (eds) *Politics and history in band societies*, pp. 61–84. Cambridge: Cambridge University Press.

Wiessner, P. (2002). Hunting, healing and *hxaro* exchange: a long-term perspective in !Kung (Ju/'hoansi) large-game hunting. *Evolution and Human Behaviour* 23: 407–436.

Williams, N. (1986). *The Yolngu and their land*. Canberra: Aboriginal Studies Press.

Wilson, M., Wallauer, W. & Pusey, A. (2004). New cases of intergroup violence among chimpanzees in Gombe National Park, Tanzania. *Evolutionary Anthropology* 5: 46–57.

Winterhalder, B. (1990). Open field, common pot. In: E. Cashdan (ed.) *Risk and uncertainty in tribal and peasant economies*, pp. 67–87. Boulder, CO: Westview Press.

Winterhalder, B. (1996). Social foraging and the behavioural ecology of intragroup resource transfers. *Evolutionary Anthropology* 5: 46–57.

Wobst, M. (1974). Boundary conditions for Palaeolithic social systems: a simulation approach. *American Antiquity* 39: 152–178.

Woodburn, J. (1972). Ecology, nomadic movement and the composition of the local group. In: P. Ucko, R. Tringham & G. W. Dimbleby (eds) *Man, settlement and urbanism*, pp. 193–206. London: Duckworth.

Woodburn, J. (1982). Egalitarian societies. *Man (n.s.)* 17, 431–451.

Wrangham, R. W. (2000). Why are male chimpanzees more gregarious than mothers? A scramble competition hypothesis. In: P. Kappeler (ed.) *Primate males*, pp. 248–258. Cambridge: Cambridge University Press.

Wrangham, R. W., Gittleman, J. L. & Chapman, C. A. (1993). Constraints on group size in primates and carnivores: population density and day-range as assays of exploitation competition. *Behavioral Ecology and Sociobiology* 32(3): 199–209.

Yellen, J. (1976). Settlement patterns of the !Kung: an archaeological perspective. In: R. B. Lee & I. DeVore (eds) *Kalahari hunter-gatherers: studies of the !Kung San and their neighbours*, pp. 47–72. Cambridge, MA: Harvard University Press.

6

Constraints on Social Networks

SAM G. B. ROBERTS

THE STRUCTURE OF PERSONAL NETWORKS

HUMAN BEINGS OPERATE in a social network made up of family, friends and acquaintances. There are two broad approaches to studying these social networks (Wellman 2007a). Personal network analysis starts with an individual (an 'ego'), and looks at that individual's set of ties to other people ('alters'). By studying the social networks of a number of egos, personal network researchers analyse issues such as the size and composition of the network, the types of support they get from alters, how relationships are maintained over time and how individual characteristics of the ego (e.g. gender, age, socio-economic status, personality) affect the size and composition of the network (e.g. Degenne & Lebeaux 2005; Fischer 1982; McPherson et al. 2006; Marsden 1987; Milardo 1992; Morgan et al. 1997; Plickert et al. 2007; Roberts et al. 2008; Wellman & Wortley 1990). The network is defined from the point of view of the ego, and thus is not bounded by a particular geographic or organizational entity such as a neighbourhood or workplace.

This approach is in contrast to the more common form of whole-network analysis, where a bounded population is first identified (e.g. an academic department, a football team, a classroom), and then the ties within that bounded population are examined (e.g. Ennett et al. 2008; Kossinets & Watts 2006; Onnela et al. 2007; see Watts 2004 for a review). This leads to a detailed understanding of the structure of the network, as typically all ties between individuals within that population are examined, but it does not consider ties lying outside the pre-determined population (e.g. ties researchers may have with academics outside the department). Thus whole-network analysis is a top-down approach, whereas personal network analysis is a bottom-up approach.

Studies of personal social networks (henceforth 'social networks') have demonstrated that they consist of a series of subgroupings arranged

Proceedings of the British Academy **158**, 115–134. © The British Academy 2010.

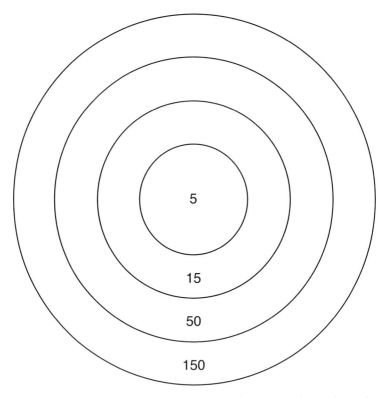

Figure 6.1. Hierarchical structure of personal networks in humans. The numbers refer to the approximate mean network size of each of the layers—the support clique (5), the sympathy group (15), the band (50) and the active network (150). The layers are hierarchically inclusive, so that the size of each layer includes all inner layers. There are further layers beyond the active network, not shown here.

in a hierarchically inclusive sequence (Dunbar 1998; Hill & Dunbar 2003). In effect, an individual ego can be envisaged as sitting in the centre of a series of concentric circles of acquaintanceship (Figure 6.1). These circles of acquaintanceship are organized according to a geometric series with a scaling ratio close to three (Zhou et al. 2005).

This hierarchical structure, with a scaling ratio of between three and four, has been shown to apply on a population level to hunter-gatherer societies (Hamilton et al. 2007) and also to four mammalian taxa that live in multi-level social systems (Hill et al. 2008). Determining why a diverse array of both human and non-human populations should be structured in this way is an important question, both in terms of understanding how social networks operate, and in guiding theorizing about how social networks may have been structured through hominin evolution.

In human social networks, the first layer of acquaintanceship surrounding the ego is the support clique, which can be defined as all those individuals from whom one would seek advice, support or help in times of severe emotional or financial distress (Dunbar & Spoors 1995) and which averages about five members (Milardo 1992). The next layer is the sympathy group, those alters whom an individual contacts at least monthly, and averages 12 to 15 members (Buys & Larson 1979; Dunbar & Spoors 1995). The layers are inclusive, so the sympathy group includes the five or so members of the support clique. Most personal network analysis has focused on these two 'inner' layers of the network, examining only the relatively small number of alters the ego is emotionally closest to (Wellman 2007b).

However, it is widely acknowledged (Hammer 1983; Pool & Kochen 1978; Wellman & Frank 2001), that these closest ties only form a small fraction of those alters that are significant to ego, and with whom ego has at least some contact. Zhou et al. (2005) found distinct groupings at around 50 alters (a 'band') and 150 alters (the active network). In personal networks, the band layer is not well understood in terms of the types of alters found in this layer, or the ties that ego has with these alters. The active network consists of all those individuals that ego feels that they have a personal relationship with, and makes a conscious effort to keep in contact with (Hill & Dunbar 2003).

As the number of alters in each layer of the network increases, the level of emotional intimacy and the level of interaction between ego and alter decreases (Hill & Dunbar 2003; Mok et al. 2007). This suggests that there are constraints on the number of relationships that ego can maintain at any given level of intensity (Dunbar 1998; Hill & Dunbar 2003; Mok et al. 2007). Exploring the operation of these constraints may lead to a greater understanding of why social networks have the distinctive hierarchical structure described above. In this chapter, I will examine the nature of these constraints, how they impact on the composition of social networks, affect individual social relationships and interact with kinship. Finally, I will consider the implications of these constraints for our understanding of human evolution.

CONSTRAINTS ON NETWORK SIZE

The notion of constraints on network size has its origins in two divergent areas of research. First, the social brain hypothesis (Byrne & Whiten

1988; Dunbar 1992a, 1998; Dunbar & Shultz 2007a, 2007b; Whiten & Byrne 1997) argues that the complexity of primate social relationships is the reason that primates have an unusually large brain for their body size. According to this hypothesis, the upper limit on the size of primates groups is set by the cognitive abilities of primates—specifically their ability to manipulate information about both direct and indirect social relationships, in order to enable large groups of individuals to be maintained as stable, functional, coherent units (Dunbar & Shultz 2007b; Kudo & Dunbar 2001; Lehmann et al. ch. 4 this volume). This suggests that human cognitive abilities may also set a limit on the maximum size of human groups, and, based on the relationship between group size and brain size in primates, this was predicted to be around 150 in modern humans (Dunbar 1993).

Second, as detailed above, the structure of human social networks suggests that there are limits to the number of people that can be maintained at each layer of the network (support clique, sympathy group, band, active network). The notion of constraints on network size was raised early in the study of social networks (Bernard & Killworth 1973; Pool & Kochen 1978), but has not received a great deal of systematic attention from network researchers. One reason for this may be that whole-network analysis is a top-down approach and thus the primary interest is often describing the properties of the network itself, rather than the cognitive processes involved at the individual level. Further, much personal network analysis is cross-sectional, examining the network at one particular point in time (Suitor et al. 1997). A more dynamic approach to networks, recognizing that networks change over time, leads to more consideration of constraints on maintaining relationships at each layer of the network.

Two broad types of constraints on network size may be identified. First, cognitive constraints refer to the fact that it is cognitively demanding to keep track of a large number of relationships simultaneously. The close relationships at the inner layers of the relationships are demanding, as 'the partner is important as a unique individual and is interchangeable with none other' (Ainsworth 1989, 711). Thus each relationship has to be individually managed, rather than treated as a category. At the outer layers of the network, the relationships are less emotionally intense and have less frequent contact (Hill & Dunbar 2003) but still need to be maintained if they are not to decay over time (Burt 2000).

One of the reasons that relationships are so cognitively demanding is that they are not fixed, static entities like physical objects, but are dynamic and thus an ego must constantly update representations of their relationships with other individuals. Further, an ego can use the information they have about individual A's relationship with individual B to adjust their behaviour towards both A and B (Dunbar 2008a). This understanding of third party relationships is present in primates as well as humans (Bergman et al. 2003; Cheney et al. 1995; Silk 1999). Calculating the effect of third party relationships on ego's own relationships becomes increasingly complex with larger groups, especially if, as in the human case, the ego also has to contend with the knowledge that the third parties themselves will also be performing similar calculations. Modern humans seem to be limited to five or six levels of intentionality (Kinderman et al. 1998), and this may place an upper limit on the number of close, intimate relationships an individual can maintain. The size of an individual's support clique is correlated with the number of levels of intentionality that an individual can process, while the size of their sympathy group is related to performance on a working memory task (Stiller & Dunbar 2007).

The second major constraint on network size is time. Time constraints have been extensively studied with relation to primate socio-ecology, and this work provides an insight into how they may affect human relationships. Primates have to invest time in grooming to create social bonds of sufficient intensity to provide them with reliable allies and buffer them from the effects of group living (Lehmann et al. 2007; Wittig et al. 2008). There are competing demands for primate time—notably feeding, resting and moving (Dunbar 1992b). Thus the proportion of time available for socializing is limited, and this may ultimately limit the size and cohesion of primate groups (Dunbar 1996; Dunbar & Shultz 2007b; Henzi et al. 1997a, 1997b; Lehmann et al. 2007).

Humans also have a finite time budget, and only have so much time to devote to maintaining social relationships (Johnson & Leslie 1982; Slater 1963; Tooby & Cosmides 1996). Thus, if it takes a certain amount of time to maintain a relationship at a given level of emotional intensity, time constraints may be predicted to limit network size. Cross-sectional studies show that network size decreases as romantic relationships become more committed—moving from occasional dating, regular dating, exclusive dating, being engaged and being married (Johnson & Leslie 1982). Detailed longitudinal work shows a decrease in the frequency and duration of actual interactions with other network members across these levels of romantic relationships (Milardo et al. 1983), demonstrating that spending increasing amounts of time with the new relationship partner leads to spending less time with other alters in the network and, over time, to a decrease in network size. A similar drop in network size occurs during the transition to motherhood, with the arrival of a dependent child reducing the amount of time available for socializing (McCannell 1988).

In a detailed analysis of how constraints affect network size and composition, Roberts et al. (2009) found a large variation in female active network sizes, with a range of 10–168. Egos with large networks were, on average, less emotionally close to the alters in their network than egos with small networks. Thus, in a sense there was a trade-off between having large networks, but being less close to each alter in the network, and having a small network of stronger ties. A similar effect has been found at the level of the support clique, in that those with a smaller support clique are more likely to receive support from each member of the support clique, as compared to those with larger cliques (Wellman & Frank 2001). This is may be due to the fact that 'persons with smaller intimate networks may have more time to attend to each alter and hence would be more apt to evoke support from each of them' (Wellman & Frank 2001, 13).

Further, there are constraints on the maximum number of individuals that can be maintained in the network—i.e. there are only so many 'slots' or 'friendship niches' (Tooby & Cosmides 1996) available to be filled. There is a distinct upper bound on network size, where egos with large related networks have smaller unrelated networks, and vice versa (Roberts et al. 2009). Effectively, egos born into large families fill many of the slots in their network with family members (on average, the women contacted 75% of their entire family within a 12-month period), leaving fewer slots left over for friends. This upper bound emerged both at the level of the active network and, in a re-analysis of data from Dunbar and Spoors (1995), at the level of the sympathy group (Roberts et al. 2009).

An important point to emerge from this analysis is that both time and cognitive constraints are likely to set an *upper limit* on the number of relationships that can be maintained at each layer of the network (Stiller & Dunbar 2007). In a similar way, cognitive limitations set a upper limit on the number of individuals that can coexist as a stable group in primates (Dunbar 1996), but due to a range of ecological factors (e.g. low predation risk) observed group sizes may be below this upper limit (Lehmann et al. 2007). In human social networks, due to social and/or environmental factors, we can expect a wide range of variation in sizes below this upper limit (Roberts et al. 2009). For example, not everyone will spend all their spare time socializing, and thus may have a network size below what they are able to sustain both cognitively and in terms of time investment.

It is also important to note that network size and composition, and the support that egos seek from their network, is likely to vary across countries and cultures. For example, there is some evidence that personal networks in Mexico are smaller and more kin-oriented than those in the USA (Bernard et al. 1990), although there is little systematic work in this area. There is stronger evidence that the support egos seek from their personal networks varies considerably by the level of economic development of the country. In developed countries, individuals are generally not coping with shortages of consumer goods or food, and often healthcare and schooling are provided by the state. The insecurities people have therefore come largely from physical and emotional stresses in their personal lives and social relations. Thus they turn to their social network to provide them with support for emotional problems, household chores and domestic crises (Wellman 1999). In contrast, in developing countries, where there may be less state support, social networks are relied upon to provide more basic functions such as providing access to child-care, food and clothing, financial assistance, house upgrades and job searches (Espinoza 1999).

HOW DO CONSTRAINTS AFFECT SOCIAL RELATIONSHIPS?

There is thus strong evidence that time and cognitive constraints affect network size and composition. But how do these constraints actually operate, and how do they affect how individual social relationships form, are maintained and decay over time? Relationships are not fixed, static entities, but are dynamic and require active maintenance if they are to survive. If no effort is made by the relationship partners, relationships tend to decay over time (Cummings et al. 2006; Dindia & Canary 1993). To prevent this decay, the individuals in the relationship need to engage in 'maintenance behaviours' that keep the relationship at a satisfactory, committed level. Maintenance behaviours—including emotional support, openness to meaningful conversation and behavioural interaction— occur more frequently in close as compared to casual friends (Oswald & Clark 2006). Further, relationship maintenance is a dyadic, dynamic process—it takes two people working together to maintain a relationship (Oswald et al. 2004).

The need for these maintenance behaviours is especially apparent when the two relationship partners are geographically separated. Longitudinal studies following students as they move from school to college have demonstrated that frequent communication and engaging in other maintenance behaviours can offset the decay in relationships and the loss of psychological closeness that can result from geographical distance (Cummings et al. 2006; Oswald & Clark 2003). In contrast, simply feeling psychologically close to friends at the time of the move to college does not prevent the friendship decaying in the absence of communication (Cummings et al. 2006). During the first year of college, around half of best friendships from school become merely close or casual relationships (Oswald & Clark 2003).

Thus, all relationships could be said to have a natural rate of decay — a decay function (Burt 2000). If no effort is made by the relationship partners to maintain the relationship, the relationship will tend to weaken over time. To offset this decay, egos need to invest both cognitive resources and time to keep the relationship at a particular level of emotional intensity. If the relationship is not maintained, it is unlikely to end abruptly (except perhaps in the case of romantic relationships), but instead the alter will drift outwards through the layers of the social network (Figure 6.1), becoming less emotionally close and having less frequent contact with ego.

EFFECT OF KINSHIP ON THE OPERATION OF CONSTRAINTS

The decay function of relationships will vary according to the nature of relationship. For example, the rate of decay in a relationship with an old friend with whom you have a long history of interaction is likely to be slower than with a newer friend whom you are just getting to know (Degenne & Lebeaux 2005).

A particularly important dimension along which decay functions may vary is kinship. Kin and non-kin relationships vary in two important, and related, respects. First, there are norms and expectations that assistance will be provided to kin, regardless of the personal relationship between the two individuals. Emotional and financial support, as well as social companionship, comes primarily from those closest to ego, with alters in the support clique providing a greater degree of support than alters in the sympathy group (Wellman & Wortley 1990). However, this relationship is mediated by kinship, with support provided by immediate kin being less conditional on the strength of the personal relationship than that provided by friends (Kruger 2003; Neyer & Lang 2003; Wellman & Wortley 1990).

The second important difference between kin and non-kin relationships is the network structure in which they are embedded. By their nature, kin alters will have many ties amongst themselves, as well as ties with ego, simply due to the fact that they are part of the same family (Wellman & Wortley 1990). Although not all kin members in an ego's network will have direct ties with other kin, enough of them will have direct ties to give the kin network a high degree of 'structural embeddedness' — the extent to which individuals relate to the same others (Granovetter 1985; Wellman 1982). By contrast, the non-kin network is typically much less dense, with a lower degree of structural embeddedness. Although some friends will have ties to each other as well as ego, the proportion of friends having ties to each other will on the whole be lower than the proportion of kin having ties to each other (see Figures 6.2a and 6.2b).

This difference in structural embeddedness has important implications for the costs of maintaining the relationship over time. From ego's point of view, if a friend in their network does not have ties to any other friends (alter 3 in Figure 6.2b), the emphasis is on ego and that friend to actively maintain the relationship. Otherwise the relationship will decay, and the friend will drift out through the layers of the personal network. There is no other way of ego finding out about significant events in that friend's life, other than directly through the friend.

In contrast, even if ego does not actively maintain a relationship with, for example, a cousin (alter 3 in Figure 6.2a) they will still be linked to that cousin, and hear about significant events, through the wider kin network —

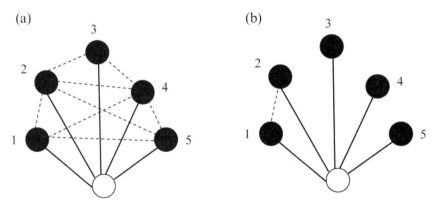

Figure 6.2. Network structure of kin (a) and non-kin (b) personal networks. White circle is ego, black numbered circles are alters. Solid lines between circles indicate ties between ego and alter, dashed lines between circles indicate ties between alters. Both networks are of equal size, but the kin network has more ties between alters than the non-kin network

parents, uncles and aunts. Thus the relationship with the cousin is less costly—in terms of both cognitive effort required to keep track of the relationship, and time spent maintaining the relationship—than the relationship with the friend, due in part to the different network structures in which the relationships are embedded. This may be especially true of the more numerous distant kin, with whom ego may not have a close personal relationship, but whose support can be activated when needed in a way that may not be possible for friends.

The extent to which egos can call upon this extended network of kin for support—and the type of support they are able to ask for—may vary by country and level of economic development. For example, in a study of personal networks in Canada, it was found that extended kin provided very little emotional aid, practical help, financial aid or companionship, as compared to the amount of support provided by immediate kin or friends (Wellman & Wortley 1990). In contrast, a study of personal networks in Chile demonstrated that the network of extended kin was extremely useful in providing financial assistance and providing access to jobs, even if the personal relationship between ego and the extended kin member was relatively weak (Espinoza 1999). The role of 'kinkeepers' may be significant in maintaining these links between kin, especially between extended kin. The position of kinkeepers tends to be filled by one of the older—usually female—members of the family, who adopts the role of passing significant news on to other family members, organizing family events and helping to keep the extended family functioning (Leach & Braithwaite 1996; Rosenthal 1985).

These 'weak ties' (Granovetter 1973)—extended kin and more distant friends—are situated in the outer network layers of the personal network beyond the sympathy group and are important in providing ego with access to a greater variety of information and ideas as compared to the strong ties at the inner layers of the network. This is partly because they are more numerous and more heterogeneous than the strong ties, but crucially because they are less likely to be connected to each other than strong ties (Granovetter 1973). Weak ties are important for obtaining information about jobs, in the spread of ideas, for obtaining advice about financial decisions or finding a place to live (Boase et al. 2006; Burt 2002; Granovetter 1983; Lin et al. 1999).

An important point about weak ties is that the degree to which they are willing to help ego with a particular request is likely to be related to the strength of the relationship between ego and the weak tie. Weak ties are not cost-free, but still need a degree of maintenance if they are to sur-

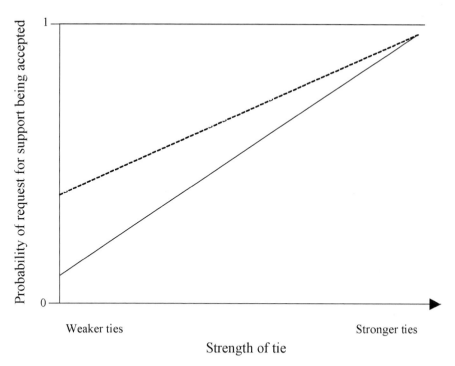

Figure 6.3. Hypothetical probability of request for support from ego being accepted by alter by strength of tie between ego and alter. Solid line is for non-kin alters, dashed line is for kin alters. The probability of request being accepted probably never reaches zero (even for very weak ties) or 1 (even for very strong ties).

vive; like stronger ties, they also show decay over time (Burt 2000, 2002; Feld 1997; Krackhardt 1998). As suggested in Figure 6.3, this maintenance is likely to be less costly for kin than non-kin relationships, both because of the norms and obligations that go with kinship, and the higher degree of structural embeddedness of kin as compared to non-kin relationships.

IMPLICATIONS OF CONSTRAINTS ON NETWORK
SIZE FOR HUMAN EVOLUTION

Given the relationship between neocortex size and group size in primates (Dunbar 1992a, 1993), hominin brain size can be used to predict hominin group size. The trend is for increasing group size, with a particularly rapid increase from around 500,000 years ago (Aiello & Dunbar 1993; Coward & Gamble 2008; Gamble ch. 2 this volume). A different method of estimating hominin group size, based directly on archaeological data, has independently shown that hominin group size is likely to have increased through evolutionary time (Grove ch. 19 this volume), in a pattern broadly congruent with that predicted by Aiello and Dunbar (1993). The assumption is that through evolutionary time hominins benefited from living in larger communities, and that these benefits selected for increasing brain size.

Increasing group size provides benefits in terms of predation defence (from animal or human threats), and in access to dispersed resources such as water holes or food resources, but also increases the costs of group living (Aiello & Dunbar 1993). Group members must be able to build and maintain social relationships of sufficient strength to buffer them from the effects of group living, keeping the group stable and avoiding permanent fission (Henzi et al. 1997a, 1997b; Lehmann et al. 2007). Thus understanding the constraints on network size—the number of relationships that can be maintained at any given level of intensity—plays a crucial role in understanding how this increase in group size could have been achieved.

Both primate (Kudo & Dunbar 2001) and human (Hamilton et al. 2007; Zhou et al. 2005) groups are hierarchically structured, and it is likely that hominin groups would have had a similar hierarchical structure (Gamble 1998, 2008). Thus the challenge for early hominins would be to manage both a small number of close ties with whom they are likely to have frequent face-to-face interaction, plus a larger number of more distant and indirect ties with whom they would have much less frequent face-to-face interaction, especially if the larger community had a fission-fusion type structure (Aureli et al. 2008; Gamble 2008; Gowlett 2008; Lehmann et al. ch. 4 this volume). In fission-fusion systems, found in chimpanzees and hunter-gatherer societies, individuals must retain and manipulate information about individuals that they do not see for substantial periods of time, which imposes a greater cognitive load than in monkey societies, where group members are out of view for much shorter periods of time (Barrett et al. 2003).

Layton and O'Hara (ch. 5 this volume) demonstrate that modern-day hunter-gatherers have both a lower population density and a larger community size (250–500) as compared to chimpanzees, suggesting that a key challenge in human evolution may have been management of an increasing number of relationships in the large extended network, numbering 100–400 people (Gamble 2008). This is especially the case if the human community, rather than the band, is the appropriate parallel with the chimpanzee community (Aureli et al. 2008; Dunbar 1998; Layton and

O'Hara ch. 5 this volume). Rather than having to keep track of around 30 relationships in the band (Marlowe 2005), early hominins would have had to keep track of a much larger number of relationships in the wider community, many of which would have involved only limited and occasional face-to-face interaction.

The nature of the constraints hominins faced was likely to be similar to that of those both primates and humans face—constraints arising from the time needed to devote to servicing social relationships, and constraints arising from the cognitive complexity of managing social relationships. As group size increases, it becomes increasingly difficult to maintain relationships using grooming, and this may lead to evolutionary pressures for more efficient bonding mechanisms, such as language (Aiello & Dunbar 1993; Dunbar 1993).

In terms of how constraints may have operated on hominin networks, two points can be made. First, as demonstrated above, the network structure in which a relationship is embedded can have significant effects on the time and cognitive costs needed to maintain that relationship. In hominin communities it is likely that, from an ego's point of view, many of the alters would have ties between themselves, as well as with the ego. Although different hominin communities may well have had some contact with each other—as evidenced by the transport of objects such as hand-axes over long distances (Gowlett 2008)—it seems safe to assume that the majority of personal interaction and social relationships would be contained within a particular community. Thus the network would be dense, in that many of the alters in the network would have ties with each other.

In contrast, in Western societies advances in communication (e.g. letters, phones, email) and transportation (e.g. cars, trains, planes), as well as increased personal mobility mean that people's personal networks are not dominated by local groupings of neighbours and kin, but are widely dispersed across and between countries. The median density of personal networks (including only alters *outside* the household) in Toronto, Canada is 0.33, meaning that on average only one-third of alters have ties with each other. The median distance between ego and alter is 9 miles, with only 22 per cent of the network living within one mile (Wellman et al. 1988). Thus modern networks are sparsely knit and loosely bounded. However, it should be noted that there is individual variation in this pattern within Western societies, with lower levels of personal mobility and living in rural areas tending to result in less dispersed personal networks with a higher density (Ferrand et al. 1999; Thomése & van Tilburg 2000).

The probable high degree of structural embeddedness in hominin networks means that hominin relationships may have been scaffolded by the network structure in which they were embedded, reducing the time and cognitive effort involved in maintaining the network. This may especially be true of the indirect ties—the extended network—which may be cognitively costly to maintain in that the alters are only seen occasionally (Barrett et al. 2003; Barton 2006; Gamble 2008; Coward ch. 21 this volume). Due to the dense network structure, these indirect ties may not have had to be maintained individually, but could be maintained through individuals known to both ego and alters. The existence of this extended network is evident in the transport of hand-axes routinely over distances of 10–15 km and up to 100 km by *Homo erectus*—transport over such a distance must have been socially mediated (Gowlett 2008).

The number of people modern humans can have a genuinely personal relationship with—that is, know one another as individual people rather than broader categories—is around 150 (Dunbar 1993, 1998; Hill & Dunbar 2003; Roberts et al. 2009). Thus to maintain a community of several hundred people, where movement between different bands within the community is accepted (Layton & O'Hara ch. 5 this volume), indirect ties—distant kin or 'friends of friends'—would have been essential (Read ch. 10 this volume). Material culture may also have been an important way of extending social networks in the absence of frequent face-to-face interaction (Coward ch. 21 this volume; Coward & Gamble 2008; Gamble 1998; Layton & O'Hara ch. 5 this volume).

The second mediating factor in the operation of constraints on network size is kinship. Early human kinship is a difficult area to study, but progress has been made in recent years in testing alternative theories as to what early human kinship systems may have looked like (Allen et al. 2008). As well as the dense network structure discussed above, kinship provides a way of reducing the costs of maintaining *individual* social relationships by 'labelling' individuals with particular kinship categories which can then be used to guide behaviour towards that person (Barnard 1978, 2008; Gamble 2008). This relaxes the costs both of maintaining the personal relationship over time, and also in determining what the appropriate behaviours, norms, trust and reciprocity levels should be on encountering another individual. Instead of calculating these social rules individually and dynamically for each relationship, a set of rules can simply be applied to all individuals in the given category (Dunbar 2008b; Read ch. 10 this volume).

Thus, it is important to realize that, as group size increased through hominin evolution, individual hominins would not necessarily have to treat each relationship within the group on an individual basis. The combination of a high level of structural embeddedness and, once language evolved, kinship labels to guide behaviour, would reduce the time and cognitive constraints on network size, allowing for larger group sizes— and possibly more extensive trading networks—than would otherwise be the case.

CONCLUSION

Time and cognitive constraints play a significant role in placing an upper bound on the number of social relationships an individual can maintain at a given level of intensity. This is true both for non-human primates (Dunbar 1992b; Lehmann et al. 2007) and for humans (Hill & Dunbar 2003; Roberts et al. 2009; Stiller & Dunbar 2007). Similar constraints are thus likely to have operated through hominin evolution, shaping the structure and size of social networks. One of the important trends through hominin evolution, alongside the increase in brain size, is likely to have been an increase in group size (Aiello & Dunbar 1993; Gamble 2008, Grove ch. 19 this volume). This could have taken the form both of an increase in community size (Aiello & Dunbar 1993), and also the development of increasingly sophisticated trading networks of 'weak ties' to other groups (Coward ch. 21 this volume).

Maintaining an increasing number of social relationships results in increasing costs, both in the time required to service the relationships, and cognitively keeping track of complex, dynamic relationships. From the analysis of time and cognitive constraints on personal networks in modern humans, two main implications emerge for our understanding of hominin social evolution. First, relationships should not be viewed as dyadic ties between two individuals, but as embedded within a larger network of relationships. This network can act as a scaffold to the dyadic tie, reducing the cognitive and time costs of maintaining the relationship. Second, and related, are the differences between kin and non-kin relationships. Kin relationships have a high degree of structural embeddedness—that is kin, are more likely to know each other than non-kin. This again reduces the cognitive and time costs of maintaining dyadic ties, allowing both for large groups and more numerous weak links to be maintained. Further, once language is in place, kin relationships can be labelled and treated as a category, so rather than managing lots of individual relationships, egos can instead use categories of kin relationships to guide behaviour. Exploring further how constraints operate to affect network size, structure and composition in non-human primates and modern humans will lead to a greater understanding of just how these constraints affected the development of social networks through hominin evolution.

Note. Sam Roberts is supported by funding from the EPSRC and ESRC as part of the 'Developing Theory for Evolving Socio-cognitive Systems' (TESS) project.

REFERENCES

Aiello, L. C. & Dunbar, R. I. M. (1993). Neocortex size, group size and the evolution of language. *Current Anthropology* 34: 184–193.
Ainsworth, M. D. S. (1989). Attachments beyond infancy. *American Psychologist* 44: 709–716.
Allen, N. J., Callan, H., Dunbar, R. & James, W. (eds) (2008). *Early human kinship: from sex to social reproduction*. Malden, MA: Royal Anthropological Institute and Blackwell.
Aureli, F., Schaffner, C. M., Boesch, C., Bearder, S. K., Call, J., Chapman, C. A. et al. (2008). Fission-fusion dynamics. *Current Anthropology* 49: 627–654.
Barnard, A. (1978). Universal systems of kin categorization. *African Studies* 37: 69–81.
Barnard, A. (2008). The co-evolution of language and kinship. In: N. J. Allen, H. Callan, R. Dunbar & W. James (eds) *Early human kinship: from sex to social reproduction*, pp. 232–245. Malden, MA: Royal Anthropological Institute and Blackwell.
Barrett, L., Henzi, P. & Dunbar, R. (2003). Primate cognition: from 'what now?' to 'what if?' *Trends in Cognitive Sciences* 7: 494–497.
Barton, R. A. (2006). Primate brain evolution: integrating comparative, neurophysiological, and ethological data. *Evolutionary Anthropology* 15: 224–236.
Bergman, T. J., Beehner, J. C., Cheney, D. L. & Seyfarth, R. M. (2003). Hierarchical classification by rank and kinship in baboons. *Science* 302: 1234–1236.
Bernard, H. R. & Killworth, P. D. (1973). On the social structure of an ocean-going research vessel and other important things. *Social Science Research* 2: 145–184.
Bernard, H. R., Johnsen, E. C., Killworth, P. D., McCarty, C., Shelley, G. A. & Robinson, S. (1990). Comparing four different methods for measuring personal social networks. *Social Networks* 12: 179–215.
Boase, J., Horrigan, J. B., Wellman, B. & Rainie, L. (2006). The strength of internet ties. *Pew Internet and American Life Project.* Retrieved 10 July 2008, from http://www.pewinternet.org/pdfs/PIP_Internet_ties.pdf
Burt, R. S. (2000). Decay functions. *Social Networks* 22: 1–28.
Burt, R. S. (2002). Bridge decay. *Social Networks* 24: 333–363.

Buys, C. J. & Larson, K. L. (1979). Human sympathy groups. *Psychological Reports* 45: 547–553.

Byrne, R. W. & Whiten, A. (1988). *Machiavellian intelligence: social expertise and the evolution of intelligence in monkeys, apes and humans.* Oxford: Oxford University Press.

Cheney, D. L., Seyfarth, R. M. & Silk, J. B. (1995). The responses of female baboons (*Papio cynocephalus ursinus*) to anomalous social interactions—evidence of causal reasoning. *Journal of Comparative Psychology* 109: 134–141.

Coward, F. & Gamble, C. (2008). Big brains, small worlds: material culture and the evolution of the mind. *Philosophical Transactions of the Royal Society: Series B* 363: 1969–1979.

Cummings, J. N., Lee, J. B. & Kraut, R. (2006). Communication technology and friendship during the transition from high school to college. In: K. Kraut, M. Brynin & S. Kiesler (eds) *Computers, phones and the internet: domesticating information technologies*, pp. 265–278. New York: Oxford University Press.

Degenne, A. & Lebeaux, M. O. (2005). The dynamics of personal networks at the time of entry into adult life. *Social Networks* 27: 337–358.

Dindia, K. & Canary, D. J. (1993). Definitions and theoretical perspectives on maintaining relationships. *Journal of Social and Personal Relationships* 10: 163–173.

Dunbar, R. I. M. (1992a). Neocortex size as a constraint on group-size in primates. *Journal of Human Evolution* 22: 469–493.

Dunbar, R. I. M. (1992b). Time—a hidden constraint on the behavioral ecology of baboons. *Behavioral Ecology and Sociobiology* 31: 35–49.

Dunbar, R. I. M. (1993). Coevolution of neocortical size, group-size and language in humans. *Behavioral and Brain Sciences* 16: 681–694.

Dunbar, R. I. M. (1996). Determinates of group size in primates: a general model. In: J. Maynard Smith, G. Runciman & R. Dunbar (eds) *Evolution of culture and language in primates and humans*, pp. 33–57. Oxford: Oxford University Press.

Dunbar, R. I. M. (1998). The social brain hypothesis. *Evolutionary Anthropology* 6: 178–190.

Dunbar, R. I. M. (2008a). Cognitive constraints on the structure and dynamics of social networks. *Group Dynamics: Theory, Research and Practice* 12: 7–16.

Dunbar, R. I. M. (2008b). Early human kinship. In: N. J. Allen, H. Callan, R. Dunbar & W. James (eds) *Early human kinship: from sex to social reproduction*, pp. 131–151. Malden, MA: Royal Anthropological Institute and Blackwell.

Dunbar, R. I. M. & Shultz, S. (2007a). Evolution in the social brain. *Science* 317: 1344–1347.

Dunbar, R. I. M. & Shultz, S. (2007b). Understanding primate brain evolution. *Philosophical Transactions of the Royal Society B: Biological Sciences* 362: 649–658.

Dunbar, R. I. M. & Spoors, M. (1995). Social networks, support cliques, and kinship. *Human Nature* 6: 273–290.

Ennett, S. T., Faris, R., Hipp, J., Foshee, V. A., Bauman, K. E., Hussong, A. et al. (2008). Peer smoking, other peer attributes, and adolescent cigarette smoking: a social network analysis. *Prevention Science* 9: 88–98.

Espinoza, V. (1999). Social networks among the urban poor: inequality and integration in a Latin American city. In: B. Wellman (ed.) *Networks in the global village*, pp. 147–184. Boulder, CO: Westview Press.

Feld, S. L. (1997). Structural embeddedness and stability of interpersonal relations. *Social Networks* 19: 91–95.

Ferrand, A., Mounier, L. & Degenne, A. (1999). The diversity of personal networks in France: social stratification and relational structures. In: B. Wellman (ed.) *Networks in the global village*, pp. 185–224. Boulder, CO: Westview Press.

Fischer, C. S. (1982). What do we mean by friend—an inductive study. *Social Networks* 3: 287–306.

Gamble, C. (1998). Palaeolithic society and the release from proximity: a network approach to intimate relations. *World Archaeology* 29: 426–449.

Gamble, C. (2008). Kinship and material culture: implications of the human global diaspora. In: N. J. Allen, H. Callan, R. Dunbar & W. James (eds) *Early human kinship: from sex to social reproduction*, pp. 27–41. Malden, MA: Royal Anthropological Institute and Blackwell.

Gowlett, J. A. J. (2008). Deep roots of kin: developing the evolutionary perspective from prehistory. In: N. J. Allen, H. Callan, R. Dunbar & W. James (eds) *Early human kinship: from sex to social reproduction*, pp. 41–59. Malden, MA: Royal Anthropological Institute and Blackwell.

Granovetter, M. (1973). The strength of weak ties. *American Journal of Sociology* 78: 1360–1380.

Granovetter, M. (1983). The strength of weak ties: a network theory revisited. *Sociological Theory* 1: 201–233.

Granovetter, M. (1985). Economic action and social structure—the problem of embeddedness. *American Journal of Sociology* 91: 481–510.

Hamilton, M. J., Milne, B. T., Walker, R. S., Burger, O. & Brown, J. H. (2007). The complex structure of hunter-gatherer social networks. *Proceedings of the Royal Society B: Biological Sciences* 274: 2195–2202.

Hammer, M. (1983). Core and extended social networks in relation to health and illness. *Social Science and Medicine* 17: 405–411.

Henzi, S. P., Lycett, J. E. & Piper, S. E. (1997a). Fission and troop size in a mountain baboon population. *Animal Behaviour* 53: 525–535.

Henzi, S. P., Lycett, J. E. & Weingrill, T. (1997b). Cohort size and allocation of social effort by female mountain baboons. *Animal Behaviour* 54: 1235–1243.

Hill, R. A. & Dunbar, R. I. M. (2003). Social network size in humans. *Human Nature* 14: 53–72.

Hill, R. A., Bentley, R. A. & Dunbar, R. I. M. (2008). Network scaling reveals consistent fractal patterns in hierarchical mammalian societies. *Biology Letters* 4: 748–751.

Johnson, M. P. & Leslie, L. (1982). Couple involvement and network structure—a test of the dyadic withdrawal hypothesis. *Social Psychology Quarterly* 45: 34–43.

Kinderman, P., Dunbar, R. & Bentall, R. P. (1998). Theory-of-mind deficits and causal attributions. *British Journal of Psychology* 89: 191–204.

Kossinets, G. & Watts, D. (2006). Empirical analysis of an evolving social network. *Science* 311: 88–90.

Krackhardt, D. (1998). Simmelian ties: super strong and sticky. In: R. M. Kramer & M. Neale (eds) *Power and influence in organisations*, pp. 21–38. Thousand Oaks, CA: SAGE.

Kruger, D. J. (2003). Evolution and altruism—combining psychological mediators with naturally selected tendencies. *Evolution and Human Behavior* 24: 118–125.

Kudo, H. & Dunbar, R. I. M. (2001). Neocortex size and social network size in primates. *Animal Behaviour* 62: 711–722.

Leach, M. S. & Braithwaite, D. O. (1996). A binding tie: supportive communication of family kinkeepers. *Journal of Applied Communication Research* 24: 200–216.

Lehmann, J., Korstjens, A. H. & Dunbar, R. I. M. (2007). Group size, grooming and social cohesion in primates. *Animal Behaviour* 74: 1617–1629.

Lin, N., Ye, X. L. & Ensel, W. M. (1999). Social support and depressed mood: a structural analysis. *Journal of Health and Social Behavior* 40: 344–359.

McCannell, K. (1988). Social networks and the transition to motherhood. In: R. M. Milardo (ed.) *Families and social networks*, pp. 83–106. Beverly Hills, CA: SAGE.

McPherson, M., Smith-Lovin, L. & Brashears, M. E. (2006). Social isolation in America: changes in core discussion networks over two decades. *American Sociological Review* 71: 353–375.

Marlowe, F. W. (2005). Hunter-gatherers and human evolution. *Evolutionary Anthropology* 14: 54–67.

Marsden, P. V. (1987). Core discussion networks of Americans. *American Sociological Review* 52: 122–131.

Milardo, R. M. (1992). Comparative methods for delineating social networks. *Journal of Social and Personal Relationships* 9: 447–461.

Milardo, R. M., Johnson, M. P. & Huston, T. L. (1983). Developing close relationships—changing patterns of interaction between pair members and social networks. *Journal of Personality and Social Psychology* 44: 964–976.

Mok, D., Wellman, B. & Basu, R. (2007). Did distance matter before the Internet? Interpersonal contact and support in the 1970s. *Social Networks* 29: 430–461.

Morgan, D. L., Neal, M. B. & Carder, P. (1997). The stability of core and peripheral networks over time. *Social Networks* 19: 9–25.

Neyer, F. J. & Lang, F. R. (2003). Blood is thicker than water: kinship orientation across adulthood. *Journal of Personality and Social Psychology* 84: 310–321.

Onnela, J. P., Saramäki, J., Hyvonen, J., Szabó, G., Lazer, D., Kaski, K. et al. (2007). Structure and tie strengths in mobile communication networks. *Proceedings of the National Academy of Sciences of the United States of America* 104: 7332–7336.

Oswald, D. L. & Clark, E. M. (2003). Best friends forever? High school best friendships and the transition to college. *Personal Relationships* 10: 187–196.

Oswald, D. L. & Clark, E. M. (2006). How do friendship maintenance behaviors and problem-solving styles function at the individual and dyadic levels? *Personal Relationships* 13: 333–348.

Oswald, D. L., Clark, E. M. & Kelly, C. M. (2004). Friendship maintenance: an analysis of individual and dyad behaviors. *Journal of Social and Clinical Psychology* 23: 413–441.

Plickert, G., Cote, R. R. & Wellman, B. (2007). It's not who you know, it's how you know them: who exchanges what with whom? *Social Networks* 29: 405–429.

Pool, I. D. & Kochen, M. (1978). Contacts and influence. *Social Networks* 1: 5–51.

Roberts, S. G. B., Wilson, R., Fedurek, P. & Dunbar, R. I. M. (2008). Individual differences and personal social network size and structure. *Personality and Individual Differences* 44: 954–964.

Roberts, S. G. B., Dunbar, R. I. M., Pollet, T. V. & Kuppens, T. (2009). Exploring variation in active network size: constraints and ego characteristics. *Social Networks*
31: 138–146.

Rosenthal, C. J. (1985). Kinkeeping in the familial division of labor. *Journal of
Marriage and the Family* 47: 965–974.

Silk, J. B. (1999). Male bonnet macaques use information about third-party rank
relationships to recruit allies. *Animal Behaviour* 58: 45–51.

Slater, P. E. (1963). On social regression. *American Sociological Review,* 28: 339–364.

Stiller, J. & Dunbar, R. I. M. (2007). Perspective-taking and memory capacity predict
social network size. *Social Networks* 29: 93–104.

Suitor, J. J., Wellman, B. & Morgan, D. L. (1997). It's about time: how, why, and when
networks change. *Social Networks* 19: 1–7.

Thomése, F. & van Tilburg, T. (2000). Neighbouring networks and environmental
dependency: differential effects of neighbourhood characteristics on the relative
size and composition of neighbouring networks of older adults in the Netherlands.
Ageing and Society 20: 55–78.

Tooby, J. & Cosmides, L. (1996). Friendship and the banker's paradox: other pathways to the evolution of adaptations for altruism. *Proceedings of the British
Academy* 88: 119–143.

Watts, D. J. (2004). The 'new' science of networks. *Annual Review of Sociology* 30:
243–270.

Wellman, B. (1982). Studying personal communities. In: P. V. Marsden & N. Lin (eds)
Social structure and network analysis, pp. 61–80. Beverly Hills, CA: SAGE.

Wellman, B. (1999). The network community. In: B. Wellman (ed.) *Networks in the
global village*, pp. 1–47. Boulder, CO: Westview Press.

Wellman, B. (2007a). Challenges in collecting personal network data: the nature of
personal network analysis. *Field Methods* 19: 111–115.

Wellman, B. (2007b). The network is personal: introduction to a special issue of
Social Networks. *Social Networks* 29: 349–356.

Wellman, B. & Frank, K. (2001). Network capital in a multilevel world: getting support from personal communities. In: N. Lin, K. S. Cook & R. S. Burt (eds) *Social
capital: theory and research*, pp. 233–275. New York: Aldine Transaction.

Wellman, B. & Wortley, S. (1990). Different strokes from different folks: community
ties and social support. *American Journal of Sociology* 96: 558–588.

Wellman, B., Carrington, P. J. & Hall, A. (1988). Networks as personal communities.
In: B. Wellman and S. D. Berkowitz (eds) *Social structures: a network approach*,
pp. 130–184. Cambridge: Cambridge University Press.

Whiten, A. & Byrne, R. W. (eds) (1997). *Machiavellian intelligence II: extensions and
evaluations*. Cambridge: Cambridge University Press.

Wittig, R. M., Crockford, C., Lehmann, J., Whiten, P. L., Seyfarth, R. M. & Cheney,
D. L. (2008) Focused grooming networks and stress alleviation in wild female
baboons. *Hormones and Behaviour* 54: 170–177.

Zhou, W. X., Sornette, D., Hill, R. A. & Dunbar, R. I. M. (2005). Discrete hierarchical organization of social group sizes. *Proceedings of the Royal Society B:
Biological Sciences* 272: 439–444.

7

Social Networks and Community in the Viking Age

ANNA WALLETTE

SOCIAL NETWORKS AMONG THE VIKINGS

THE 17TH-CENTURY PHILOSOPHER Thomas Hobbes argued that a strong central authority was necessary to avoid societal chaos. In the Viking Age, the use of private violence was a precondition for social power. All (free) men had the right to their freedom and property, but the enjoyment of this right was uncertain as long as it was vulnerable to others. Viking Age Scandinavia consisted of law-making communities; but even if the rules were commonly recognized, the executive power that Hobbes thought necessary to put the laws into effect was lacking. Politics throughout the region was therefore based on strong personal relations.

In this chapter I discuss how solidarity in a pre-modern society is always associated with obligations—notably the obligation to defend and avenge those allied with you. Even blood kinship has to be activated and nurtured, and we see the need for strong bonds not only with family and kin, but also with neighbours and friends. In short, a medieval Scandinavian had to create alliances, and forged new relationships by marriage, business arrangement, fosterage and friendship.

This chapter is intended as a general discussion of collective under-standings and attitudes in political culture, and as an introduction to a study of the cultural implications of networks in a medieval society where few political institutions existed. Asking questions about what people accepted as a good way of regulating their relationships, and in what way they described these relations, allows us to explore the structure and dynamics of social networks.

Proceedings of the British Academy **158**, 135–152. © The British Academy 2010.

A SHORT HISTORICAL BACKGROUND

Viking Age Scandinavia has traditionally been regarded as a society of kinship. In a society where few central authorities existed, kinship is crucial to consolidate one's position. Viking Age Scandinavia was not unique in being a stateless society in which individuals resolved disputes for themselves. Scholars have looked for well-defined clans of either matrilinear or patrilinear groups that collectively owned land, or had a clear-cut system of blood feuds. The assumption that Germanic areas had a unilineal clan system has been challenged (e.g. Gaunt 1983). Viking Age and medieval Scandinavia reckoned kin bilaterally; as a result, one individual's relations may not themselves have been related.

During this period, new areas were settled, and new self-regulating communities established. Between AD 800 and 1100, Scandinavians settled Iceland and Greenland, ruled parts of the British Isles, and were also known to travel to Russia, Constantinople, Greece, Africa and North America. Foreigners identified three groups of people in Scanidnavia: Norwegians, Dani and the so-called Sveones. The Scandinavians described themselves as *norrænir menn*, Northmen or Danes. We often call the medieval culture of Scandinavia 'Old Norse', and a common language can trick us into believing that there were no differences in politics, social order, culture or religious beliefs. Scandinavia is a very large region in which there was considerable diversity. Today, archaeologists concentrate not only on finding similarities in the grave material, but also on mapping out the differences within the region (e.g. Svanberg 2006).

Most medievalists pay particular attention to Iceland. There are two reasons for this: first, the textual sources from the island are still seen as representative for the whole region. Second, this was a society without a king. A group of people moved to the island and needed to adjust to new conditions. They formed assemblies of free men to settle disputes and stipulate laws. Such assemblies provide us with the idea of freedom as a characteristic of Scandinavia. The political arrangements of the Icelanders often become symbolic of the whole of Scandinavian culture.

It is true that Scandinavia had less political centralization; the individual had much economic and political freedom. During the early phase of the colonization of Iceland, there were neither military leaders, nor central authority. But society was nonetheless hierarchical: farmers stood in a dependent relationship to local leaders, chieftains or petty kings, and there were various degrees of free men, from leader of household to lord. The presence of overlordship in Scandinavia is known from Frankish sources in the 9th century. An overlordship is always easier to create with good communications, which is probably why it was seen earlier in Denmark and along the 'Northern Way' (the coastline of Norway) than in the rest of the Nordic countries. There was a population increase and new forms of cultivation led to larger communities. Since it was easier to support and defend a concentrated population, these areas were easier for an overlord to administer (Sawyer & Sawyer 1993, 41–47). Besides a concentration of power in Norway in the late 9th century, Haraldr Blátönn (or Black-tooth) proclaimed the unification of Denmark in runes on a large stone in Jelling around the year 980. A handful of circular forts in Denmark and in the southern part of modern Sweden are also credited to his name, and the enormous amount of manpower necessary for their construction suggests an effective level of political organization over a wide geographical area.

Scandinavians were also in service to lords elsewhere. The literature tells us that the kings in England made the Norsemen petty rulers in Northumbria to protect the land against 'Danes' (i.e. Scandinavians), and to defend the land against the Scots and the Irish. The saga of Egill Skallagrímssonar recounts travels around Europe, Viking raids in the Baltic and Scandinavian area, and Icelanders joining the army of Anglo-Saxon King Athelstan at the battle of Brunanburgh in the early 900s: 'When Thorolf and Egil came before the king, he thanked them generously for their courage they had shown and the victory they had won, and he promised them his constant friendship.' Egil's brother Thorolf dies at Vin Moor, as it is called in the saga, and the king gives him silver to bring home to his father 'in compensation for his son's life' (*Egil's saga* 1976, chs 54–55). Apart from leading to further raiding and even conquests, this policy led to a huge inflow of silver coinage into Scandinavia. At the same time, Western ideas were also flooding into Scandinavia. The ideas of Christianity, together with ideas of kingship, coincided with the gradual unification of the smaller kingdoms into what we now know as Denmark, Norway and Sweden.

Traditionally, Scandinavians were probably used to the *þing* (thing) institution as their social organization. Big meetings during the summers, and smaller local things in spring and autumn, provided meeting places for social gatherings and economic trade. Since every farmer had to defend himself, his family, his labour, his belongings and his slaves, he did his best to follow a strong leader. Thus large groups of farmers were led by chieftains or petty kings, who took charge of these assemblies and the military organization. Wealth or family connections might not have been

the most important factor in choosing a leader, but riches would be helpful in being a good one. All Scandinavian chieftains would exchange
gifts and hold feasts in order to retain formal alliances. The overlord
was the person who could provide stability and, even in Iceland, it would
have been expensive to be the first among equals, to call on support from
others.

> To his friend
> a man should be a friend,
> and gifts with gifts requite.
> Laughter with laughter
> men should receive,
> but leasing with lying.
> (*Hávamál* 1866, 42)

We do know that Scandinavians experienced changes in the social
order during this period. This was a time when church and king consolidated their power. Alongside the development of church and kingdom we
see an overall integration into a more complex political system (Sawyer &
Sawyer 1993). Little is known about the political and social organization
of the eastern part of Scandinavia, especially if we are searching for local
cultures rather than one regional culture. We know more about the settlement of Iceland. Most settlers came from Norway, bringing their local
customs with them. In *Landnámabók* (*Book of settlements* 1972) we find
descriptions of over 3,000 people, and 1,400 different residences. It is a
book with many contradictions—at least 200 years had passed since the
settlement. Although archaeological findings confirm the dates given,
Landnámabók was reworked several times, becoming longer each time.
The same difficulty occurs with many of the sources we use for this
period. What we can say regarding the *Landnámabók* is that even if the
settlers of Iceland came from different places, the fact that they compro-
mised on a political and social organization suggests that the variations
in mainland Scandinavia might not have been that big. *Íslendingabók*
(*Book of the Icelanders* 2006) was written in the 1120s as a brief survey of
Icelandic history. It contains an account of the settlement of the country,
the discovery of Greenland and stories of the first bishops, but also provides information on the administrative system. It tells us that the farmer
was legally obliged to be an assembly man for the local chieftain, and had
a duty to ride with him to the assemblies. The local leaders presided at the
smaller meetings, protected their followers and solved disputes on their
behalf. But in the Iceland setting it was not necessary to follow a chieftain
in the vicinity; and in theory every farmer had the right to choose who to

follow. However, even if local leaders had no automatic geographical authority, scholars have pointed out that it would not be practical to show loyalty to a strong man further away without moving closer to him (Jón Viðar Sigurðsson 1999).

LITERARY SOURCES

After this short account of the historical background of the political order, we turn to the issue of social relations in an early medieval Scandinavian setting. But, apart from archaeology, we have only two contemporary sources for the Viking Age: the skaldic verse composed in honour of Scandinavian leaders and preserved in Icelandic and Norwegian texts, and runic inscriptions. Before we can say anything about the societal dimensions, we need to consider the other sources that can tell us about social networks in a pre-modern society.

Political organization was not the only part of life that had undergone changes during the Viking Age. The import of parchment and the knowledge of how to prepare vellum influenced the ideology and world-view of the region's inhabitants. The new technology made it possible to produce one of the largest collections of vernacular narratives from medieval times. The first texts produced were of Christian origin, usually translations from other languages, but soon vernacular stories were written down as well.

The Icelandic sagas are compelling stories of dramatic events and the everyday life of kings, chieftains and farmers. The subgenre of family sagas, *Íslendingasögur*, are set in the period from the end of the 9th century to 1000. In over 30 sagas of different lengths, the texts tell of the first generations of settlers in Iceland. Other subgenres include the contemporary sagas, telling the stories of Icelandic chieftains and their feuding from the 1100s to 1264, and stories of Scandinavian kings. Furthermore, we have legendary and chivalric sagas, more easily dismissed as pure fiction since they include the presence of dragons, enchanted swords, etc.

The sagas were first written down between the 1100s and the 1400s, and there have been several debates as to how one should treat them as historical sources. The problem is that they claim to describe events that occurred well before they were composed. These sagas surely drew from traditions that were passed down orally over the centuries, but they are the products of medieval writers. In the climate of stern source criticism that has dominated most of the 20th century, only a few fragments of facts from these texts have been considered reliable. However, the saga writers' own analyses of human actions can be considered useful. Therefore, even if the sagas may not be historical, they can claim historical reality all the same. They provide the social and moral codes of a society, since they could have been written during an adjustment of local practices to more continental European ideals (Torfi H. Tulinius 2003). During a political transformation, a confusion of loyalty is inevitable. Jón Viðar Sigurðsson (1999, 7–38) suggests that the saga literature served the purpose of illustrating the historical social change that led to the Icelanders becoming subject to the Norwegian king in 1262–1264. The differences between the backward-looking family sagas and the contemporary sagas would make more sense in this context.

The sagas are still difficult to use as source material, and it is questionable whether they are representative for the whole of Scandinavia. It is difficult to use the sagas as sources for political events, indeed even for reliable family history. The anthropologist Victor Turner (1971) called the sagas 'social dramas', and we can use them, carefully, to investigate themes and tendencies in social structures and value systems.[1]

We should be aware that the description of an event could be presented in opposite ways, depending on the opinion of the author. The saga actors are literary characters, but their connection with the saga writer and his work of writing history gives the sagas relevance within social history. The actors may or may not have existed. However, this may be less important than the fact that they are *seen* to have existed, and were important to medieval people as forefathers. The events may or may not have happened, but the fact that what is happening was plausible for the audience is the important part. The speeches are probably fiction, but again it is their plausibility that is important. The actors' characteristics—or the nodes' characteristics, to use network terminology—are of interest if this relates to her/his contacts with others, and in the Icelandic sagas characterization always matters, otherwise the event or person would not be included. The sagas, then, are fiction realistic enough to allow the study of human behaviour in a social setting, even if they do not contain historical truth in a political sense. The main characteristic of the narrative technique of the sagas is that the stories are realistic, a reflection of expected norms of behaviour in medieval Iceland. In most cases, how-

---

[1] Several scholars dispute the use of sagas as sources: Guðrún Nordal (1988, 19) says that family sagas 'are literary compositions rather than historical documents' and that the contemporary sagas provide a contrast to this.

ever, the characters of the sagas are well known and the place names accurate.[2]

The suggestion is that the sagas provide us with information on social networking. But what was the relationship between kin and non-kin according to these texts? Why was it at all-important to use kin or friendship terminology for a pre-modern Scandinavian?

KINSHIP

Network analysis can provide explanations for the structure and functions of how individuals or groups of individuals interact, but it cannot explain change. The alliance patterns described in the sagas can still shed light on the political and social change in an Icelandic setting in their capacity of being written as history. Medieval politics was based on strong personal relations, and we need to study the political culture, that is, the interaction amongst various groups and individuals. Guðrún Nordal (1998) argues that scholars have unanimously recognized the role of kinship in governing human behaviour in Scandinavia. However, there were no deeper investigations into how and why kinship matters in the practice of alliance building until William Ian Miller's book on feuding in 1990 (see Guðrún Nordal 1998, 31, 41).

Frændi is a term for kin, while *frændsemi* is an acknowledgement of a kin relation—someone who is a kinsman and with whom there is a feeling of solidarity: Miller (1990, 167) found this expression was used for a mother's father's sister's husband. The term *náfrændi* could be used for near affinity: 'There was a man called Thorkel the Black who was a member of Illugi's household; he was a close relative [*náfrændi*] as well and had grown up at Gilsbakki' (*Saga of Gunnlaug Serpent-Tongue* 1957, ch. 5).

Most of the approximately 3,000 rune inscriptions in mainland Scandinavia carved between 800 and 1100 are considered commemorative monuments. Besides being memorials to the dead, the rune-stone texts can be seen as legal documents that tell us about inheritance patterns in nuclear families, according to Sawyer (2000). They depict nuclear families (Sawyer & Sawyer 1993, 168). Similarly, the Icelandic *Grágás* (1980–2000) is a collection of legal statements, or advice, given on how to apply the law. *Grágás* is divided into chapters, such as an inheritance section

---

[2] Meulengracht Sørensen (1993) has argued that this historicity is mainly a technique used by the authors to increase the realism.

(*Erfðaþáttur*) or a wergild ring list (*Baugatal*) that gives us insights into kin-based alliance building. The wergild list of blood money does not appear in any other text, and here we can see the discrepancy between sagas and *Grágás* (Guðrún Nordal 1998, 32). The saga writers wrote about and for themselves, for an audience that was familiar with the social organization and thus knew the norms and what was socially acceptable (Gunnar Karlsson 2000, 23). Miller (1990, 164) suggests that paying blood money to the counterpart was meaningful even if this was not formally stated in the sagas—otherwise it would not have been mentioned in *Grágás*. It is by combining these texts, therefore, that we learn the terminology and meaning of kinship and friendship situations.

'IT IS NOT PROPER FOR KINSMEN TO COME TO BLOWS'[3] — KIN AND NETWORK

Kin-based support in legal actions had to be actively sought out and activated in a network-recruiting fashion. Relations needed to be emphasized, especially if the issue was one of vengeance killing. Miller (1983, 98) argues that recruiting was done primarily in the narrow kin group. People in the sagas expanded their personal support network to distant parts of the country, perhaps because they had already entwined themselves in alliances with people close by. But Richard Gaskins (2005, 203) suggests that these 'weak links' could serve as bridges between otherwise disparate centres of power, and are therefore useful to study in a network analysis.

Within the narrow kin group, a son should care for his mother, and, if possible, for his father, and—if it was within his power—for his children, according to *Grágás*. He should go into debt bondage for his parents, but not necessarily for his children. A son's duty was towards the father, not the other way around. The father administered the children's fortunes, and loyalty was naturally a social expectation in both directions (Percivall 2005, 58). Although the family circle might be seen as the most likely place for individuals to seek comfort, even blood kin needed to maintain their bonds of kinship for them to matter.

Uncles seem to present a specific problem in alliance building. Scholars have proposed that maternal uncles had a special duty of soli-

---

[3] *Laxdæla saga* (1969, ch. 37).

darity. Guðrún Nordal (1998, 86) says that a brother should provide for his sister and her children if his brother-in-law disappears. She proposes there were more quarrels between paternal uncles and nephews than between family members on the maternal side. Johnson and Johnson (1991, 216), however, refer to Miller in arguing that maternal uncles had weaker obligations than paternal uncles. This would be due to more beneficial ranking in terms of blood compensation and inheritance. The distinction between the stable bonds of solidarity between maternal uncles and their nephews, or paternal uncles having stronger obligations may come from the fact that Guðrún Nordal's work deals with contemporary sagas covering 12th- and 13th-century Icelandic affairs, while Johnson and Johnson include family sagas as well as sagas from other subgenres. Or it may be the case that the maternal side entailed less responsibility, but the narrators of the sagas wanted to enforce the importance of actively upholding these relations. A third alternative could be that this illustrates a change in the value systems, between the retrospective family sagas and more current times presented in the contemporary sagas.

Of 365 different social events (such as feuding, gift-giving and asking for marriage or advice) in the two family sagas *Laxdæla saga* (1969) and *Egil's saga* (1976), 25 concern uncles and nephews, of which 15 are affirmative and 10 involve conflict. Among the positive interactions, 11 are between maternal blood kin, 2 between paternal blood kin, 2 between maternal social kin and none between paternal social kin (where social kin are defined as foster or step relations). The uncles travel together with their nephews, offer support or give inheritances. Of the 10 negative interactions, 7 are among paternal blood kin, 2 maternal blood kin and 1 paternal social kin. These events involve fighting, feuding or simply the expression of hostile feelings.

By showing these examples from just two of the family sagas it is obvious that, by going beyond the genetic relationships to include ties between social kin, we can see a more flexible social configuration. Johnson and Johnson could not find a single incident where a nephew was killed by an uncle or vice versa, and are therefore inclined to see this kin relation as a strong alliance. By adding in the constructed relationships we get a different picture. For example, in the *Laxdæla saga* (1969, ch. 37) Hrut is targeted by his half-brother's son, his step-nephew Thorkel, when his (Hrut's) 12-year-old son is killed as a way to humiliate him for a perceived insult.

SOCIAL KIN

Even if a feeling of solidarity was present among kinsmen, the alliances were not easily upheld. Kin and marriage systems are the main organization form for people, but it is the cultural norms that regulate these relationships. The aim of marriage is reproduction and the parties will share a common bloodline through their children. But there is more at stake in making good marriage alliances. Marriage was not a private affair in Scandinavia, and it was often the father's decision.[4] In-laws were strong alliances, and we can easily find loyalty between in-laws in the family sagas as well as in the contemporary sagas. This is the case not only between current *mágr* (brothers-, fathers- or sons-in-law), but also taking account of future arrangements. For example, in the *Laxdæla saga* (1969, ch. 59), Thorgil takes part in avenging the death of Guðrún's husband, believing that he will receive her hand in marriage in return.

People need companions, and there is strength in numbers. But it can be dangerous to create alliances. The sagas are full of examples of people being tricked into marriage alliances. The historian Eva Österberg (1991, 1995, 2003, 2007) uses the story of Hen Thorir to illustrate the fact that alliances were not always the best thing for all parties. A good example of the complicated bonds and the dangers of a liaison is offered by the case of Blund-Ketil's son, who needs allies to avenge his father's death. He tricks an unmarried girl's father into a marriage arrangement, without disclosing that the reason for the proposal is that the girl's mother's brother is a powerful chieftain named Thorð Gellir. By giving the girl away in marriage the uncle is bound to aid the new son-in-law: 'Thorð was as angry as he could be, for he thought that they had made a fool of him' (*Hønsa-þoris saga* 1953).

In the *Grágás* it is clearly stated that vengeance for social kin is equivalent to that for blood-related kin. We see values and norms in the law, but human action may run counter to this and in the literary sagas life could be quite risky. Guðrún Nordal emphasizes this even more with the contemporary sagas: if the choice is between brother or in-laws, choose neither (1998, 130).

---

[4] This social obligation included illegitimate sons; Nic Percivall (2005) and Auður Magnúsdóttir (2001) demonstrate that Guðrún Nordal is wrong in assuming that legitimacy was a big issue when it came to inheritance, since there was no social stigma associated with not being married. This situation changed in the 13th century, when it became more common for one son to inherit everything.

These socially constructed relationships may seem fragile compared to kinship patterns. Guðrún Nordal (1998, 199) suggests that clashes in obligations were depicted in the sagas as cautionary tales, to warn people what would happen if their kinship or neighbourhood peace is neglected. Even if we do not find any patricides or matricides in the sagas, Percivall (2005, 60) also proposes that a bad relation between father and son might be a warning to the audience. In this way, the literary texts can provide us with the cultural norms regarding social realities.

There is nothing new in declaring that alliance building is a central theme in the sagas. But studying how kinship relations interact with other social ties provides a more complex image of the network system. To emphasize a society of friendship as well as kinship shows the density of divided loyalties and entangled alliances. As Alan Barnard claims (ch. 12 this volume), no one is without a family. Furthermore, you will never find half a kinship system. Even if Scandinavians acknowledged non-kin, the fact that they used kinship terms to associate with non-relatives is noteworthy.

Besides marriage, there is a significant display of fictive kinship in the sagas through labelling people as kin. There were two kinds of fostering: fostering of a child—with the involvement of the family—or sworn brotherhood between adults, which did not involve their families. Medieval Scandinavia was a gift-giving society, like many other pre-modern societies that lacked a central authority based on bureaucracy.[5] Fostering of children can be seen as a gift-giving custom since it was a reciprocal exchange. There was a probability of further interactions taking place with the same person. The parties tended to be of different status, and the fostering created a vertical alliance: 'I want to regain your goodwill by fostering your son: for he who fosters another's son is always said to be a lesser man' (*Laxdaela saga* 1969, ch. 27).

Emotional ties did not always accompany the fostering of a child, although the love between the child and the foster parent, as well as between foster siblings, is apparent in many cases. In *Fóstbrœðra saga* two men are foster brothers from childhood, but swear an oath of loyalty as adults as well (*The sagas of Kormák and The sworn brothers* 1949). The ritual is described in *Gísla saga Súrssonar* (*The story of Gisli the Outlaw* 1866), where the implications of taking the oath of foster-brothers are well illustrated:

[5] See Österberg (2007) for the key differences between a pre-modern and a modern society. For the classic work on gift exchange, see Mauss (1954 [1922]).

> [They] cut up a sod of turf in such wise that both its ends were still fast to the
> earth, and propped it up by a spear scored with runes, so tall that a man might
> lay his hand on the socket of the spear-head. Under this yoke they were all four
> to pass—Thorgrim, Gisli, Thorkel, and Vestein. Now they breathe each a vein,
> and let their blood fall together on the mould whence the turf had been cut up,
> and all touch it; and afterwards they all fall on their knees and were to take
> hands, and swear to avenge each the other as though he were his brother, and
> to call all the gods to witness. But now, just as they were going to take hands,
> Thorgrim said: 'I shall have quite enough on my hands if I do this towards
> Thorkel and Gisli, my brothers-in-law; but towards Vestein I have no tie to bind
> me to so great a charge.' As he said this he drew back his hand. 'Then more will
> do the like,' says Gisli, and drew back his hand. 'I will be bound by no tie to the
> man who will not be bound by the same tie to my brother-in-law Vestein.' (*The
> story of Gisli the Outlaw* 1866, ch. 4)

Adult foster brothers, or blood-brotherhood, was an affair between
equals, where the participants vow to avenge one another. However, it
could have consequences for the biological kin as well. In a legendary
saga called *Þorsteins saga Víkingssonar* (in *Viking tales of the north*,
1877), one man's sons are in a feud with his sworn brother. This shows
that while there might have been a norm, reality was much more complex.

FRIENDSHIP

Kinship terminology was used as a way to increase the sense of group
belonging even towards non-relatives. Miller (1990, 157ff.) implies that it
is a narrative tool, perhaps even used with sarcasm at times, when individuals in the sagas used the word *frændi* or *frændsemi* without there
being a blood relationship. I suggest, however, that using kinship terminology for non-genetic relatedness was actually a strengthening of bonds:
'It is an ignoble deed, kinsman, that you are about to do: but I would
much rather accept death at your hands, cousin, than give you death by
mine' (*Laxdæla saga* 1969, ch. 49).

Österberg has looked closely at friendship from antiquity to modern
times, and suggests that there are three necessary concepts: friendship
should be reciprocal, voluntary, and based on trust and goodwill.
Vinfengi, or *vinátta*, is usually translated as 'friendship'. Friendship was a
political contract which implied mutual help and protection. It was the
power base of the chieftains, according to Jón Viðar Sigurðsson (1999).
A *ðingmaðr*, an assembly man, was also a *vinr*, a friend. In the *Laxdæla
saga* (1969) and *Egil's saga* (1976), we find 17 cases of declared friendship,

9 of which involve individuals who were not related at all. The rest concern more distant kin than second cousins (two cases of paternal kin), two maternal grandparents and their grandchildren, as well as foster brothers or blood siblings.

Even if friendship was not necessarily combined with affection, it was not simply a formal relationship but could also be emotional. One example of friendship of this kind is found in *Njál's saga*, or the story of Burnt Njal. Gunnar and Njáll are close friends and neighbours. They have no formal relationship, and their friendship should have been strained since their wives argued constantly. The conflict became more and more intense, escalating with the death of both Gunnar and Njáll. However, the friendship between the two men continues up till their deaths.

VIOLENCE AND HONOUR

The sagas are largely concerned with revenge and counter-revenge, which has given society in the Viking Age the reputation of being very violent. According to Andersson (1967, 4f.), it is part of the narrative structure of a family saga that there has to be a conflict. The narrative structure usually includes an introduction of the protagonists, the development of a conflict, the climax, revenge, reconciliation and, finally, the concluding remarks or the aftermath. The conflict can involve a group or just two individuals, and the motive varies (love, honour, land, etc.).

The sagas are concerned with conflicts, which is no surprise since it is fundamental for any society to maintain a balance of power. The narratives of the sagas move from balance to imbalance and back to balance. This is probably why the saga authors considered it important to explore people's relationships, and feuding can be seen as a means of preventing unnecessary violence. Violence is a relational term—it cannot stand on its own. The relationship term paired with violence should be friendship. But violence, as well as friendship, is dependent on its historical and cultural context. Even if we have the law, and the model of a bilateral kinship, the composition of the groups involved in vengeance and lawsuits depends on the situation at hand (Miller 1983, 163); hence the need to emphasize that the sagas depict a society of friendship, as well as one based on kinship.

As we have seen, obligations did sometimes clash. A man might receive support in avenging his father from the same man who participated in an attack on his great-uncle (e.g. *Njáls saga* 2001, ch. 129).

Similarly, Njáll's son kills his foster-son (*Njáls saga*, ch. 111). Another example is in *Laxdæla saga*, in which the two foster-brothers Kjartan and Bolli court the beautiful Guðrún. Guðrún is in love with Kjartan, but she marries Bolli. The climax of the story comes when Bolli, provoked by Guðrún, kills Kjartan. Bolli is later killed by Kjartan's kinsmen, and Bolli's sons are also caught up in the vengeance. Fathers had an obligation to avenge sons, including foster-sons, which puts Kjartan's father in an awkward situation. Kjartan's mother, on the other hand, sees no conflict. She hates her foster-son Bolli: '[She] thought the reward he paid for his fostering a bitter one' (*Laxdæla saga* 1969, ch. 51). The destruction of a relationship between foster-brothers, as well as a father–son relationship gone sour and sons rebelling, can be seen as providing an example of what not to do. It is worth repeating that kinship, or foster-kinship, are beneficial if the relationships are maintained, but may lead to ruin if neglected (see Parkes 2004, 601; Percivall 2005, 58).

There was no shame in violence in Viking Age Scandinavia, as long as it was conducted in the open and between equals. This was a question of honour. Honour being the unwritten rules and principles of behaviour, concerning individual prestige and gaining respect. The violence was not principally designed to destroy others but to strengthen or regain one's own status. Honour has to do with a key concept in network analysis: trust. Trust is always tested in the sagas; trust is broken by bad people, or by bad luck. Honour was seen as a real entity, something that could be owned, diminished, lost or stolen, and as such it was defended by free males (but not by women, slaves or men who were too young or too old). In the sagas, violence is very seldom uncontrolled. When a house is burnt down, women, slaves, children and the elderly are often granted permission to leave. These were the people forbidden by law to carry weapons, and who should therefore not die by the sword. The question of maintaining honour had to do with being an open and honest man. No one should do things in secret, or associate themselves with liars. Compare this with the *Grágás*, which states that any deed of killing should be announced immediately, and the slayer should not ride by three houses without telling someone of the deed. Revenging an insult with aggression was beneficial for an individual, since the sagas are concerned with maintaining honour.

There has been considerable interest in understanding violence in a historical perspective ever since the sociologist Norbert Elias's work on societal change suggested that humans had become more and more civilized though history (Elias 2000 [1939]). Elias saw this as a process of developing more rules concerning behaviour, and increased feelings of shame, for social control. Elias's theories were not appreciated before the 1970s, but have dominated discussion since. According to Elias, the change in medieval times was due to monopoly. In the 10th century, the feudal lords of Europe had a monopoly on physical and economic power. In early modern days, the division of labour increased the speed of the civilizing process. Dependence on a larger number of people and less intense contact between people increased the importance of etiquette. This led to more social control due to increasing centralization of power.

Elias's idea of the civilizing process has not gone without critique. Even when scholars agree that such a process has taken place—leading people to become more and more respectful of human life, aiding the weaker in society, promoting tolerance and individual freedom—not everyone thinks that we have seen more control of base impulses in humans over the past 1,000 years. Nor does this process follow some kind of law. The attitudes towards violence have been the stepping-stone for further discussions. Many scholars do not see medieval society as a society of uncontrolled violence; nor have humans become more able to control their impulses over the course of time. Quite the opposite. In medieval and early modern societies, the agenda was not to punish a criminal for doing the wrong thing, but to integrate the offender back into society in accordance with the social code. Fines often took into account what the offender could afford to pay, or, in the case of the Icelandic community, the punishment was to place oneself as an un-free man (temporary slave) for as long as it would take to work off the debt. Human self-control does not necessarily improve, but the attitude towards social codes is always changing (Österberg 1995, 140f.).

Feuds and violence were neither war nor anarchy, but the legitimization and mobilization of power as a result of the lack of a central authority (Miller 1990, 146). The psychological mechanism that shapes behaviour and the network of relatives' and non-relatives' interactions—how people interact when it comes to violence, and in what way kinship is related to it—has not changed significantly during evolution, but the way that instincts are interpreted and acted upon makes an historical analysis possible.

CONCLUSION

Old Norse texts, rune-stones and the medieval Icelandic sagas, in combination with burial finds and other sources, illustrate the social order in different parts of Scandinavia. The sagas in particular are concerned with conflicts, and can be used to gain knowledge of social networking in newly settled societies. The theme in this article has been alliance building, the use of alliances to expand networks of power and support, and how kinship relations interact with other social ties. The creation of networks of loyalty and support is viewed here as a means to regulate the use of violence in establishing a stable society in a time of change. Providing a few examples from the sagas has demonstrated how network models can explain social dynamics.

During this period, new areas were being settled by people from different places, and ideas of Christianity and the concept of kingship coincided with the gradual unification of Scandinavian countries. By studying how kinship relations interact with other social ties, a more complex image can be formed of divided loyalties and entangled alliances. One basic theme in the sagas has to do with maintaining a balance of power, and the texts can be used to illustrate how Scandinavians themselves depicted the problems with alliance building.

REFERENCES

Andersson, T.M. (1967). *The Icelandic family saga: an analytical reading.* Cambridge, MA: Harvard University Press.

Auður Magnúsdóttir (2001). *Frillor och fruar. Politik och samlevnad på Island 1120–1400*. Göteborg: Historiska institutionen.

Egil's saga, trans. with an introduction by H. Pálsson & P. Edwards (1976). Harmondsworth: Penguin.

Elias, N. (2000 [1939]). *The civilizing process*, rev. edn, trans. E. Jephcott with some notes and corrections by the author, edited by E. Dunning, J. Goudsblom & S. Mennell. Oxford: Blackwell.

Gaskins, R. (2005). Network dynamics in saga and society. *Scandinavian Studies* 2: 201–216.

Gaunt, D. (1983). *Familjeliv i Norden*. Stockholm: Gidlund.

Grágás (1980–2000). *Laws of early Iceland: the Codex Regius of Grágás with material from other manuscripts 1–2*, ed. A. Dennis. Winnipeg: University of Manitoba.

Guðrún Nordal. (1998). *Ethics and action in thirteenth-century Iceland*. Odense: Odense University Press.

Gunnar Karlsson (2000). *Iceland's 1100 years: the history of a marginal society*. London: C. Hurst.

Hávamál, trans. B. Thorpe (1866). *Edda Sæmundar Hinns Froða: the Edda of Sæmund the Learned*. London: Trübner & Co.

Hønsa-þoris saga (1953). Halle: Altnordische Textbibliothek.

Íslendingabók. Kristni saga/The book of the Icelanders. The story of the conversion, trans. S. Grønlie (2006). London: Viking Society for Northern Research.

Johnson, S.B. & Johnson, R.C. (1991). Support and conflict of kinsmen in Norse earldoms, Icelandic families and the English royalty. *Ethnology and Sociobiology* 12: 211–220.

Jón Viðar Sigurðsson (1999). *Chieftains and power in the Icelandic Commonwealth*. Odense: Odense University Press.

Karlsson, see Gunnar Karlsson.

Landnámabók—The book of settlements, trans. with an introduction and notes by H. Pálsson and P. Edwards (1972). Winnipeg: University of Manitoba Icelandic Studies.

Laxdæla saga, trans. M. Magnusson & H. P. M. Magnusson (1969). Harmondsworth: Penguin Books.

Magnúsdóttir, see Auður Magnúsdóttir.

Mauss, M. (1954 [1922]). *The gift: forms and functions of exchange in archaic societies*, trans. I. Cunnison. London: Routledge.

Meulengracht Sørensen, P. (1983). *The unmanly man: concepts of sexual defamation in early northern society*. Odense: Odense University Press.

Miller, W. I. (1983). Choosing the avenger: some aspects of the bloodfeud in medieval Iceland and England. *Law and History Review* 1/2: 159–204.

Miller, W. I. (1990). *Bloodtaking and peacemaking: feud, law and society in saga Iceland*. Chicago: University of Chicago Press.

Njal's saga, trans. with an introduction and notes by R. Cook (2001). London: Penguin.

Nordal, see Guðrún Nordal.

Österberg, E. (1991). Tystnadens strategi. Miljö och mentalitet i de isländska sagorna. *Historisk tidskrift* 2: 165–185.

Österberg, E. (1995). *Folk förr. Historiska essäer*. Stockholm: Atlantis.

Österberg, E. (2003). Vänskap—hot eller skydd i medeltidens samhälle? En existentiell och etisk historia. *Historisk tidskrift* 4: 549–573.

Österberg, E. (2007). *Vänskap. En lång historia,* Stockholm: Atlantis.

Parkes, P. (2004). Fosterage, kinship, and legend: when milk was thicker than blood? *Comparative Studies in Society and History* 46: 587–615.

Percivall, N. (2005). *Ideals, masculinity and inheritance: a study of father/son relationships presented in the narrative sources of Iceland and Normandy in the eleventh to thirteenth centuries*. Unpublished PhD thesis, Liverpool University.

Saga of Gunnlaug Serpent-Tongue, trans. R. Quirk (1957). London: Nelson.

The sagas of Kormák and The sworn brothers, trans. with introduction and notes by L. M. Hollander (1949) New York: Princeton University Press for the American-Scandinavian Foundation.

Sawyer, B. (2000). *The Viking Age rune-stones: custom and commemoration in early medieval Scandinavia*. Oxford: Oxford University Press.

Sawyer, B. & Sawyer, P. (1993). *Medieval Scandinavia from conversion to Reformation, circa 800–1500*. Minneapolis: University of Minnesota Press.

Anna Wallette

Sigurðsson, see Jón Viðar Sigurðsson.

The story of Gisli the Outlaw, trans. G. W. Dasent (1866). Edinburgh: Edmonston & Douglas.

Svanberg, F. (2006). Death rituals, identity and religion. In: A. Andrén & P. Carelli (eds) *Odin's eye, between people and powers in the pre-Christian north*, pp. 144–153, 299–301. Helsingborg: Dunkers Kulturhus.

Torfi H. Tulinius (2003). The matter of the North: fiction and uncertain identities in thirteenth-century Iceland. In: M. Clunies Ross (ed.) *Old Norse myths, literature and society*, pp. 242–266. Odense: University Press of Southern Denmark.

Tulinius, see Torfi H. Tulinius.

Turner, V. (1971). An anthropological approach to the Icelandic saga. In: T. O. Beidelman (ed.) *The translation of culture: essays to E. E. Evans-Pritchard*. London: Tavistock Publications.

Viking tales of the North: the sagas of Thorstein, Viking's son, and Fridthjof the Bold, trans. R. B. Anderson and J. Bjarnason (1877) Chicago: S. C. Griggs & Co.

PART III

EVOLVING BONDS OF SOCIALITY

8

Deacon's Dilemma:
The Problem of Pair-bonding
in Human Evolution

ROBIN DUNBAR

AT THE END OF HIS BOOK *The symbolic species*, Deacon (1997) drew attention to the fact that humans are unusual in having a form of pair-bonded
monogamy set within a large multimale/multifemale social system. The
difficulty this creates is that whenever the mated individuals are apart,
they are at risk of rivals who might either steal the mate or effect extra-
pair copulations (Baker & Bellis 1995; Davies 1992). This is a particular
problem for males because they are always vulnerable to paternity uncertainty: among mammals, a female always knows that the offspring she
gives birth to are hers, but a male can never be 100 per cent certain.
Deacon argued that humans face this problem in a particularly intrusive
way because of two key features of human sociality. One is the large size
of their communities, which means that they are always surrounded by
many rivals; the other is the sexual division of labour, which means that
individuals are often obliged to leave their mates for long periods of time
(e.g. while away hunting).

The solution, Deacon suggested, was overt social statements of ownership such as marriage ceremonies and symbolic badges (e.g. wedding
rings, titles, changes of name, styles of dress or coiffure) that signal marital status. He argued that, being symbolic, these all required language,
and he thus saw symbolic contracts of this kind as being the key selection
pressure behind the evolution of language—hence the title of his book.
If monogamy evolved early (and he followed Lovejoy [1981] in assuming
that it did), then language necessarily evolved early too—and by early, he

Proceedings of the British Academy **158**, 155–175. © The British Academy 2010.

meant with the appearance of *Homo erectus* around 1.5–2.0 Ma. Irrespective of when either pair-bonds or language evolved, the steady increase that apparently occurred in community size during the course of hominin evolution (Aiello & Dunbar 1993; Dunbar in press), and its large terminal size in modern hunter-gatherer communities (Dunbar 1993), combined with their characteristically dispersed, fission-fusion nature (Aureli et al. 2008; Dunbar 2003; Grove ch. 19 this volume), must significantly exacerbate the problem of maintaining pair-bonds.

Deacon is surely right to identify the formation of pair-bonds in humans as a major anomaly that requires explanation. And I emphasize the word 'pair-bonds' here rather than 'monogamy', because it is pair-bonds that are the substantive issue: pair-bonds seem to be universal among humans irrespective of whether their marital arrangements are monogamous, polygamous, polyandrous or promiscuous (Fisher 2004; Jankowiak & Fischer 1992). The issue I want to highlight is the fact that human's pair-bonds are underpinned by a very peculiar mechanism that we refer to as 'falling (or being) in love'. At least in the more relaxed atmosphere of modern Western society, this state is usually associated with a number of characteristic traits: attention focused almost to exclusion on the object of one's desire, heightened affect (often associated with glazed eyes, a faraway look and a 'smiley' face) and roused (but not turbulent) emotions (Fisher 2004; Fisher et al. 2006), a suite of behaviours sometimes referred to as 'besotted'. The kind of besottedness that we associate with romantic love can be both intense and, compared to mate attraction in most other animals, relatively long lasting (this early intense phase of a human relationship typically lasts 12–18 months, but often extends for several years beyond that in attenuated form: Marazzitti et al. 1999). It is associated with a distinctive set of behaviours (focused attention, obsessive following, goal-oriented behaviours and motivation to win a particular preferred partner) that are widely common to mammalian mating behaviour (Fisher 1998; Fisher et al. 2006). Notwithstanding occasional claims to the contrary, some form of romantic attachment of this kind seems to be a very widespread phenomenon that transcends historical and cultural boundaries (Fisher 2004; Jankowiak & Fischer 1992), and may well be a human universal (accepting that there are degrees of expression in this trait even within the same culture).

This phenomenon is clearly designed (in the evolutionary sense) to create, and then maintain, a pair-bond. Functionally, at least, it may not be too different from the equivalent mechanisms that seem to occur in at least some other anthropoid primates (triadic differentiation in hamadryas baboons: Kummer et al. 1974; pair-bond defence in titis: Cubicciotti & Mason 1978), although in humans we obviously know a great deal more about how it 'feels'. In so far as its purpose is to protect the pair-bond (at least for a limited period of time), it suggests that social contracts, symbolic markers and language may not in themselves be essential for protecting pair-bonds in social environments where they are inevitably under threat. What it might suggest, instead, is that pair-bonds (and the processes that underpin them) evolved well before language, and that language was later co-opted to the business of reinforcing whatever natural mechanisms already existed to protect pair-bonds.

FUNCTIONAL EXPLANATIONS FOR PAIR-BONDING

In general, pair-bonds are likely to evolve for just three reasons: (1) to allow males to protect mating access to a female so as to ensure paternity certainty; (2) to reduce the risk of offspring mortality through predation or infanticide; and (3) to facilitate biparental care where this is essential for successful rearing. The first is likely to be asymmetric and biased toward the male (males should be more attentive/besotted than females because they have more at stake), the second more evenly balanced (both parties have an interest in achieving a mutual reproductive objective), while the third is more likely to be asymmetric toward the female (females will be more concerned to ensure that they benefit from their male's protection).

Because maternity certainty is always less of an issue for mammals than paternity certainty is, there is no reason why females would wish to monopolize males for this reason alone. In effect, sperm competition obliges males to find ways to minimize the risk that the females they have mated are inseminated by other males. Males will thus be more interested in protecting their access to mates, especially if they make a significant investment in parental care. If paternal investment in offspring is minimal, males might care less about paternity certainty and may instead prefer to opt for promiscuity and a siring lottery. Mate defence has been explicitly identified as a selection factor in the evolution of pair-bonding in small monogamous antelope (Brotherton & Komers 2003) and some communal-living birds (notably the little bee-eater: Hegner et al. 1982).

Male antelope maximize their fecundity by ensuring that they are around when the female comes into oestrus (under circumstances where oestrus is concealed and males have few distance cues they can rely on to identify when females are fertile): pair-bonded monogamy is in effect a best-of-a-bad-job strategy when females are solitary and widely dispersed, such that males cannot easily ensure they can monopolize matings with more than one female. In primates, however, males never seem to be forced into such a situation, since, in all cases where this has been investigated, male day-journey length is more than long enough to allow him to defend a territory of sufficient size to encompass the ranges of several (typically 4–5) females and their dependent young (gibbons: van Schaik & Dunbar 1990; marmosets and tamarins: Dunbar 1995a). Yet they mate monogamously and stay close to their female partner. Even though a male's active breeding lifetime may be much shorter in promiscuous mating systems due to competition from rivals (and this may offset the advantages of mating with several females each year), there is still a very considerable opportunity cost for a male, suggesting that the benefit to be gained from monogamy in terms of numbers of offspring successfully reared must be very considerable.

In callitrichid primates, males may benefit from pair-bonded monogamy because its evolution appears to have allowed females to increase their reproductive rate by a factor of about four above that likely if males opted for roving polygamy: this is because when males help with rearing (and they do so heavily in callitrichids), females are able to produce twins twice a year, whereas without male help they would probably only be able to manage singleton litters once a year (Dunbar 1995a). This may well be a unique outcome of the way a number of key life history traits converge in very small primates (Leutenegger 1973). Even so, a game theoretic analysis suggests that males had to be pair-bonded first before females would have been willing (in an evolutionary sense) to take the risk of increasing their reproductive rate (Dunbar 1995a). Indeed, Dunbar (1995b) showed that when female reproductive rates decline in poor-quality habitats (thereby making monogamy less advantageous for males), male callitrichids switch to a form of roving male polygyny.

However, this cannot explain all cases of monogamy in primates: male gibbons do not benefit in this way, yet are still monogamous, suggesting that the conditions favouring pair-bonded monogamy in larger-bodied primates may have more to do with offspring survival. The most likely causes of reduced survival, at least in the case of large-bodied primates like gibbons with slow reproductive rates, is infanticide by other males (van Schaik & Dunbar 1990). In this case, mortality from more conventional predators could be ruled out, although this might still be a significant issue in the case of some small-bodied open country antelope

(Dunbar & Dunbar 1980). Infanticide risk has also been argued to be the main reason why female great apes are social, and specifically why they associate with males (the 'hired gun' hypothesis: Harcourt & Greenberg 2001).

Dunbar (2000) modelled ape mating systems as an optimal foraging problem, and showed that, across extant great ape populations, males adjust their willingness to associate with groups of females as a direct function of female grouping patterns and male search rates. Figure 8.1

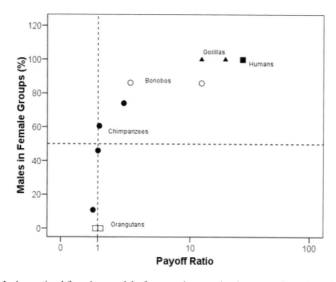

Figure 8.1. An optimal foraging model of ape male reproductive strategies: when should males prefer roving polygamy to being social? The ape male mating strategies model of Dunbar (2000) is here extended to include humans, based on parameter values for !Kung San (from Lee 1979). The model estimates the number of sirings that a male would achieve if he opted for roving polygamy versus staying permanently with one group of females during the average female reproductive cycle (defined by the interbirth interval) (plotted as the X-axis). The payoff for roving male polygamy is a function of the size of female groups, the length of the female reproductive cycle, the number of days for which an average female is fertile within that cycle (assumed to be a five-day conception window in each of three menstrual cycles to conception), the distance that a male typically travels each day and the radius either side of that path of travel that a male can locate groups of females (assumed to be 0.05 km). The payoff for a social male is simply the number of females in the group (each would become fertile once during the focal time interval and the focal male is assumed to sire offspring with all of them). The X-axis plots the ratio of payoffs (social/roving) and the Y-axis plots the proportion of males that are social (attached to a female group) for individual hominoid populations. As optimal foraging theory predicts, males are ambivalent about whether to stay with a female group (percent of males in groups = 50%) when the payoffs of the two strategies are equally balanced (payoff ratio ≈ 1). Note that increasing detection distance to 1.0 km either side of the path of travel for humans would not change the male's decision. Study sites are (left to right within taxa): orangs—Tanjung, Kutai; chimpanzees—Mahale, Kibale, Bossou, Tai, Lomako, Wamba; gorilla—Lope, Virunga.

shows these same data with an added data point for humans based on !Kung San demographic and ecological characteristics. With female grouping patterns like those found among the Dobe !Kung, human males would do their best to attach themselves permanently to female groups rather than opt for roving male polygamy. By doing so, they would on average gain more successful sirings than males who attempted to range widely in search of further females with whom to mate. More importantly, Figure 8.1 suggests that, for humans, female group sizes and/or male search rates (a function of day-journey length and population density) would have to be around an order of magnitude lower for it to be worth a male's while opting for roving polygamy.

Note that these results suggest that males pay little if any attention to the potential impact of rivals (something that has also been shown in feral goats: Dunbar et al. 1990). This may simply be because in polygamous mating systems a male's tenure as a breeding male is short and there is little point in worrying too much about what rivals might be doing: it is best just to do the best you can. Note also that these results only imply that males should be social and remain with groups of females: they do not commit males to pair-bonded monogamy, except in the special case where females live alone. In large social groups, a male might nonetheless benefit by being monogamous if rivals have a significant negative impact on his fecundity, either through infanticide or because paternity certainty is greatly reduced if his female mates with rival males. Infanticide is a particular problem for primates because of their long reproductive cycles and relatively low lifetime reproductive output (Henzi & Barrett 2006; van Schaik & Dunbar 1990). In humans, the risk of sirings by other males is significant, if modest (Baker & Bellis 1995).

In these kinds of situations, we would expect males to be the more proactive sex in soliciting and maintaining the pair-bond. This is certainly true in both klipspringer (where it is typically the male that tends to follow and maintain close contact with the female rather than vice versa: Dunbar & Dunbar 1980; Roberts & Dunbar 2000), in at least some monogamous prosimians (Fuentes 2002) and in gibbons (Palombit 1999).

However, if there is significant risk of infanticide or sexual harassment of the female by males, females may have most to gain by strategies that reduce this (e.g. acquiring a male protector), and the pattern of attachment should therefore be female-biased unless there is significant male parental care. Hegner et al. (1982; Emlen 1984) argued that little bee-eaters are pair-bonded, despite living in large communal roosts, precisely because communal roosting exposes females to the risk of forced copulations by non-pair males: unpaired males often cluster around burrow entrances and harass females that emerge alone. To ensure paternity certainty, paired males remain close to their mates, especially when the females leave and return to the colony on foraging trips. In effect, bee-eaters suffer from Deacon's Dilemma, and might thus provide a possible analogy for why humans should pair-bond—and, perhaps, how it can be done without the benefit of language. Indeed, Harcourt and Greenberg (2001) have explicitly argued that the risk of infanticide explains why gorillas (but not chimpanzees) attach themselves to individual males who then act as protectors or 'hired guns' (Smuts & Smuts 1993).

Among animals in general, sexual harassment seems to be most common among those species that have promiscuous mating systems (Clutton-Brock & Parker 1995). Both chimpanzee and orang-utan males commonly harass females in oestrus and attempt to coerce them into sex (Muller et al. 2007; Newton-Fisher 2006; Stumpf et al. 2008) and, at least among chimpanzees, males gain more copulations with those females they harass most (Muller et al. 2007). These attacks usually result in disrupted foraging, and occasionally even in injury (Newton-Fisher 2006), and females who are subject to repeated attack have greatly elevated cortisol levels, and thus incur significant physiological stress (Muller et al. 2007). Since stress is usually associated with reduced fertility (Abbott et al. 1986), females may incur a significant disadvantage from being the focus of males' (or, indeed, females') attention. One solution is to form a bond with a particular male so as to minimize the overall amount of attention received. Cercopithecine primate females use grooming-based coalitions with both other females (Dunbar in press; Wittig et al. 2008) and, occasionally, individual males (gelada: Dunbar 1984, 1989; baboons: Smuts 1986) to buffer themselves against the stresses of group-living. Such coalitions reduce the frequency of harassment and, as a result, significantly improve fertility (Dunbar 1989, in press).

The importance of hired guns in protecting females' sexual and reproductive interests is given added support by evidence from modern humans. Among the Ache of eastern Paraguay, for example, a man who takes over a woman after the death or disappearance of her previous 'spouse' will frequently kill her dependent offspring on the explicit grounds that he is not willing to pay the costs of rearing another man's child (Hill & Kaplan 1988).

Finally, pair-bonds may arise where biparental care is crucial for the successful rearing of offspring. The most familiar example is, of course, birds, where biparental care is particularly associated with species that have especially large brains, and for whom rearing costs are significantly elevated. Biparental care is rare outside selected bird orders (notably raptors, geese, some sea birds, corvids, parrots and songbirds) and, in mammals, among the canids, though it does occur in some primate genera besides humans (e.g. callitrichids). However, the key caveat in all these cases is whether pair-bonding occurred in order to facilitate biparental care, or biparental care was made possible once pair-bonding had occurred for some other reason (mate defence or infanticide avoidance). It is not always obvious which of these is correct.

One unresolved issue here that might guide us to the right explanation is the precise form of the human pair-bond. There has been an implicit assumption that it is mutual rather than one-sided because both parties cooperate in child-care, and both parties experience the process of 'falling in love'. However, it is not entirely obvious that this is so. Although there are surprisingly few studies of this aspect of relationships in humans, what evidence there is tends to suggest that, even though males may exhibit more jealousy when relationships are threatened (Baumeister & Bratslavsky 1999), it is females that may be more strongly committed to pair-bond relationships and more proactive in pursuing them.

Although it has often been assumed that the most likely benefit of human pair-bonds is some form of biparental care (Quinlan 2008), the evidence is in fact somewhat equivocal. Although Quinlan (2008) showed, in a cross-cultural analysis, that human pair-bonds are most stable in those societies where parental care is equal between the sexes, Hawkes (1991) has argued that, in traditional hunter-gatherers, big game hunting (the exclusive prerogative of males and the main focus of their foraging effort) is a form of male mate advertising rather than a form of paternal investment. Indeed, among hunter-gatherers in general, the proportion of the diet derived from hunting is negatively related to habitat productivity, with a correspondingly greater proportional contribution from women (Belovsky 1987). Even when males hunt, their contribution to the rearing process may often be quite limited because, unlike the products of female foraging, most of a male's output from hunting is shared with all members of the band rather than being invested in his mate(s) and her offspring (Kaplan & Hill 1985).

Further support for this conclusion comes from a consideration of the energetic costs of large brains. Foley and Lee (1991) calculated the additional energetic costs (relative to chimpanzees) of rearing hominid offspring with progressively larger brains. As we might anticipate, the total costs are very considerable (approximately three times those incurred by a chimpanzee), and Foley and Lee (1991) argued that these costs could not have been offset either by male provisioning or by a shift to a higher quality diet (e.g. meat). Rather, they argue that the only way these costs could have been accommodated is by spreading them out over a proportionately longer period of time—in other words, by slowing down the rate of growth and extending the period of parental care (just as we find in humans).

If the evidence for the need for biparental care is weak, then the benefits that *females* gain from being pair-bonded may have had much more to do with reducing harassment levels and/or the risk of infanticide. Some support for this suggestion is provided by ethnographic studies of tourism, which report that lone young Western women tourists commonly find it convenient to attach themselves to individual males in a relationship that, in strictly functional terms, trades sex for protection from excessive harassment by other males (Zinovieff 1991; see also Bowman 1989). If a stable relationship is a *sine qua non* for effective reproduction in humans for essentially personal security reasons, this would imply that human pair-bonding processes are female-biased. Folk psychology has, in fact, always tended to suggest that not only may women effectively control which relationships are allowed to blossom, but also that they tend to work harder at building and servicing romantic relationships than men do. The fact that women are more demanding than men in the criteria they expect prospective partners to satisfy (Grammer 1989; Pawłowski & Dunbar 2001; Waynforth & Dunbar 1995) and typically require more intimacy and other cues of affection in order to reach the same level of passion as men (Baumeister & Bratslavsky 1999) offers some support at least to the first of these claims.

That said, however, the evidence as to whether human romantic relationships are symmetrical or asymmetrical is surprisingly sparse, and certainly not good enough to allow us to draw any firm conclusions either way. Unfortunately, it seems that these behavioural aspects of relationships have simply not been a focus of interest among those who have studied this phenomenon. Once again, we need better behavioural data on the symmetry and functions of human romantic relationships.

ORIGINS OF PAIR-BONDED RELATIONSHIPS

Despite the limitations outlined in the previous two sections, we can still consider the implications of the issues these have raised for the timing of the evolution of pair-bonds in human evolutionary history. The alternative functional hypotheses inevitably suggest different evolutionary pathways, and at least allow us to spell out exactly what kinds of data we need to test between them.

Pair-bondedness has conventionally been equated with biparental care, and the need for biparental care has in turn been equated with the sudden increase in brain size (and the associated changes in life history traits required to accommodate this: Robson & Wood 2008). It has thus inevitably been assumed that pair-bonds/monogamy must have arisen at the time when these anatomical changes are first recorded in the archaeological record around the time of the appearance of archaic humans (*Homo heidelbergensis* and contemporaries) some 500,000 years ago. The classic view, then, is that the massive increase in brain size that begins around this time (Figure 8.2) placed such pressure on rearing costs for females that biparental care (and hence pair-bonded monogamy) became essential—although some authors have assumed a much earlier origin for monogamy, associated with the first significant increase in brain size that occurred with the appearance of the *Homo ergaster/erectus* lineage (Lovejoy 1981).

Large brains/neocortices are widely characteristic of monogamous species throughout the mammals and birds (Shultz & Dunbar 2007), irrespective of whether or not biparental care is involved. This relationship seems to have been overridden in primates by its generalization to include non-reproductive relationships (i.e. friendships). However, we have yet to test whether, beneath this generalized quantitative relationship between group size and brain size, a pair-bonded effect can still be detected in primates. Figure 8.3 tests this for primates, by plotting residual absolute neocortex volume (partialling out mean social group size) for individual primate species as a function of mating system. The main taxonomic groups (prosimians, tarsiers, monkeys and apes) are shown separately. Pair-bonded (i.e. monogamous) species have significantly larger neocortices for group size than promiscuously or polygamously mating species, irrespective of taxonomic group (ANOVA: $F_{1,30} = 4.58$, p = 0.041, with taxon as a covariate; humans, callitrichids and tarsiers excluded from this analysis). We get the same result using neocortex ratio (neocortex volume divided by the rest of the brain), and if we use taxon-specific regressions equations to obtain residuals.

Two points should be noted. First, callitrichids—the one group of primates characterized by a significant level of male parental care, but rather loose 'pair-bonds'—do not have an especially large neocortex

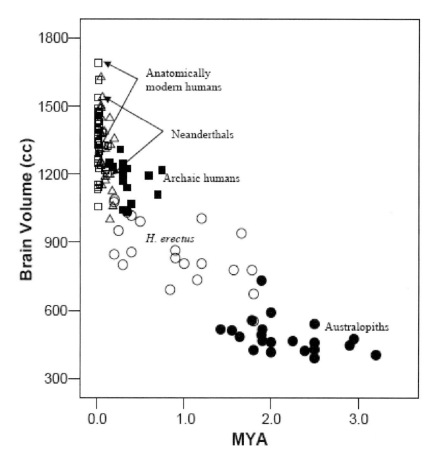

Figure 8.2. Brain volume for individual populations of fossil hominids (defined as individual skulls present at particular sites within a 50,000-year time period), plotted against time. Data are based on brain volumes averaged for individual specimens from De Miguel and Henneberg (2001).

when group size is partialled out. This would seem to suggest that it is pair-bonding that is cognitively demanding and requires a large brain, not the need for biparental care in the development of large-brained off-spring. If this is so, then the causal arrow must run in the reverse direction: the evolution of pair-bonding is dependent on having a large brain to manage the relationships involved, rather than pair-bonding having evolved to facilitate the rearing of large-brained offspring. The second point is that humans do not differ significantly from the other polygamous primates in this respect. If anything, they seem to resemble cal-litrichids, who are characterized by a mating system that is fluid and perhaps best described as a loose form of facultative monogamy (i.e. monogamy when it is convenient).

In fact, the analogy with callitrichids involves a number of unexpected parallels. Dunbar (1995a) found that callitrichids differed from other small platyrrhine primates in having a high fecundity rate (typically twins twice a year), concealed ovulation (absence of visible signs of oestrus), an oestrous phase that covers most of the menstrual cycle and local female reproductive synchrony. These are all features that are shared by modern humans (Table 8.1). The fact that humans seem to share with the callitrichids an unusually flexible mating/social system may add another point of convergence. The fact that both taxa—uniquely among the primates—exhibit accelerated reproductive rates compared to the other members of their respective families (twinning twice a year in callitrichids, greatly shortened interbirth intervals in the case of humans) can be interpreted as females' attempts to manipulate male behaviour so as to persuade males to remain with them and continue parental investment.

If human pair-bonding evolved to solve a problem of infanticide risk or male sexual harassment, the timing of the transition from the ancestral state of ape-like polygamy to pair-bonded monogamy probably hinges around the size of female foraging groups in the successive stages of hominid evolution and the consequences female group size has for attracting males searching for matings. Aside from a tripling in community size (Aiello & Dunbar 1993; Dunbar in press; Grove ch. 19 this volume), the one key difference between human and chimpanzee communities is the fact that human communities are structurally more cohesive: at least part of the community (the band) reconvenes each night, whereas chimpanzee foraging parties do not coalesce at night (Aureli et al. 2008). We do not know when this transition occurred, but it must surely have ramped up the problems females faced when it did, and this could well have precipitated a hired-gun strategy by the females (Harcourt & Greenberg 2001).

If brain size selecting for biparental care is not the functional explanation for the evolution of pair-bondedness, it may instead be that the increase in brain size after about 500 kyrs ago is actually the *consequence* rather than the cause of pair-bonded monogamy, analogous to the increase in female fecundity brought on by male parental care in callitrichids. If so, then this is likely to have been a consequence of the fact that the cohabiting group (the foraging or overnight camp group, as opposed to the wider dispersed community) had increased significantly above that found in chimpanzees (and probably the australopiths) and greatly increased the stresses involved. Why group size increased so dra-

Table 8.1. Analogies in the reproductive biology of humans and callitrichid primates

Trait	Callitrichids *	Humans *
High reproductive output	Females twin twice a year (other platyrrhines: singletons once a year)	Short interbirth intervals for an ape (ca 4 years vs ca 5 years in great apes)
Concealed ovulation	No external signals of oestrus	No external signals of oestrus
Duration of 'oestrous' phase§ (% of menstrual cycle)	Median 100% (range 23–100%, N = 5 species) (other platyrrhines: median 14%, N = 4 species)	100% (other apes: median 22%, N = 4 species)
Female reproductive synchrony	Local synchrony in 66.7% of species (vs 6.7% in other platyrrhines)	Both menstrual and conception synchrony occur
Mating system	Unusually variable (facultative monogamy)	Extremely variable (facultative monogamy)

*Sources: callitrichids and other platyrrhines, Dunbar (1995a); humans, Dixson (1998); apes: Hrdy and Whitten (1997), Campbell et al. (2007).
§ Technically, anthropoid primates all have menstrual rather than oestrous cycles (Dixson 1998). I use the term 'oestrus' here to refer to that proportion of the menstrual cycle during which mating is (mostly) confined.

matically towards the end of the *H. erectus* phase remains to be determined. However, given that pair-bonding evolved to counteract these stresses, the sudden increase in brain size facilitated by that may have unlocked a further increase in group size that made new ecological opportunities possible (see also Grove ch. 19 this volume; Lehmann et al. ch. 4 this volume).

It may be relevant here that, although Wrangham (1979, 1980) argued cogently that apes in general are not female-bonded, a plausible case can be made for suggesting that all the great apes are female-to-male bonded in some form (Figure 8.4). The one exception is the lesser apes, the gibbons (*Hylobates*): these are universally and uncontroversially monogamous (allowing for a small amount of polygamy), and data on grooming patterns and approach/retreat frequencies between the pair consistently suggest that the pair-bond is mainly maintained by the male (Fuentes 2002; Palombit 1999). In this respect, they seem to be typical of a wider mammalian pattern where pair-bonds are primarily maintained by the male (lemurs: Fuentes 2002; klipspringer antelope: Dunbar & Dunbar 1980). This seems to set the gibbons apart from the other apes, where female-to-male bonds arguably seem to be the rule (Figure 8.4).

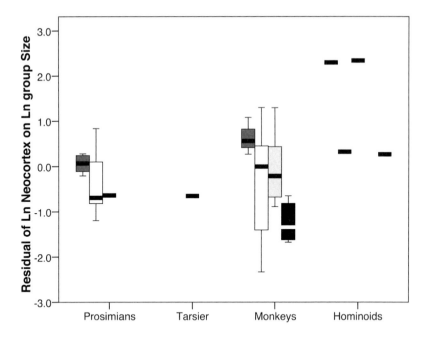

Figure 8.3. Median (±50% and 95% range) residual log$_e$ neocortex volume (residualized from the RMA regression equation of ln[neocortex] on ln[group size]) for primate species as a function of mating system. Species are differentiated by major taxonomic groupings, with callitrichids (black bar) separated within the monkeys. Mating systems are distinguished as follows (L to R): dark grey bars, pair-bonded monogamy; open bars, promiscuous; light grey bars, harem-based polygyny. The tarsier species represented is monogamous. Among the hominoids, the species are (L to R): gibbon (monogamous), chimpanzee (group-living promiscuity), gorilla (harem-based polygyny), humans (pair-bonds within groups). Brain size data are from Stephan et al. (1981), and group size data from Dunbar (1998). Prosimian group sizes are updated using data from Kappeler and Heymann (1996) and Bearder (1987), with nest-group sizes being used for 'semi-solitary' species. The lorisids have been excluded on the grounds that their social systems are not well understood.

Orang-utans (*Pongo*) now live in a dispersed social system that has often been interpreted as effectively semi-solitary, even though distinctive communities clearly exist (e.g. MacKinnon 1974). More importantly in the present context, it has often been noted that orang females tend to stay within the (non-overlapping) ranges of particular large, dominant ('flanged') males who effectively protect them from harassment and attempted forced copulations by other (usually younger) males (Knott & Kahlenberg 2007; MacKinnon 1974; Stumpf et al. 2008). In effect, females maintain a form of spatially based pair-bonding that may not

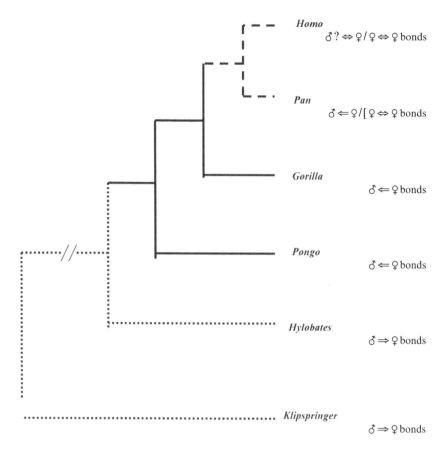

Figure 8.4. Hominoid phylogeny with putative bonding patterns. Klipspringer antelope (*Oreotragus oreotragus*) are given as an outgroup which has pair-bonds.

have quite the intensity of conventional pair-bonds, but certainly has the functional effect of protecting the females from harassment. It is worth noting that adult male orang-utans seem to be able to live quite content-edly in all-male social groups, and become deeply antagonistic towards each other only when females are present (Gilloux 1997). Harcourt and Greenberg (2001) have argued that gorillas are female-to-male bonded as a consequence of females' need to reduce the risk of harassment from males. In effect, they seem to provide a more social version of the orang-utan system, differing only by the fact that the community members move as a coordinated group. The orang social system looks suspiciously like what we might expect the gorilla social system to become if females were unable to forage in groups. Finally, chimpanzees (*Pan*) have usually been described as being male-bonded (Wrangham 1980), with females living within the ranges of male brotherhoods (seemingly, a communal version of the orang-utan social system?). In effect, these males protect the females from harassment by males from neighbouring communities. However, there is now clear evidence that females do form coalitions and maintain longer-term bonds (Boesch & Boesch-Aschermann 2000; Newton-Fisher 2006), often between closely related females (de Waal 1982).

This pattern leads me to suggest, at least by way of a tentative hypothesis, that the evolution of pair-bonds within the hominoids may have been a three-step process. The evidence suggests male-to-female pair-bonds (reflecting conventional mate defence, widely typical of mammals) in the lesser apes and, on the grounds of its occurrence in an outgroup like the klipspringer, the ape common ancestor. These underwent a reversal into female-to-male pair-bonds (hired gun mode) with the emergence of the great apes, because of the greater risks of infanticide in the larger communities characteristic of these species. A similar female-to-male bond can be found in gelada (Dunbar 1984) and hamadryas baboons (Kummer 1968), both of which are characterized by very large social groups. Although this may be a consequence of male punishment in the case of the hamadryas, in the gelada they are a consequence of decisions made by some females to have male rather than female coalition partners to reduce the risks of harassment by other females (Dunbar 1989). Among pair-bonded South American cebid monkeys (e.g. titis, *Callicebus* spp.), pair-bond maintenance may also be largely female driven (Anzenberger 1988).

The second step-change may have happened in the common ancestor of humans and chimpanzees, and seems to have involved a generalization of female-to-male pair-bonds into female-to-female pair-bonds, in the latter case perhaps in response to the need for significantly greater protection against males within much larger communities that contained several reproductively active males. The final step-change seems to have involved an intensification of the female-to-male pair-bond and the incorporation of a male-to-female component to yield the kind of intense semi-mutual pair-bond we find in modern humans. The latter step may have occurred very late (with the appearance of archaic humans after 500,000 years ago), and might in turn have been responsible for releasing some of the constraints on further evolution in brain size (and hence group size), thereby opening the way for the kinds of dramatic changes in human social organization that are associated with the Neolithic and later periods (see Coward ch. 21 this volume; Knappett ch. 11 this volume).

CONCLUSIONS

I make three claims in this chapter. First, following Deacon (1997), the existence of pair-bonds within a large multimale/multifemale community in humans is an evolutionary conundrum and needs explanation. Second, I suggest that only one of the suggested explanations for the evolution of monogamy seems to apply to humans, and this is defence against infanticide and/or sexual harassment by other males. The conventional explanation for pair-bonding in humans (biparental care or provisioning through sexual division of labour) is more likely to be a consequence rather than a cause of pair-bonding. Third, putting these two components together, and mapping the patterns of pair-bond behaviour onto the ape phylogenetic tree suggests that male-biased pair-bonding may be ancestral, with female-biased bonding emerging with the great apes, perhaps as a consequence of increased community size.

REFERENCES

Abbott, D. H., Keverne, E. B., Moore, G. F. & Yodyinguad, U. (1986). Social suppression of reproduction in subordinate talapoin monkeys, *Miopithecus talapoin*. In: J. Else & P. C. Lee (eds) *Primate ontogeny*, pp. 329–341. Cambridge: Cambridge University Press

Aiello, L. C. & Dunbar, R. I. M. (1993). Neocortex size, group size and the evolution of language. *Current Anthropology* 34: 184–193.

Anzenberger, G. (1988). The pair bond in the Titi monkey (*Callicebus moloch*): intrinsic versus extrinsic contributions of the primates. *Folia Primatologica* 50: 188–203.

Aureli, F., Schaffner, C., Boesch, C., Bearder, S., Call, J., Chapman, A. et al. (2008). Fission-fusion dynamics: new research frameworks. *Current Anthropology* 49(4): 627.

Baker, R. R. & Bellis, M. A. (1995). *Human sperm competition: copulation, masturbation and infidelity*. London: Chapman & Hall.

Baumeister, R. F. & Bratslavsky, E. (1999). Passion, intimacy, and time: passionate love as a function of change in intimacy. *Personality and Social Psychology Review* 3: 49–67.

Bearder, S. (1987). Lorises, bushbabies and tarsiers: diverse societies in solitary foragers. In: B. Smuts, D. Cheney, R. R. Seyfarth, R. Wrangham & T. Struhsaker (eds) *Primate societies*, pp. 11–24. Chicago: University of Chicago Press.

Belovsky, G. E. (1987). Hunter-gatherer foraging: a linear programming approach. *Journal of Anthopological Archaeology* 6: 29–76.

Boesch, C. & Boesch-Aschermann, H. (2000). *The chimpanzees of the Taï Forest.* Oxford: Oxford University Press.

Bowman, G. (1989). Fucking tourists: sexual relations and tourism in Jerusalem's Old City. *Critique of Anthropology* 9: 77–93.

Brotherton, P. N. M. & Komers, P. E. (2003). Mate guarding and the evolution of social monogamy in mammals. In: U. H. Reichard & C. Boesch (eds) *Monogamy: mating strategies and partnerships in birds, humans and other mammals*, pp. 59–80. Cambridge: Cambridge University Press.

Campbell, C. J., Fuentes, A., MacKinnon, K. C., Panger, M. & Bearder, S. K. (2007). *Primates in perspective*. New York: Oxford University Press.

Clutton-Brock, T. C. & Parker, G. A. (1995). Sexual coercion in animal societies. *Animal Behaviour* 49: 1345–1365.

Cubicciotti, D. D. & Mason, W. A. (1978). Comparative studies of social behaviour in *Callicebus* and *Saimiri*: heterosexual jealousy behaviour. *Behavioral Ecology and Sociobiology* 3: 311–322.

Davies, N. B. (1992). *Dunnock behaviour and social evolution*. Oxford: Oxford University Press.

Deacon, T. (1997). *The symbolic species: the co-evolution of language and the human brain*. London: Allen Lane.

De Miguel, C. & Henneberg, M. (2001). Variation in hominin brain size: how much is due to method? *Homo* 52: 3–58.

de Waal, F. (1982). *Chimpanzee politics.* London: Unwin.

Dixson, A. F. (1998). *Primate sexuality: comparative studies of prosimians, monkeys, apes and human beings*. New York: Oxford University Press.

Dunbar, R. I. M. (1984). *Reproductive decisions: an economic analysis of gelada social strategies*. Princeton, NJ: Princeton University Press.

Dunbar, R. I. M. (1989). Reproductive strategies of female gelada baboons. In: A. Rasa, C. Vogel & E. Voland (eds) *Sociobiology of sexual and reproductive strategies*, pp. 74–92. London: Chapman & Hall.

Dunbar, R. I. M. (1995a). The mating system of Callitrichid primates I: conditions for the coevolution of pairbonding and twinning. *Animal Behaviour* 50: 1057–1070.

Dunbar, R. I. M. (1995b). The mating system of Callitrichid primates II: the impact of helpers. *Animal Behaviour* 50: 1071–1089.

Dunbar, R. I. M. (1998). The social brain hypothesis. *Evolutionary Anthropology* 6: 178–190.

Dunbar, R. I. M. (2000). Male mating strategies: a modelling approach. In: P. Kappeler (ed.) *Primate males*, pp. 259–268. Cambridge: Cambridge University Press.

Dunbar, R. I. M. (2003). *The human story: a new view of mankind's evolution*. London: Faber & Faber.

Dunbar, R. I. M. (in press). Brain and behaviour in primate evolution. In: P. H. Kappeler & J. Silk (eds) *Mind the gap: tracing the origins of human universals.* Cambridge, MA: MIT Press.

Dunbar, R. I. M. & Dunbar, P. (1980). The pairbond in klipspringer. *Animal Behaviour* 28: 251–263.

Dunbar, R. I. M., Buckland, D. & Miller, D. (1990). Mating strategies of male feral goats: a problem in optimal foraging. *Animal Behaviour* 40: 653–667.

Emlen, S. T. (1984). Cooperative breeding in birds and mammals. In: J. R. Krebs & N. B. Davies (eds) *Behavioural ecology*, 2nd edn, pp. 305–339. Oxford: Blackwell.

Fisher, H. E. (1998). Lust, attraction and attachment in mammalian reproduction. *Human Nature* 9: 23–52.

Fisher, H. E. (2004). *Why we love: the nature and chemistry of romantic love*. New York: Holt.

Fisher, H. E., Aron, A. & Brown, L. L. (2006). Romantic love: a mammalian brain system for mate choice. *Philosophical Transactions of the Royal Society, London* 361B: 2173–2186.

Foley, R. A. & Lee, P. C. (1991). Ecology and energetic of encephalization in hominid evolution. *Philosophical Transactions of the Royal Society, London* 334B: 223–232.

Fuentes, A. (2002). Patterns and trends in primate pairbonds. *International Journal of Primatology* 23: 953–978.

Gilloux, I. (1997). *Social intelligence and dynamics in group-living orang-utans,* Pongo pygmaeus pygmaeus. Unpublished PhD thesis, University of London.

Grammer, K. (1989). Human courtship behaviour: biological basis and cognitive processing. In: A. E. Rasa, C. Vogel and E. Voland (eds) *The sociobiology of sexual and reproductive strategies*, pp. 147–169. London: Chapman & Hall.

Harcourt, A. H. & Greenberg, J. (2001). Do gorilla females join males to avoid infanticide? A quantitative model. *Animal Behaviour* 62: 905–915.

Hawkes, K. (1991). Showing off: tests of another hypothesis about men's foraging goals. *Ethology and Sociobiology* 11: 29–54.

Hegner, R. E., Elmen, S. T. & Demong, J. (1982). Spatial organisation of the white-fronted bee-eater. *Nature* 298: 264–266.

Henzi, S. P. & Barrett, L. (2006). Evolutionary ecology, sexual conflict, and behavioural differentiation among baboon populations. *Evolutionary Anthropology* 12: 217–230.

Hill, K. & Kaplan, H. (1988). Trade-offs in male and female reproductive strategies among the Ache. In: L. Betzig, M. Borgerhof-Mulder & P. Turke (eds) *Human reproductive behaviour*, pp. 277–305. Cambridge: Cambridge University Press.

Hrdy, S. B. & Whitten, P. L. (1997). Patterning of sexual activity. In: B. B. Smuts, D. L. Cheney, R. M. Seyfarth, T. T. Struhsaker & R. W. Wrangham (eds) *Primate societies*, pp. 370–384. Chicago: University of Chicago Press.

Jankowiak, W. R. & Fischer, E. F. (1992). A cross-cultural perspective on romantic love. *Ethnology* 31: 149–155.

Kaplan, H. & Hill, K. (1985). Food sharing among Ache foragers: tests of explanatory hypotheses. *Current Anthropology* 26: 233–245.

Kappeler, P. M. & Heymann, E. W. (1996). Nonconvergence in the evolution of primate life history and socio-ecology. *Biological Journal of the Linnean Society* 58: 297–326.

Knott, C. D. & Kahlenberg, S. M. (2007). Orangutans in perspective: forced copulations and female mating resistance. In: C. J. Campbell, A. Fuentes, K. C. MacKinnon, M. Panger & S. K. Bearder (2007). *Primates in perspective*, pp. 290–305. New York: Oxford University Press.

Kummer, H. (1968). *Social organisation of Hamadryas baboons*. Bern: Karger Verlag.

Kummer, H., Goetz, W. & Angst, W. (1974). Triadic differentiation: an inhibitory process protecting pair bonds in baboons. *Behaviour* 49: 62–87.

Lee, R. B. (1979). *The !Kung San: men, women and work in a foraging society*. Cambridge: Cambridge University Press.

Leutenegger, W. (1973). Maternal-fetal weight relationships in primates. *Folia Primatologica* 20: 280–293.

Lovejoy, O. (1981). The origin of man. *Science* 211: 341–350.

MacKinnon, J. (1974). The behaviour and ecology of wild orang utans (*Pongo pygmaeus*). *Animal Behaviour* 22: 3–74.

Marazziti, D., Akiskal, H. S., Rossi, A. & Cassano, G. B. (1999). Alteration of the platelet serotonin transporter in romantic love. *Psychological Medicine* 29: 741–745.

Muller, N. M., Kahlenberg, S. M., Emery Thompson, M. & Wrangham, R. W. (2007). Male coercion and the costs of promiscuous mating for female chimpanzees. *Proceedings of the Royal Society, London* 274B: 1009–1014.

Newton-Fisher, N. (2006). Female coalitions against male aggression in wild chimpanzees of the Budongo Forest. *International Journal of Primatology* 27: 1589–1599.

Palombit, R. A. (1999). Infanticide and the evolution of pairbonds in nonhuman primates. *Evolutionary Anthropology* 7: 117–129.

Pawłowski, B. & Dunbar, R. I. M. (2001). Human mate choice strategies. In: J. van Hooff, R. Noë & P. Hammerstein (eds) *Economic models of animal and human behaviour*, pp. 187–202. Cambridge: Cambridge University Press.

Quinlan, R. J. (2008). Human pair-bonds: evolutionary functions, ecological variation, and adaptive development. *Evolutionary Anthropology* 17: 227–238.

Roberts, S. C. & Dunbar, R. I. M. (2000). Female territoriality and the function of scent-marking in a monogamous antelope (*Oreotragus oreotragus*). *Behavioural Ecology and Sociobiology* 47: 417–423.

Robson, S. L. & Wood, B. (2008). Hominin life history: reconstruction and evolution. *Journal of Anatomy* 212: 394–425.

Shultz, S. & Dunbar, R. I. M. (2007). The evolution of the social brain: anthropoid primates contrast with other vertebrates. *Proceedings of the Royal Society, London* 274B: 2429–2436.

Smuts, B. B. (1986). *Sex and friendship in baboons*. New York: Aldine.

Smuts, B. B. & Smuts, R. W. (1993). Male aggression and sexual coercion of females in nonhuman primates and other mammals: evidence and theoretical implications. In: P. Slater, J. Rosenblatt, C. Snowdown & M. Milinski (eds) *Advances in the study of behavior*, pp. 1–63. New York: Academic Press.

Stephan, H., Frahm, H. & Baron, G. (1981). New and revised data on volumes of brain structures in insectivores and primates. *Folia Primatologica* 35: 1–29.

Stumpf, R. M., Emery Thompson, M. & Knott, C. D. (2008). A comparison of female mating strategies in *Pan troglodytes* and *Pongo* spp. *International Journal of Primatology* 29: 865–884.

van Schaik, C. P. & Dunbar, R. I. M. (1990). The evolution of monogamy in large primates: a new hypothesis and some critical tests. *Behaviour* 115: 30–62.

Waynforth, D. & Dunbar, R. I. M. (1995). Conditional mate choice strategies in humans: evidence from 'Lonely Hearts' advertisements. *Behaviour* 132: 755–779.

Wittig, R. M., Crockford, C., Lehmann, J., Whitten, P., Seyfarth, R. M. & Cheney, D. L. (2008). Focused grooming networks and stress alleviation in wild female baboons. *Hormones and Behavior* 54: 170–177.

Wrangham, R. W. (1979). On the evolution of social systems. *Social Science Information* 18: 335–368.

Wrangham, R. W. (1980). An ecological model of female-bonded primate groups. *Behaviour* 75: 262–300.

Zinovieff, S. (1991). Hunters and hunted: *Kamaki* and the ambiguities of sexual predation in a Greek town. In: P. Loizos & E. Papataxiarchis (eds) *Contested identities: gender and kinship in modern Greece*, pp. 203–220. Princeton, NJ: Princeton University Press.

9

The Evolution of Altruism
via Social Addiction

JULIE HUI & TERRENCE DEACON

THE 'PROBLEM OF ALTRUISM' has remained a thorn in the side of evolutionary biology since Darwin. In *On the origin of species* (1859), Darwin clearly recognized that the widespread existence of altruistic behavioural adaptations was a potential problem for his theory of natural selection. The general problem is that, if nature is 'red in tooth and claw' and natural selection produces adaptations by virtue of competitive elimination of the less fit, how could it produce the many examples of cooperation found in nature in which individuals sacrifice some degree of fitness for another? Since Darwin's time, evolutionary biologists have tried to explain altruism within the natural selection framework. This has resulted in many different efforts to explain how altruism could be maintained under selection. These many theories all appear to successfully demonstrate ways that altruistic behaviours might be sustained against 'invasion' by non-altruistic alternatives. These are relevant to our approach, but only as *post hoc* adaptive consequences of the emergence of altruism. We will argue below that the standard natural selection approach does not do an adequate job of explaining the origins of such adaptations.

The selection framework itself is an incomplete explanation for the evolution of altruism because it necessarily avoids answering the question of how altruistic behaviours initially arise in a non-altruistic context, and instead explains how they might be stabilized or modified with respect to alternatives in a given environment. This is because natural selection theory is intrinsically agnostic to how a given trait initially arises. Nevertheless, this does not mean that the question of how modification of traits is generated is entirely irrelevant. This agnosticism can lead to the expectation that random mutation, recombination and genetic drift are sufficient mechanisms to explain the creativity that is evident in evolution. It has been easy to avoid addressing the question of the source of variant forms in contexts where a new adaptation can be traced to prior

Proceedings of the British Academy **158**, 177–198. © The British Academy 2010.

trait states that could have been incrementally modified to reach the known end state. There are, however, adaptive transitions where certain directions of modification should have been blocked by countervailing factors, apparently requiring a discontinuous jump. In such cases, it is common for evolutionary theorists simply to imagine that the transition occurred due to a 'hopeful monster' mega-mutation or some other accidental radical reorganization of the genome. This can strain the dependency on accident as an explanation, especially as the adaptive complexity of the transition increases. This is most obviously problematic in the case of what Maynard Smith and Szathmáry (1995) have described as major transitions in evolution, such as the transition to multicellularity in plants, animals and fungi (e.g. Buss 1987). In such transitions, there has been a shift from autonomy to codependence, with the result that a higher-order unit of evolution emerges, organized around a novel synergy of multiple lower-order units that previously would have been in competition. Both the combinatorial complexity of hitting upon a sufficient complementarity of interdependencies and the dangers due to loss of autonomy in the process pose a high barrier to achieving such a transition.

In general terms, the problem of explaining the origin of an altruistic adaptation is a paradigm case of such a major transition. First we will argue that a shift to codependence maintained by altruistic adaptations cannot be fully explained by natural selection alone. Natural selection acts as a limitation on variety, but does not account for the generation of the variant forms that are its substrates. Since the form of the relevant variation in the case of altruism involves potentially high costs, incremental transition is more problematic. Second, we will suggest instead that relaxation of selection may be an important factor due to the degradation of autonomy that can result, and because this creates conditions which both allow for and aid in the emergence of new potential interdependencies.

To exemplify the general mechanism involved we will examine two cases of reorganization effects due to relaxation of selection: an increase in the complexity and neural control of song in a domesticated bird and the evolution of dependency on dietary vitamin C in anthropoid primates and its consequences for other adaptations. Both examples demonstrate how relaxation of selection may lead to a degradation of autonomy, and how this may contribute to the emergence of functional codependence. Neither matches the problem of altruism exactly, but both are informative in different ways. Borrowing insights from these two examples, we extrapolate a novel approach to the origins of altruism.

OVERVIEW OF THE PROBLEM

Darwin himself recognized that examples of evolved altruism, such as that of hive bees, posed problems for his theory (1860). His solution was to suggest that a form of 'community selection' might occur when traits that undermine an individual's reproduction turn out to be adaptive in terms of the reproduction of a group, which is likely to contain family members of the altruistic individual. This explanation was developed by Petr Kropotkin who, based on his observations of wildlife communities in Siberia (1902), argued that limited resources would select for a tendency to cooperate rather than compete. Subsequent work drew further links between environmental structure and social behaviour; Wynne-Edwards (1962), for example, argued that if resources are clumped and can only be obtained or protected by multiple individuals working in concert, then selection pressures are likely to favour cooperative behaviours over selfish individual behaviours.

However, some difficulties with group selection approaches remained, notably the assumption that groups can be treated as a type of individual with respect to natural selection. Critics pointed out that in fact many groups tend to have rather fluid memberships (e.g. Williams 1966), and that group selection arguments lacked an explanation for how group benefits may arise.

The discovery of DNA and its integration with Darwinian theory allowed Hamilton (1964a, 1964b) to solve Darwin's problem with eusocial insects by demonstrating that the close genetic relatedness of bees explained the altruism of sterile workers. Subsequent work attempted to generalize from kin altruism among genetically related individuals to a broader theory of evolved altruistic behaviour, showing that reliably reciprocated altruistic behaviours between unrelated individuals could also serve to maintain social cooperation (e.g. Trivers 1971). More recent developments generalized this work still further by considering direct reciprocity as a special case of *indirect* reciprocity within a population of two (Nowak 2006), as aid given within groups is not necessarily limited to pairs of individuals engaging in repetitive or exclusive interactions.

Such indirect reciprocity may also include more complex forms of interaction; language, for example, allows gossip and the exchange of information about cooperators and cheaters alike, so that individuals are able to weigh the likely costs of giving against both direct and indirect benefits. In this scenario, natural selection should favour cooperation (as groups of cooperators do better than their cheating counterparts) as well as better forms of communication, as offsetting the costs of group living.

However, language and communication more generally must themselves be the result of a complicated evolutionary history; thus indirect reciprocity approaches require that a whole slew of elements come together to form both a cohesive system of behavioural predispositions for maintaining group cohesion and expelling cheaters, some of which (such as language) are symbolic processes probably restricted to human cooperative groups.

Indirect reciprocity also generally assumes that interactions among group members are relatively equiprobable. However, this is generally not the case in actual biological systems as inter-individual distance is usually quite variable and non-symmetric, and more recently network reciprocity theory has used graph theory to take into account the statistical nature of interactions limited by spatial constraints (Nowak 2006). In this approach, each individual communicates/interacts with a limited number of other members of the population who may be either cooperators or defectors (cheaters). It is assumed that when members gain direct knowledge of a cheater they will attempt to shift their interactions to a different neighbour. As neighbouring cooperators discover one another in this manner they begin to share information amongst themselves, i.e. in a local sub-network within the group that will have a better overall fitness than the sub-networks of cheaters.

In recent decades such approaches have been complemented by work investigating the issue from a standard economic perspective which attempts to explain how cooperators can maintain their populations against cheaters. Organisms do better as cheaters only if they subsequently avoid associating with the organism they cheated: if information on cheaters' reputations is available, cheaters are forced into drifting. Cooperators, however, repeat cooperative interactions with other cooperators and thereby eventually benefit from the occasional costs of being cheated, thus maintaining their populations through group selection.

This perspective has been used in several different game theory approaches that pre-date many network reciprocity approaches, including the 'Prisoner's Dilemma' and 'Stag Hunt' type games which alter the relative costs and benefits of cooperating or defecting (cheating). Research on which algorithms of play did best at the Prisoner's Dilemma (PD) game (Axelrod 1984) established several stable solutions: briefly, groups of cooperators can maintain group cohesion and keep out cheaters if they maintain a strategy of cooperating until the other player cheated, as well as occasionally cooperating even when the strategy dictated cheating. In this way, mistakes that throw the interaction into a series of cheating interactions can be corrected.

Thus far, work on the problem of altruism has suggested several mechanisms through which cooperation, when it occurs, can be maintained in a variety of populations of cooperators and defectors. More recent co-evolutionary approaches have also investigated aspects of altruism that are transmitted socially, or that involve niche construction effects influencing subsequent generations. These co-evolutionary approaches differ primarily in their addition of non-genetic components that are transmitted independent of an organism's biological lineage and which may affect an organism's genetic reproduction. We will return to these human-specific variants on the altruism problem below, but first we consider some special circumstances that aid the evolution of pro-social behaviour in animals.

Social spiders offer an interesting case in which cooperation can emerge due to advantages of maintaining proximity. Sociality has arisen in several different groups of spiders, and researchers have been concerned with why this might be the case. Generally all populations of animals must balance the dual constraints of population density and its link to the distribution and accessibility of environmental resources. Thus spiders working together can capture larger prey than solitary individuals (Nentwig 1985), but how spiders become habituated to social living so that they can take advantage of this synergistic benefit provides additional insight into conditions favouring the evolution of altruism. The Allee effect, named for Warder Clyde Allee (1951), examines conditions under which population density and the resulting proximity of individuals can have a positive correlation with survival and reproduction of that population. Living in groups can be advantageous under certain conditions, and if there are collective effects through which cooperating individuals can gain access to special resources, then generally the larger your numbers the better off you are. But there are usually costs to group membership as well, due to the need to share resources. Allee was primarily concerned with group effects such as predatory protection and group hunting, but the theory also suggests that if a group is brought together there could be multiple ways in which maintaining the group could be reinforced. For instance, if group size is correlated with better survival, then selection for sex ratios would heavily bias the production of females so that the optimal population size can be reached at a faster rate than a population without this bias.

A recent study (Bilde et al. 2007) shows that in one social spider group, *Stegodyphu dumicola*, reduced female body size and correspondingly smaller clutch sizes would seem to be a cost to group living. However, overall lifetime reproductive success in these same individuals increases with colony size due to the greater percentage of offspring that survive the juvenile to adult transition and persist to form the basis of the next generation. Other examples from social spiders show some of the integrated functions that can occur with prolonged group living. Matriphagy (eating the mother) occurs at the end of each season so that the offspring from the previous year now have a source of food upon which to begin the new season of colony development. In addition, there appears to be shared care for offspring. Presumably, non-cooperative behaviours that benefit individuals at the expense of other members of the group do not arise because the benefit of cooperative behaviour always outweighs any benefits that would arise due to defection. Thus social spiders demonstrate that cooperative group living can provide many benefits accruing from population density effects, such as collective resource acquisition and reproductive support, and that these benefits can be a source of selective advantages which will also select against non-cooperative and defecting behaviours.

Turning our attention to the role of social transmission on the evolution of altruism, there have been a number of approaches that demonstrate how processes of social transmission can augment the stabilization of altruistic behaviours in social groups. Many have been motivated by the evolutionary analogy drawn between genes and social traits, such as the concept of memes introduced by Richard Dawkins (1976). Despite criticisms with respect to how to categorize memes and whether or not discrete units of socially transmitted information are obtainable or transmissible, there are aspects of these general principles that are relevant to our discussion. With respect to evolution, an advantage of social transmission, and particularly cultural evolution (memetic or otherwise), is that it can occur at rates that are orders of magnitude faster than biological evolution due to its de-coupled relationship from genetic material that has to be passed from parents to offspring. Social transmission is also not limited to related individuals, but can travel across individuals. Co-evolutionary theories share this blending of behaviour and biological evolution, and work to understand their relationships to one another.

One example of an account of the evolution of altruism that depends on social transmission effects is Lehmann's (2007) notion of transgenerational altruism. Lehmann argues that, by assuming that the altruism is occurring among contemporaries, we tend to ignore the role of behaviours that provide altruistic benefits (as well as potential costs) across generations. This is particularly relevant with respect to niche construction effects (e.g. Laland et al. 1996, 2000), where an environmental modification may persist across generations. In the extreme case of humans, extensive man-made modifications of both local living environments and the global socio-economic context of social life over the past century have radically altered the conditions affecting social behaviours of future generations in both beneficial and deleterious ways. But even in more typical cases, such as nests that are maintained across generations, trans-generational altruism and selfish behaviours are possible. Consider the example of matriphagy (discussed above), in which mothers die to leave a carcass for their offspring to eat. Thus, not only can an altruistic benefit be paid forward to future generations, but selfish behaviours such as resource depletion can also have cross-generational effects. These considerations greatly enlarge the scope of the evolutionary problem of determining what constitutes an evolutionary stable altruistic strategy.

Heylighen (1992) argues that theories restricted to biological evolution are incapable of explaining true unselfish altruism, and that only memetic or dual inheritance approaches can achieve this result. Although we will not pursue this hypothesis below, the role of biologically uncoupled cultural processes is not incompatible with the approach we will pursue. An evolutionary mechanism that can achieve some degree of altruistic behaviour even at the cost of individual or kin selection advantage would provide a foundation for the evolution of socially transmitted biologically disadvantageous altruistic behaviours.

CODEPENDENCY

These co-evolutionary and niche construction considerations demonstrate that the problem of the evolution of altruism is far more general than merely sacrificial and helpful interactions between pairs of interacting organisms. Formulated more abstractly, they demonstrate that the underlying issue is whether higher-order synergistic interdependencies with distributed advantages can emerge and be maintained in the face of costs imposed by breakdowns in this synergy, either because of a failure to maintain an equal distribution of costs and benefits or because of invasion by non-cooperative elements. Framing the problem in these more general terms, however, highlights the fact that this is not merely an issue concerning animal social behaviour, but also a more general problem concerning the evolution of synergistic codependency relationships in biology at all levels.

Of course, explaining the *maintenance* of such synergies and the *emergence* of *novel* synergies are distinct evolutionary problems. Identifying the classes of stable interactive strategies that maintain such higher-order synergistic social organizations does not necessarily provide insight into how they could form in the first place. Nevertheless, perhaps exploring cases in which higher synergistic relationships have emerged in physiological systems can shed light on how analogous relationships can emerge socially.

Below we describe two examples in which synergistic physiological interactions have emerged from previously non-interacting components. Although physiological mechanisms are not in reproductive competition with each other as social interactions are, one similarity between social and physiological cooperation is that, in both circumstances, synergistic interactions emerge from statistically unlikely combinatorial relationships before any functional advantage is exhibited. The relevance of these cases to our present problem is that functions depending on the interaction of distributed components require those components to co-occur reliably. Therefore, irrespective of whether the problem is the prevention of a synergistic combination of phenotypes from becoming dissociated, or the defence of codependent individuals in a social group from defectors, the combinatorial interdependency itself must come under selection. For this to happen, the synergistic interaction must emerge and persist in a sufficiently robust manner.

This poses what we will call the 'Secretariat problem' (named for a horse that was a spectacular Triple Crown winner a few generations back). Though bred from the same stock as many of the horses he competed against, Secretariat seemed to run effortlessly away from the competition. The traits brought together in his breeding had produced an unprecedented synergy, resulting in just the right balance of strength, body proportions, metabolism and coordination to be an ideal racehorse—every breeder's dream. But breeding Secretariat would not produce an offspring with this same synergy of traits, because sexual reproduction reshuffles the combination and passes on only 50 per cent of the relevant genes to be mixed with those from a mate in his progeny. So, whether in groups or in individuals, the emergence and evolution of high-level synergistic functions depends on the possibility not merely of 'discovering' a reciprocal complementarity among traits, but having this condition occur with sufficient reliability for selection to emerge with respect to it.

Thus, while we do not dispute the importance of natural selection for the stabilization of the synergistic interdependency of cooperatively acting individuals in a group, we will argue that such interdependencies must arise and be regularly present *before* natural selection can begin to shape and stabilize their supportive conditions. We hypothesize that—counter-intuitively—this requires a relaxation of selection. Below we will show how relaxing selection pressures, as demonstrated in the 'evolution' of socially acquired song in a domesticated finch and in the evolution of dietary vitamin C dependency in primates, can lead to the emergence of complex functional interdependencies that may become subject to stabilization and further shaping by natural selection. In these cases relaxation of selection produces degradation of the autonomy of some function which leads spontaneously to dependency on a more distributed realization of that function—a kind of addiction—and out of this a complex and codependent function can arise. Invoking a similar mechanism of relaxed selection, self-organization of current behaviours, and a reintroduction of natural selection, we will suggest a possible mechanism for the generation of altruistic-like behaviours.

COMPLEXIFICATION OF BIRD SONG

Recent work examining the neuroanatomy of song-learning in birds has shown some unexpected effects that we believe exemplify the results of relaxed selection (Deacon 2009). Kazuo Okanoya (2004) has studied the singing behaviour of the Bengalese finch, which has been domesticated for 250 years in Japan. Breeders have kept documents of their breeding process, showing that this bird was not domesticated for its song but was bred for traits such as coloration and ability to breed in captivity. Okanoya has also studied the finch's wild cousin, the White-backed Munia. One of the major differences between the two species is that the White-backed Munia has a very stereotypic song, which means that its song structure is very predictable in that song element A is always followed by song element B. In other words, the transition probability between song elements is nearly 1.0 (completely predictable). The Bengalese finch has a song that is more complex than its wild cousin in three ways. First, the transition probability between song elements has equalized, which means that the predictability of the next song element in a singing bout has decreased significantly, resulting in considerable variability. Second, the song of a Bengalese finch is strongly influenced by songs sung by other Bengalese finches during its development, whereas White-backed Munia songs are produced irrespective of social influence. Third, Okanoya found that the number of forebrain structures and the complexity of the neural connections involved in song production in the Bengalese finch is greater than the relatively simple motor output found in the White-backed Munia. The White-backed Munia has essentially one forebrain nucleus (the nucleus RA) providing the motor output controlling song production. The Bengalese finch, by contrast, depends on several different forebrain nuclei in addition to the nucleus RA for the acquisition and control of song.

It has generally been assumed that bird song complexity, like other display behaviours, increases as a function of the importance and intensity of sexual selection in a species. Likewise, it is believed that complex functional organization of a physiological function—such as a complex, context-sensitive, coordinated behaviour and its neurological substrates—can only result from intense selection favouring this capacity. But in the case of Bengalese finch domestication, there appears to have been neither artificial nor sexual selection on singing behaviour, nor selection favouring complex reorganization of this brain function. This poses a conundrum for more traditional neo-Darwinian accounts: how might the Bengalese finch's abilities have arisen so rapidly (250 years is a mere blink in evolutionary time) without intense and specific artificial or natural selection favouring these consequences? We suggest that the breeding process shielded singing behaviour from the effects of selection that were present in the wild (a 'masking' of selection), causing its highly constrained structure and motor control to degrade by a process of genetic drift (Deacon 2009). This degradation is what we believe to be responsible for allowing song complexity to increase, song structure to become dependent on experience, and brain control of song to become more distributed.

Much of the background research on the song development and its neural control was pioneered by Fernando Nottebohm and colleagues (Nottebohm 1970, 1980, 1996). He found that if birds with stereotyped songs were deafened at hatching so that they could hear neither their own singing nor the singing of their conspecifics, they would still sing a crude version of their species' subsong at puberty. The notes were distorted and in some cases only vaguely resembled the appropriate note, but there was still some resemblance to the species-typical song. Thus these birds have an internal bias to sing particular notes in particular sequences. The motor template of their song is highly constrained and is under strong stabilizing selection that requires little outside influence to maintain, though being able to hear oneself sing does matter. This is supported by comparison of deafened birds' singing to that of normal birds raised in isolation. While isolated birds could not hear other birds, they could hear themselves sing and as a result they produced notes and song sequences that were much more like those of normal, socialized birds, demonstrating that the innate song template is effectively distributed to both auditory and motor systems. In species that depend more on social learning for normal song development, still other forebrain nuclei are critical. These include brain structures contributing pre-motor and striatal-like motor learning functions (including most critically, the nuclei designated HVc, iMAN and Area X). While these structures play a small or nonexistent role in species with stereotyped song, they increase in importance in species engaging in complex song learning and song production. So although all these brain structures and their interconnections exist in both social learners and stereotypic singers, they only seem to play a significant role in song behaviour in the species that acquire a normal song by listening to other singers. In these latter species, often there are also differences in these brain structures and their connections that appear to be correlated with selection augmenting their functioning.

How could relaxation of selection, at the hands of breeders interested in feather coloration, have produced effects analogous to those undergone by complex song-learning birds? We are not suggesting that new brain structures emerge, that these many nuclei become augmented in their functionality, nor that a series of new neural connections is made in this process. We merely argue that the existing structures and their direct and indirect inputs to the nucleus RA can begin to have an increased influence on this song output nucleus as its specificity of function degrades.

We suggest that this change in brain function is a result of a shift from a template-based song that is highly constrained to mechanisms intrinsic to the nucleus RA to a learned song with many more inputs affecting the nucleus RA. Learning is a distributed function that requires strong links across sensory and motor modalities and their memories. For this reason, learning cannot reside in a single nucleus. We suggest that relaxation can occur in multiple ways, one of which is through domestication as in the Bengalese finch example. Due to the effects of long-term breeding that masked the selection pressures typical of life in the wild, the song template of the Bengalese finch was no longer under strong stabilizing selection. In the wild, we would expect that aspects such as predation and sexual selection play a role in stabilizing the song template, and the relative autonomy of nucleus RA control of song. With breeding comes a relaxation of those constraints so that selection no longer plays a role in maintaining tight constraints on the functional autonomy of the nucleus RA. As the integrity of the RA-based template degrades due to the effects of drift, the inputs to RA from other structures change their effective weighting and can begin to exert influence on the song template. With weakened intrinsic constraints on song structure, various extrinsic influences, both from other brain functions and from indirect environmental influences, can begin to influence song. Thus both the flexibility and the conditionality of song structure with respect to other factors can begin to emerge.

Since these other systems are themselves serving complex functions that have evolved for various other reasons, these influences are not merely random but carry with them some trace of these functional consequences. As a result, novel coupling between singing and other functions becomes more likely. Therefore, despite emerging irrespective of selection on any synergistic function, synergistic interactions may be more likely to result than by chance alone. The tendency for epigenetic processes to compensate for changes in organization due to damage or mutation altering typical anatomical features may also play a role in ensuring that the resulting neural outcome is functionally well integrated.

The point of this example is to show how relaxation of selection pressures can allow for the generation of variation through drift that can lead to self-organizing effects with organized functional consequences, even though functional correspondence of these changes with the environment is not shaped by selection (for more details see Deacon 2009).

LOSS OF ENDOGENOUS VITAMIN C PRODUCTION

Another way that this relaxation effect can occur in the wild is through a functional duplication. As an exemplar of this, we turn to something relevant to us—our addiction to fruit. Among mammals, anthropoid apes are some of the few that lack the ability to endogenously produce ascorbic acid or vitamin C (Chatterjee 1973). To better understand this, researchers in Japan examined the gene for the final catalyst in the production of ascorbic acid, called L-gulano-lactone oxidase (GULO), in rats (Nishikimi et al. 1994). They used this gene sequence as a probe to search for a homologous GULO gene in humans, and demonstrated its existence, albeit in a greatly degraded form. In humans, this once-functioning gene has accumulated many loss-of-function mutations such as the deletion of coding segments (exons) and the insertion of 'stop' codons, making it a pseudogene.

This poses an interesting problem. How can the degeneration of a gene with a necessary functional product, gain a foothold within a lineage? Selection on the essential ascorbic acid in the body is maintained, so how can mutations that occur which render the GULO homologue useless not only occur, but spread throughout the lineage?

In part, the answer lies in the evolutionary timing of this genetic degeneration. We know from phylogenetic research that the GULO mutations date back to approximately 35 million years ago. A series of other primate morphological changes began to take place at roughly the same time, such as the development of colour-vision and changes in tooth structure to better handle frugivory. We suggest that if primates, 35 million years ago, are able to eat foods rich in vitamin C regularly, then genetic mutations that result in loss-of-function of their GULO catalyst will not affect their survival and reproduction (Deacon 2003; Wiles et al. 2005). In other words, the change to frugivory does not begin as a functional adaptation because fruit is not necessary to the diet, although it may be a plentiful resource. In this sense, the early stage of fruit-eating can be considered facultative. However, as frugivory becomes habitual and is maintained over evolutionary time, it will mask selection that would otherwise maintain the genetic mechanisms necessary for endogenous production of ascorbic acid. This will allow the GULO gene to accumulate loss-of-function mutations, and consequently the lineage will become forced into maintaining frugivory in compensation. Currently, primates obtain vitamin C from dietary sources such as fresh fruits and vegetables. Transport and storage of foodstuffs are not significant factors when vitamin C is endogenously produced, as it is available at steady levels. If, however, it must be obtained purely from dietary sources, then the lack of storage means that the external sources of vitamin C must be relatively constant throughout the year. Given the importance of vitamin C, we can be fairly certain that there has been continuous selection on its antioxidant function. Therefore, when the gene for GULO became a pseudogene in the anthropoid primate lineage, primates became forced to maintain a frugivorous diet because of the negative reproductive consequences for those that do not maintain healthy levels of ascorbic acid.

In this example, something that was entirely endogenous to the organism has become fully 'off-loaded' onto the environment. An animal must ether produce vitamin C endogenously, or acquire it extrinsically. Unlike bird song, vitamin C foragers are entirely dependent on acquiring vitamin C from their environment. In this sense there is a dependency roughly analogous to an addiction. It is an addiction in that it is reached while under constant selection. Unlike the relaxation of selection on Bengalese finch song, the function of ascorbic acid is not made irrelevant by its availability in fruit. There is merely a redundant way that this function can be fulfilled, one endogenous and one extrinsic. This redundancy could be the source of relaxation of selection on either source, but one— endogenous synthesis—is more susceptible than the other as mutations to the primate GULO gene do not negatively affect health and reproduction if the function can be met by eating enough fruit to maintain appropriate ascorbic acid levels in the body. Therefore it is not relaxation of selection on ascorbic acid function, but on the maintenance of constraints on endogenous ascorbic acid production that is occurring. Furthermore, whereas, periodic irregularities of frugivorous foraging behaviours can be easily redeveloped, functional degradation of the GULO genetic sequence can only be recovered with a very low probability inverse sequence of point mutation changes.

Unlike the complexification of song structure and control in the Bengalese finch, which was a spontaneous side-effect of degradation, the persistence of function in the case of the degradation of vitamin C synthesis creates a context for unmasking selection on other functions. Because extrinsic vitamin C is not as reliable as endogenously produced vitamin C, breakdown of endogenous synthesis and dependence on a dietary source can be a source of reintroduced selection affecting any adaptations that help to maintain this extrinsic source. These probably include the evolution of three-colour vision, changes in tooth structure, digestive adaptations, metabolic changes and probably many other primate-specific adaptations, all of which would have increased the reliability of access to and utilization of dietary vitamin C (Deacon 2009). Thus evolutionary addiction to extrinsic vitamin C probably unmasked selection on a variety of phenotypes not previously under selection for anything to do with this function, but which have subsequently come to function as an integrated suite.

The phenomenon of relaxation of selection is relevant to the evolution of altruism because it provides an evolutionary mechanism whereby codependent relationships can develop and become integrated. Below we argue that reciprocally altruistic behaviours can also be understood as a form of codependence, and that the logic of relaxation of selection, degeneration and addiction, and re-distribution of selection can be applied to the problem of altruism in a way that complements earlier theories.

IMPLICATIONS FOR ALTRUISM

Taking the relationship between relaxed selection, reorganization and natural selection into account, let us reconsider the problem of explaining the evolution of altruism and its co-evolution with cheating behaviours. Earlier studies assuming the ubiquity of natural selection have demonstrated a number of ways that altruism can be maintained across generations despite being faced with cheating strategies. Presumably these various strategies evolved to overcome the challenge of cheating and so would have evolved as a consequence of a prior rise in altruistic behaviours and the presence of cheaters. The question that is not well addressed by these theories is how altruistic and pro-social behaviour can arise and become widespread in a population prior to the evolution of mechanisms to defend against non-cooperative and cheating behaviours.

What evolutionary mechanism can lead progressively from a non-cooperative state to cooperation before there are mechanisms for its maintenance via selection? Unless we invoke the unprecedented and sudden population-wide appearance of cooperation, we are forced to show how every incremental move towards increasing levels of cooperation within a population is more effective than prior non-cooperative behaviours. This raises a particularly difficult problem, because the shift from autonomy to codependence is at every stage susceptible to invasion by non-cooperators, and at any one moment the two strategies are mutually exclusive.

We argue that there is another way of dealing with the problem of competition, by removing the source of the competition. This is because cheating and various forms of cheating defence have evolutionary consequences only if they provide reproductive advantage over not doing so. When selection is removed, so are the adaptive values previously placed on these behaviours, and cheating, hoarding, competing over resources etc. due to a lack of differential reproductive consequences. Selection gives value to phenotypes by determining their fitted-ness with the world. Relaxing selection decreases the constraints on what counts as fitted-ness.

Although there are probably multiple ways that relaxation of selection can lead to the diminution of non-cooperative behaviours we will explore only two: a change in environment that masks selection on certain competitive traits and the appearance of a redundant substitute for a competitive adaptation.

Consider a situation where individuals must compete over resources because they are insufficient to sustain the entire population. If there is a change in the environment such that food becomes over-abundant, there will be relaxation of selection on competition over food. In this case, individuals who remain competitive over food do not gain with respect to reproduction and health over those who are non-competitive. The result of prolonged reduction in the stabilizing selection that previously maintained genetic predispositions to engage in food competition will be degradation and drift of those traits and their genetic supports. Thus, over time, relaxation of this selection pressure would cause the behaviour patterns of individuals to tend towards less and less competition with respect to food. Resource-defence behaviours such as hoarding, territory defence, aggressive displacement of competitors and so forth, would no longer confer any reproductive advantage. Although relaxation of selection only has an indirect effect on the possibility of the emergence of cooperative behaviours, by removing the advantages of maintaining competitive behaviours it significantly increases the likelihood of cooperation emerging and spreading in a population. Furthermore, relaxation of selection on resource competition could potentially also be an indirect source of selection *against* competitive adaptations if these diverted time and energy from other reproductively important tasks and exposed the actor to possible damage.

Though degradation and drift are probably more likely than specific selection against competitive adaptations under these conditions, neither mechanism explains how new pro-social behavioural tendencies might be predisposed to emerge: they merely relax selection against them. Is there reason to expect more than just a permissive effect? In the examples of finch song and vitamin C adaptations discussed above, we observed that synergistic interactions were actually facilitated. Is something analogous possible in the case of social behaviour?

In the example of prolonged relaxation of food competition, competitive predispositions and related adaptations will devolve to a degraded state, while the variety of non-competitive behaviours would proliferate in the population. We can imagine that this would also include various degrees of egalitarian behaviours related to food, such as food sharing among both kin and non-kin, and tolerance of multiple individuals feeding side by side without threat. Even if none of these behaviours makes any reproductive difference, the generation of 'new' behavioural variants can in effect 'explore' potential functional possibilities that could not be sampled previously. For example, adaptive options that were previously blocked or limited by the need to compete may now become subject to selection. There might be advantages for individuals who want to be near others for predator defence or temperature maintenance, for example. Such advantages would have been unrealizable in a context of intense competition over resources, but masking selection on this one feature will tend to unmask an array of selective differences in the population that were effectively 'below the radar' as long as competition was important. In other words, if new domains of selective advantages are unmasked by the removal of this competing selection pressure, then variations in social predispositions within the population that tended to be suppressed in the context of competition can now provide a source of variation upon which novel forms of fitted-ness can emerge. Moreover, since many of these variants will share in common features that were to some degree or other incompatible with competitive strategies, they will also be more likely to share non-competitive attributes in common and in this way be more likely to interrelate synergistically with one another (much as in the cases of finch brain structure interactions and vitamin-C-acquiring adaptations). So we need not merely assume that groups simply happen to be cooperative and then ask how they could maintain this state against cheaters: we can now begin to explore ways in which cooperation can incrementally emerge.

Here we have only described one context in which relaxation of selection might lead to the emergence of cooperative behaviours. There may be many others: for example, situations where social living is enforced for other reasons, such as when rookery sites are limited, food sources clumped, temperature must be maintained or predators defended against, and probably many more. However, the relaxation effect is only part of the story because selection probably never remains entirely relaxed. The degradation of competitive behaviours is only one consequence of relaxation of selection: group living may mask many other adaptations for living non-socially. So the availability of close group members can result in the degradation of the capacity to live autonomously. Analogous to the evolution of vitamin C dependency, merely the presence of multiple individuals acting as a buffer against environmental challenges such as predation can lead to degradation and an addiction to group living. Such an addiction will specifically favour adaptations for maintaining social cohesion, even if there is some reproductive cost. This can further lead to selection for behavioural adaptations to minimize or police against potential sources of group disruption.

As discussed above, there are many reasons why individuals might be brought into close proximity with one another. Moreover, changes that result in the clumping of individuals into groups that persist over many generations may relax selection on the maintenance of those adaptations critical to solitary life. One factor that is often significantly affected is the probability of being preyed upon. Where individuals tend to be near one another, a likely common side-effect is a change in strategies of predator defence. If a predator normally targets lone, isolated individuals, there will be intense selection favouring the abilities to detect, escape from and ward off the predator, resulting in individual defences against predation that can be quite well developed. For example, vigilant monitoring of the surroundings is strongly selected for, because if an animal notices the predator before it is too close it may have a better chance at escape or defence.

In highly social conditions, where individuals are constantly and reliably near one another, a predator attack has an intrinsic ambiguity and uncertainty as to the intended target. In clustered groups, when an individual animal detects a predator it cannot necessarily determine whether it is the target, and so must react to diminish the chance of being the target and of being caught. Means of doing so are likely to be quite different in a social context than when solitary. For example, solitary animals cannot rely on the possibility of others being targeted, their monitoring of the surroundings or on the startle reactions of others to serve as an alert, nor on the additive effects of many individuals' defensive behaviours. But if circumstances consistently cluster individuals together, the possibility of other individuals producing responses that are redundant to those an isolated individual would produce can lessen the selection pressure to maintain these more self-reliant predator defences.

For example, actively monitoring the surroundings for predators might be well developed in a population of independently foraging diurnal animals because those that spot predators from afar are likely to reproduce more reliably than those that do not. But in social contexts, where the target of predation is ambiguous and unclear to the prey animal, individual monitoring of the surroundings will be less critical. Many eyes periodically looking up from foraging etc. to scan the surroundings will diminish the amount of time any one individual needs to be doing so and yet increase the potential of early predator detection. In addition, the startle response and escape tendencies of other group members can be relied on when a predator is detected, and these can evolve to become surrogates for one's own constant attention to the possibility of predation. In addition, there are many more potential targets and potential defenders in a social group. We see this in examples of eagles attacking small monkeys that are feeding in trees and herd animals feeding in large numbers on the savanna. Increased prey densities will reduce the probability that any particular individual will be caught in a given attack. Higher densities allow individuals with more socially dependent predator detection or evasion abilities to enjoy both a greater degree of freedom from predation and some lessening of the costs which defensive adaptations would otherwise impose (in terms of time and energy diverted from other needs).

As we saw in previous examples, even partial masking of selection can cause degradation of phenotypes so long as the masking is relatively stable and reliable over a significant number of generations. In this sense, the side-effects of population density are similar to the effects of ubiquitous dietary vitamin C, in that partial protection from predation supplied extrinsically is analogous to an essential nutrient being available extrinsically. As masked selection for vitamin C led to degradation of intrinsic production capabilities, so masked selection on specific predation defences could lead to degradation of those most effectively masked by social conditions. Finally, degradation of the autonomous function in both cases can lead to increased dependency on the extrinsic support and an unmasking of other traits that play some role in maintenance of this offloaded function.

Consider the situation that would exist subsequent to the evolutionary degradation of autonomous predator defence capabilities as a result of long-term evolution of social foraging. Individuals with a slight reduction in the tendency to constantly monitor the presence of predators or with slightly degraded ability to physically ward off a predator, will be at a decided disadvantage if separated from the social group. This will make it extremely costly for individuals to forage outside a social group, and thus will create a context that makes group break-up a decided danger. In other words, the degradation of non-social protections can lead to a corresponding increase in need to stabilize those social contexts, and thus to selection favouring any behavioural variations that tend to minimize this possibility.

This suggests only one way in which a transition from solitary foraging to social living can lead to addiction to social living. As a result, there will be a shift from selection on individuals' predator defence behaviours to behaviours that take advantage of social redundancy and that at the same time will lead to selection on any features that contribute to group maintenance. These may include both affiliative and social monitoring behaviours such as those that have been identified in other analyses (discussed above), e.g. reciprocity, cheater defence, etc. But since the masking effect of groups affects both the development of cooperative behaviours and the degeneration of non-cooperative behaviours, it can also lead to conditions that favour other non-cooperative behaviours (e.g. cheating), which must be defended against. For this reason, it is not surprising to find both a social hierarchy and social cooperation side by side in nature. The competition found in social hierarchies can be seen as both remnant of earlier autonomous competitive behaviours (which never fully degraded and are now limited by the necessity of group living) and an evolutionary consequence of cooperation. The various forms of 'cheating' that evolve after group-living addiction will only confer selective advantage once codependent interactions amongst group members have been established. Thus the importance of degeneration of strong autonomy is that it can lead to addiction to social living, and this can contribute to the evolution of both anti-social and pro-social behaviours.

CONCLUSIONS

In this chapter, we have argued for the existence of a previously underappreciated factor in the evolution of pro-social behaviours: the degradation of functional autonomy due to relaxed selection conferred by group living. This is not proposed as a mechanism in competition with other accounts of the evolutionary stabilization of altruistic adaptations, but as a mechanism that can explain how such stable cooperative conditions might have arisen from previously non-cooperative conditions. This approach was suggested by the analogy between social cooperation and other intra-organismic synergistic functions. The demonstration that conditions of reduced selection resulting from redundancy effects can eventually lead to a redistribution of function and an increase of codependent relationships in physiological evolution is here generalized and extrapolated to apply to certain group living contexts. In other words, we argue for a parallel logic behind the evolution of synergistic interdependencies in both organismic and social domains.

What is unusual about this hypothetical mechanism is that it is not strictly Darwinian, but instead depends on the reduction of selection pressures in some domain and an ensuing degradation of function. Basically, it is an argument for the emergence of pro-social adaptations in defence of social dependency, and it explains the emergence of social dependency as a consequence of the degradation of functional autonomy. This particular account of a mechanism that can lead to the emergence of codependency from a condition of autonomy does not exclude other possible mechanisms, including the serendipitous emergence of conditions where group effort (such as in the social spiders discussed above) can provide advantage over individual effort. However, we would predict that the transition into such relationships will be more likely under conditions of relaxed selection; e.g. non-zero sum contexts. In this respect, this hypothesis is consistent with earlier theories, but additionally contributes a source of selection pressures favouring the evolution of group-maintaining adaptations via a kind of addiction to group living.

Based on these considerations, we predict more generally that higher-order units of evolutionary adaptation arise only after there has been a loss of functional or individual autonomy and consequent selection to maintain the stability of codependent synergies. This should be as true for intra-organismic synergies as inter-organismic synergies, and should even apply to the emergence of cultural adaptations supporting social cohesion which have arisen via social evolution.

REFERENCES

Allee, W. C. (1951). *The social life of animals*. Boston, MA: Beacon Press.

Axelrod, R. M. (1984). *The evolution of cooperation*. New York: Basic Books.

Bilde, T., Coates, K. S., Birkhofer, K., Bird, T., Malakov, A. A., Lubin, Y. et al. (2007). Survival benefits select for group living in a social spider despite reproductive costs. *Journal of Evolutionary Biology* 20: 2412–2426.

Buss, L. W. (1987). *The evolution of individuality*. Princeton, NJ: Princeton University.

Chatterjee, I. B. (1973). Evolution and the biosynthesis of ascorbic acid. *Science* 182: 1271–1272.

Darwin, C. (1859). *On the origin of species by means of natural selection, or The preservation of favoured races in the struggle for life*. New York: D. Appleton & Co.

Dawkins, R. (1976). *The selfish gene*. Oxford: Oxford University Press.

Deacon, T. (2003). Multilevel selection in a complex adaptive system: the problem of language origins. In: B. H. Weber & D. J. Depew (eds) *Evolution and learning: the Baldwin effect reconsidered*, pp. 81–106. Cambridge, MA: MIT Press.

Deacon, T. (2009). Relaxed selection and the role of epigenesis in the evolution of language. In: M. Blumberg, J. Freeman & S. Robinson (eds) *Handbook of developmental behavioral neuroscience*, ch. 37. Oxford: Oxford University Press.

Hamilton, W. D. (1964a). The genetical evolution of social behaviour I. *Journal of Theoretical Biology* 7: 1–16.

Hamilton, W. D. (1964b) The genetical evolution of social behaviour II. *Journal of Theoretical Biology* 7: 17–52.

Heylighen, F. (1992). Evolution, selfishness and cooperation. *Journal of Ideas* 2: 70–76, 77–84.

Kropotkin, P. A. (1902). *Mutual aid: a factor of evolution.* London: William Heinemann.

Laland, K. N., Odling-Smee, J. & Feldman, M. W. (1996). The evolutionary consequences of niche construction: a theoretical investigation using two-locus theory. *Journal of Evolutionary Biology* 9: 293–316.

Laland, K. N., Odling-Smee, J. & Feldman, M. W. (2000). Niche construction, biological evolution, and cultural change. *Behavioral and Brain Sciences* 23: 131–146.

Lehmann, L. (2007). The evolution of trans-generational altruism: kin selection meets niche construction. *Journal of Evolutionary Biology* 20: 181–189.

Maynard Smith, J. & Szathmáry, E. (1995) *The major transitions in evolution*. Oxford: W. H. Freeman/Spektrum.

Nentwig, W. (1985). Social spiders catch larger prey: a study of *Anelosimus eximius* (Araneae: Theridiidae). *Behavioral Ecology and Sociobiology* 17: 79–85.

Nishikimi, M., Fukuyama, R., Minoshima, S., Shimizu, N. & Yagi, K. (1994). Cloning and chromosomal mapping of the human nonfunctional gene for L-gulono-gamma-lactone oxidase, the enzyme for L-ascorbic acid biosynthesis missing in man. *Journal of Biological Chemistry* 269: 13685–13688.

Nottebohm, F. (1970). Ontogeny of bird song. *Science* 167: 950–956.

Nottebohm, F. (1980). Brain pathways for vocal learning in birds: a review of the first 10 years. *Progress in Psychobiology and Physiological Psychology* 9: 85–124.

Nottebohm, F. (1996). A white canary on Mount Acropolis. *Journal of Comparative Physiology A: Neuroethology, Sensory, Neural, and Behavioral Physiology* 179: 149–156.

Nowak, M. A. (2006). Five rules for the evolution of cooperation. *Science* 314: 4.

Okanoya, K. (2004). The Bengalese finch: a window on the behavioral neurobiology of birdsong syntax. *Annual of the New York Academy of Science* 1016: 724–735.

Trivers, R. L. (1971). The evolution of reciprocal altruism. *Quarterly Review of Biology* 46: 35–57.

Wiles, J., Watson, J., Tonkes, B. & Deacon, T. (2005). Transient phenomena in learning and evolution: genetic assimilation and genetic redistribution. *Artificial Life* 11: 177–188.

Williams, G. C. (1966). *Adaptation and natural selection: a critique of some current evolutionary thought*. Princeton, NJ: Princeton University Press.

Wynne-Edwards, V. C. (1962). *Animal dispersion in relation to social behavior*. Edinburgh: Oliver & Boyd.

10

From Experiential-based to Relational-based Forms of Social Organization: A Major Transition in the Evolution of *Homo sapiens*

DWIGHT READ

THE EVOLUTIONARY TRAJECTORY from non-human primate to human forms of social organization encompasses an extraordinary series of social and cultural changes that belie our close anatomical affinity with other primates. Through our capacity to transfer what is in the conscious mind of one individual to another, we have developed adaptations that incorporate collective and not just individual thinking and learning, and thereby have been able to integrate together into larger-scale social entities what would be, for our non-human primate ancestors, disparate, spatially and behaviourally differentiated social groupings such as a primate troops or communities. This trajectory is not simply one of elaboration on characteristics already present in non-human primates in nascent form, but one that initially reached a hiatus due to a cognitive constraint acting on the consequences of interaction between two trends in primate evolution. One trend has been the elaboration and intensification of social interactions, especially through alliance or coalition formation (de Waal 1992). The other is a phylogenetic trend towards increased individualization of behaviour, which places exponentially greater cognitive demands on individuals having to cope with a social unit composed of behaviourally individualized members (Read 2004, 2005). The difficulty that individualization poses for social coherence was graphically described almost a century ago by the sociologist F. H. Hankins:

> Social life would become utterly impossible because of the utter chaos of individual behaviour . . . a society of free-willers in the sense now under discussion ['an undetermined, unrelated, and uncaused factor in human action'] would be Bedlam and Babel thrown into one. (1925, 622)

Proceedings of the British Academy **158**, 199–229. © The British Academy 2010.

A more modern phrasing than 'free will' would be behavioural unpre-
dictability of a completely individualized actor, the antithesis of a necessary condition for coherent and on-going social interaction to take place
(Misztal 2000, 7).

Jointly, these two trends led to an exponential increase in the complexity of the field of social interactions with which the members of a primate social unit must cope, thereby running into a cognitive constraint.
The cognitive constraint stems from the intersection between an increase
in the complexity of social interactions and conceptual restrictions
imposed by the limited size of working memory in non-human primates
(Read 2008). The negative consequence of this intersection was identified
by the French anthropologist Claude Lévi-Strauss for the great apes:

> It seems as if the great apes, having broken away from a specific pattern of
> behaviour, were unable to re-establish a norm on any new plane. The clear and
> precise instinctive behaviour of most mammals is lost to them, but the differ-
> ence is purely negative and the field that nature has abandoned remains
> unoccupied. (1969 [1967], 8)

The great apes, in their evolutionary trajectory, found resolution to
the conflict between exponentially increasing social complexity and cognitive constraints by reverting to smaller social units (Read 2004, 2005).
In contrast, the evolutionary trajectory leading to modern *Homo sapiens*
developed a different basis for the social organization of social groups
than the ancestral, primate pattern of social learning through extensive
face-to-face interaction. This different basis, it will be argued, arose out
of a shift from experiential- to relation-based social behaviours. Relation-
based behaviours stem from categorization of individuals according to
the relation of one individual to another (such as biological mother–
biological offspring categorization among the macaques; Dasser 1988a,
1988b) and not the traits of individuals *per se* (such as a category of
aggressive males). But even more, unlike trait-based categorizations,
relation categorizations lend themselves to the formation of new relation
categories through the conceptual 'product' of relations; that is, categorizations constructed from computing the relation of a relation. This
made it possible for social integration to be freed from being primarily an
epiphenomenon of experientially based social interaction.

Though the details of the evolutionary trajectory from experiential-
to relation-based social organization are necessarily speculative, the end-
result has been extensively studied through ethnographic fieldwork
among the small-scale hunter-gatherer societies whose mode of adapta-

tion preceded the larger, more complex social systems that arose as part of the Neolithic Revolution. These precursor, small-scale societies are structured around relations among individuals that are defined through a cultural kinship system expressed concretely by a society-specific kinship terminology that both defines and structures the domain of kin for the members of that society. Whereas face-to-face interaction is a necessary component of, and precursor to, long-term, on-going and non-disruptive social interaction in non-human primates, the organization of behaviour provided by culturally constructed kinship relations is a necessary component of, and precursor to, extensive social interaction and stable organization in hunter-gatherer—and subsequent—human societies. Consequently, we can identify the outcome of the evolutionary trajectory leading to relation-based forms of social organization by considering the organizational principles embedded in a kinship terminology through which social organization is then built around kin relations defined and expressed via a kinship terminology. Once the outcome is identified, we can then consider a possible evolutionary trajectory that begins with experientially based forms of social organization, as found in non-human primates, and leads to the form of relation-based forms of social organization that we find in extant human societies. Our goal in this chapter, then, is two-fold. First, to briefly characterize the way in which kin relations in human societies are organized and structured through a kinship terminology which provides the basis for relation-based forms of social organization; and, second, to identify a plausible trajectory beginning with experientially based forms of social organization and leading to relation-based forms.

KIN RELATIONS AND KINSHIP TERMINOLOGIES

Human societies can be usefully, if not precisely, distinguished by the organizational structure of the society as a whole. Characterization of human societies in this manner led to Elman Service's (1962) long-standing typology of band, tribal, chiefdom and state level forms of organizational structure for human societies, which has provided a framework for considering evolutionary change in human societies despite its oversimplification of variability in organizational configuration (Crumley 1995; Hass 1998). In this sequence of organizational structures, social units defined through culturally defined kinship relations are integrated at higher ontological levels using criteria derived from the structural properties of kinship terminology systems. However, these structural properties do not relate in a straightforward manner to external constraints on behaviour derived from factors such as ecological conditions, interaction with other societies and the like, but are instead based on an internal logic for the form of the kinship terminology and hence to culture-specific criteria that provide the terminology with its structural form (Leaf & Read n.d.; Read 1984, 2001, 2007b). The organization of behaviour, both individual and collective, provided by the structure of a kinship terminology as a system of logically interconnected concepts is, therefore, constructed as opposed to emergent. As a consequence, it is only those whose enculturation encompasses the same cultural kinship system who will interact in a mutually understood manner as culturally determined kin, thereby enabling social interaction that does not depend on prior face-to-face interaction.

The structure of a kinship terminology can be worked out and formally expressed by eliciting from informants the way kin terms form a system of interconnected concepts (Leaf 2006; Leaf & Read n.d., ch. 4). This may be done by asking for all pairs of kin terms what kin term one person (ego) would use to refer to a third person (alter 2) when ego refers to a second person (alter 1) by one of the paired terms and alter 1 refers to alter 2 by the other. For example, in the American/English kinship terminology and for the paired terms aunt and child, if ego refers to alter 1 by the kin term 'aunt' and alter 1 refers to alter 2 by the kin term 'child', then ego (properly) refers to alter 2 by the kin term 'cousin'. Thus in the American kinship terminology, the terms 'aunt', 'child' and 'cousin' are conceptually interconnected through the use of 'cousin' as the kin term that ego would use when ego refers to alter 1 as 'aunt' and alter 1 refers to alter 2 as 'child'. The complete structure of a terminology may be elicited systematically in this manner and the structure displayed as a directed graph where the nodes are kin terms connected by arrows (see Figures 10.1A and 10.1B).

In a directed graph showing the structure of a kinship terminology, each type of arrow (with an arrow type distinguished by features such as the shape of the arrow head and the features of the shaft) corresponds to one of the primary kin terms. The primary kin terms are the terms from which all other kin terms in that terminology may be computed; e.g. the primary kin terms are 'parent', 'child' and 'spouse' in the English/American terminology, as all other terms may be generated by taking products of these primary kin terms (Read 1984; Read & Behrens 1990). An arrow points to the kin term that is the product of the primary kin

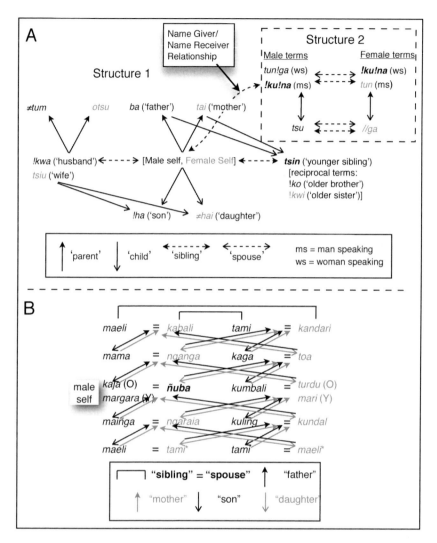

Figure 10.1. (A) Terminology structure (excluding affinal terms) for the !Kung San (hunter-gatherer group) in Botswana. Structure is based on two substructures joined by a name-giver/name-receiver (*!gu!na*) relationship activated by the parents giving the name of a close relative to a newborn child. The structure has a horizontal focus formed by spouse and sibling relations that are paralleled by residence groups strucutered bilaterally through chains of siblings and spouses of siblings. (B) Terminology structure for the Kariera (hunter-gatherer group) in western Australia from the perspective of a male speaker. Structure includes a prescriptive marriage rule for ego marrying a relative he/she refers to by the kin term *ñuba*. The terminology has a vertical structure joined by spouse links paralleled by the Kariera dividing themselves into four 'sections' structured vertically through parent/child links and horizontally through spouse links. Both groups have comparable modes of resource exploitation. Terms with black font are male-marked, terms with grey font are female-marked, and terms in bold are neutral.

term associated with the arrow and the kin term at the node where the arrow begins. Thus in Figure 10.1A, an arrow with an open arrow head corresponds to the primary kin term 'child' in the !Kung San (a hunter-gatherer group in Botswana) kinship terminology and points, for example, from the kin term *ba* ('father') to the kin term *tsin* ('younger sibling') since the product of the kin term *ba* with the kin term 'child' is the kin term *tsin* in the !Kung San terminology.

The structure of a kinship terminology may vary widely from one terminology to another as a result of internal differences in structural properties. Compare Figure 10.1A, which displays the structure of the kinship terminology for the !Kung San, with Figure 10.1B, the graph for the structure of the terminology for the Kariera (a hunter-gatherer group in Australia). Structural differences in the terminologies are evident from their respective graphs and arise from differences, in this example, from the presence of non-sex-marked primary kin terms, 'parent', 'child', 'sibling', 'spouse' and the 'name-giver/name-receiver' relation for the !Kung San kinship terminology (Read 2007a) versus the sex-marked primary kin terms 'father', 'mother', 'son' and 'daughter', and structural equations that lead to a *ñuba* ('cross-cousin') marriage rule for the Kariera terminology (Leaf & Read n.d., ch. 7). These differences in choice of primary terms and structural equations determine the structural differences between terminologies without relating to different modes of resource procurement, ecological conditions and the like. Both the !Kung San and the Kariera are hunter-gatherer groups that live in desert-like environments organized in residence groups in similar ways for tasks such as resource procurement (Leaf & Read n.d.). The structural differences in the terminologies are culture-specific, hence historically contingent, yet constrained in structural form by general, structural properties common to kinship terminologies (Leaf & Read n.d., ch. 5; Read 2001, 2007b).

Culturally constructed kinship relations are a group-, not an individual-level, phenomenon whose functionality arises through and depends upon cultural knowledge being distributed among the members of a social group through enculturation. It is only with other persons who share the same kinship terminology knowledge that kin relations may be identified and are meaningful. When one person or group encounters another person or group for the first time and the latter also share the same kinship terminology knowledge, they can determine, according to their mutually shared conceptual system of kin relations, that they are kin to one another and in so doing their status vis-à-vis each other changes from that of strangers likely to engage in unpredictable and possibly dangerous behaviour, to kin who will act in a predictable and supportive manner. This contrasts sharply with the highly aggressive and lethal encounters between males in different chimpanzee communities (despite transfer of females between communities) and was a transformation in behaviour that had a profound impact on the evolutionary trajectory of our species. The transformation overcame the cognitive barrier reached by the great apes for more encompassing patterns of social behaviours (Read 2004, 2005) by changing the basis for social behaviour from face-to-face encounters to that of a constructed, kinship relational system for determining the domain of individuals among whom social interaction may take place, along with the behaviours expected when individuals act in accordance with one's culturally constructed kinship system.

FORMS OF SOCIAL ORGANIZATION AND EVOLUTIONARY CHANGE IN SOCIAL BEHAVIOUR

In order to make evident the implications that the change from experiential to relational social behaviours had for social organization, we will distinguish four forms of social behaviour that can occur between any two individuals, and their associated form of social organization. The four forms of social behaviour are:

(1) asocial
(2) action/reaction
(3) interaction and
(4) social interaction

These forms of behaviour must be considered in the context of a temporal event consisting of the *prior* behaviour of an initiating individual and the *post* behaviour of a responding individual. The forms will be distinguished by the probabilities of a prior behaviour by the initiating individual and an associated post behaviour by the responding individual.

These four forms of social behaviour do not exhaust all possibilities, but can be related usefully to changes in the form of social organization among primate species that evolutionarily led to *Homo sapiens*. Of the four, the final is uncommon among the non-human primates and only partially incorporated among the chimpanzees. It only becomes fully central to systems of social organization with the appearance of our species, *Homo sapiens*.

Assume a repertoire of behaviours engaged in by one or more of the members of a group of individuals. We may use set notation to denote the repertoire of behaviours as a set of behaviours $B = \{b_i\}$ and to denote the group of individuals as a finite set of individuals $I = \{A, B, C \ldots\}$. For each individual, A, in I, let b_A denote a behaviour from B engaged in by individual A. (Individual A may engage in more than one behaviour from B, but for notational simplicity we will focus on a single behaviour by individual A, hence we can use the same symbol to represent an individual and to index the behaviour engaged in by that individual.) We will refer to a *dyadic behaviour episode* as a sequence of behaviours in which one individual engages in a behaviour and another individual acts in response to the behaviour of the initiating individual. The same individual may sometimes be the initiator of a dyadic behaviour episode and sometimes the responding individual. When individual A initiates the dyadic behaviour episode with behaviour b_A, we will refer to the initiating behaviour by A as the *prior* behaviour b_A by individual A. By this we mean that A does behaviour b_A prior to another individual B doing some behaviour b_B in response to the behaviour b_A. When individual A is the responding individual in a dyadic behaviour episode, we will refer to the response behaviour b_A as the *post* behaviour by individual A. By this we mean that individual A does behaviour b_A in response to the behaviour b_B of some individual B.

In general, the occurrence of particular behaviour by an individual over some time-frame and under specified conditions may be represented probabilistically. For a dyadic behaviour episode, we may say that, over a specified time-frame, an individual I has some probability of engaging in a behaviour that initiates a dyadic behaviour episode. Similarly, an individual has some probability of engaging in a specific post behaviour in response to the prior behaviour by another individual. For some behaviours, these probabilities may not be subject to learning; e.g, for genetically based, so-called instinctual behaviours. Other behaviours may be subject to learning and so the probability of a behaviour in the present will depend on the past consequences an individual has experienced when engaging in that behaviour. Our concern here is with dyadic behaviour episodes and so we will be concerned with the probabilities of prior and post behaviours. We may define the four forms of social behaviour we identified above as follows using probabilities for prior and post behaviours. Formal definitions are given in Box 10.1.

Box 10.1. Mathematical definitions

1. Asocial behaviour
Prior behaviour: Probability, $Pr(b_A)$, for behaviour b_A by individual A depends only on the behaviour, $b_{A'}$. Post behaviour: Conditional probability for behaviour b_A by individual A given prior behaviour b_B by individual B is independent of the prior behaviour b_B: $Pr(b_A \mid b_B) = Pr(b_A)$.

2. Action/reaction behaviour
Prior behaviour: Probability, $Pr(b_A)$, for behaviour b_A by individual A depends only on the behaviour, $b_{A'}$. Post behaviour: $Pr(b_A \mid b_B) \neq Pr(b_A)$.

3. Interaction behaviour
Prior behaviour: Let $\theta j = Pr(b_B)$ be a parameter whose value may be specific to B. Probability for behaviour b_A by individual A is a function of θj: $Pr(b_A) = f(\theta j)$. We will use the notation $Pr(b_A \mid \theta j = Pr(b_B))$ to denote the probability that A does the behaviour b_A knowing that B does behaviour b_B with probability $Pr(b_B)$. Post behaviour: $Pr(b_A \mid b_B)^* \neq Pr(b_A)$. (The '' indicates that the conditional probability is subject to updating by individual A through Bayesian learning.)*

4. Social interaction
Prior behaviour: Let $\varphi_{A,B} = Pr(b_B \mid b_A)$ be a parameter whose value may be specific to B and A. The probability for behaviour b_A by individual A is a function of φ_B: $Pr(b_A) = g(\varphi_{A,B})$. We will use the notation $Pr(b_A \varphi_{A,B} = Pr(b_B \mid b_A))$ to denote the probability that A does the behaviour b_A knowing that B does behaviour b_B with conditional probability $Pr(b_B \mid b_A)$. Post behaviour: $Pr(b_A \mid b_B)^* \neq Pr(b_A)$.

5. Phylogenetic trend
We can express the phylogenetic trend by the sequence of probabilities for prior behaviour: (1) $Pr(b_A)$ (solitary behaviour), (2) $Pr(b_A \mid b_B) \neq Pr(b_B)$ (action/reaction behaviour), (3) $Pr(b_A \mid \theta j = Pr(b_B))$ (learned interaction) and (4) $Pr(b_A \mid \varphi_{A,B} = Pr(b_B \mid b_A))$ (social interaction). The first three can be realized by individuals through Bayesian updating of prior probabilities in accordance with the outcomes of encounter events. Benefits obtained from these prior behaviours do not, generally speaking, depend on symmetry in behaviour between the individuals involved. The fourth behaviour depends upon a parameter value difficult to assess accurately without extensive face-to-face learning.

Asocial behaviour

For asocial behaviour, the post behaviour of one individual, *A,* is statistically independent of the prior behaviour of another individual, *B.* Hence the probability of individual *A* engaging in behaviour b_A does not take into account the prior behaviour, b_B, by individual *B.* Associated with asocial behaviour is a solitary form of social organization, hence the distribution pattern of individuals in space will tend to be random after taking into account constraints such as resource location and physical limitations on the spatial location of individuals (see Figure 10.2, solitary

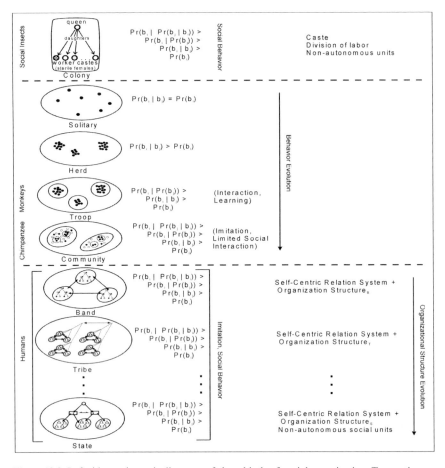

Figure 10.2. Left side—schematic diagrams of three kinds of social organization. Top section—social organization for eusocial insects. Middle section—evolutionary trend for social organization arising out behaviours between pairs of individuals. Bottom section—evolution in the organizational structure for human societies, keeping fixed the behavioural basis for social organization.

social structure). Among the primates, many of the prosimians have been characterized as displaying asocial behaviour. Asocial behaviour does not characterize any of the Old World monkeys (*Cercopithecoids*) or New World monkeys (*Ceboids*). Among the great apes, the orang utans (*Pongo pygmaeus*) provide an example of behaviour that is close to solitary social organization as there is little interaction other than chance encounters between individuals outside of copulatory behaviour. For *Pan troglodytes*, females (at least in East Africa) have been characterized as asocial in comparison to the highly social behaviour of males.

Action/reaction behaviour

The post behaviour of individual A depends, for at least some of the behaviours engaged in by A, on the prior behaviour of another individual B. For these behaviours individual A is reacting to prior behaviour by individual B. From an evolutionary perspective, the probabilities are fixed when the probabilities are genetically encoded and individuals do not yet have the cognitive capacity for updating probabilities through learning. Action/reaction behaviour may be asymmetric since an individual can react to the behaviour of another individual who acts asocially. It can directly affect the form of social organization: a response behaviour can be negative; e.g. the reaction b_A, of A to an action b_B, by individual B, may be to move away or disassociate from B, in which case the social structure is pushed in the direction of dispersal of individuals. Alternatively, a response behaviour can be positive; e.g. the reaction of A may be to move towards B, in which case the social structure is pushed towards herding or flocking behaviour, where each individual acts positively to a neighbouring individual. Group boundaries may arise from the probability values for action/reaction behaviour, thereby leading to emergent social organization in the form of herds or flocks (see Figure 10.2, herd social structure).

Interaction behaviour

Interaction behaviour differs from action/reaction behaviour in the fact that prior behaviour by individual A anticipates the behaviour of B based on experience with their behaviour pattern. Like action/reaction behaviour, interaction behaviour can be asymmetric, with individual A acting according to their experience with B while individual B may simply be acting in response to behaviour b_A by individual A.

Experience can lead to genetic encoding for a behaviour based on prior experience (the Baldwin effect [Baldwin 1896; Simpson 1953]), though the likelihood of genetic encoding depends on consistency in interaction behaviour patterns, which decreases as behaviours become more individualized and need not be consistent over long enough time periods for parameter values to become genetically encoded. Non-genetic encoding arose with evolution of the cognitive capacity for learned behaviour. Individual A can learn the likelihood of a behaviour by B through the outcomes of encounters with B, so more elaborated forms of social organization in species with more individualized behaviour can arise through interaction behaviour with increasing learning capacity. The capacity for learned behaviours also affects post behaviours, since the likelihood of doing behaviour b_A in response to behaviour b_B can be updated by taking into account the consequence of one's post behaviour in response to the prior behaviour b_B by individual *B*.

The form of social organization that arises from learned interaction among the primates will be referred to as a troop structure (see Figure 10.2). Troop structure organization is widespread among the Old World monkeys (*Cercopithecoids*) and the New World monkeys (*Ceboids*) and consists of cohesive, integrated social organization within a group and isolation of groups from one another, except for transference of individuals (typically males, except for the piliocolobines) from one troop to another around the time of sexual maturity (di Fiore & Rendall 1994, 9944). The effectiveness of a troop form of social organization can be seen in the adaptation of different species of macaques to virtually every climatic condition, as well as to coexistence with humans in India.

Social interaction

Here we use Talcott Parsons' definition of social interaction:

> . . . in the case of interactions with social objects a further dimension is added. Part of ego's expectation . . . consists in the probable reaction of alter to ego's possible action, a reaction which comes to be *anticipated in advance* and thus to affect ego's own choices. (Parsons 1964, 5, emphasis added)

Social interaction differs from interaction by virtue of individual *A* taking into account when doing behaviour b_A what they assess to be the likely response b_B by individual *B*. Interaction and social interaction behaviours also differ with respect to the consequences of asymmetric behaviour.

Asymmetric *interaction* behaviour by *A* is advantageous to *A* since *A* takes into account past behaviour by *B*, whereas *B* does not take into account the behaviour of *A*: i.e. *A* uses more information about the behaviour of *B* than *B* uses about *A* in responding to *A*'s behaviour. In contrast, asymmetric *social interaction* behaviour by *A* may be disadvantageous to *A* when *A* attempts to assess the likelihood for each of *B*'s possible responses to *A*'s behaviour, since *A*'s assessment of *B*'s likely response may be subject to error, thereby leading *A* to engage in a behaviour unrelated to *B*'s average behaviour pattern. Hence, in this scenario, *A* would do worse on average than simply acting on the basis of *B*'s average behaviour pattern based on *A*'s past experience with *B*. In addition, *B* may simply

revert to novel post action/reaction behaviour in response to the behaviour
b by A, and thereby engage in behaviour unanticipated by A.

For example, if A assesses in a Prisoner's Dilemma context that B will
act cooperatively (as jointly cooperative behaviour would have the highest payoff), and A therefore acts cooperatively, B may simply respond
with non-cooperative behaviour. Social interaction will, therefore, be
most effective when this behaviour pattern is symmetric and leads each
actor to engage in the behaviour anticipated by the other. With symmetric social interaction, A and B may be independently biasing their own
behaviour in the direction anticipated by the other individual, and therefore any updating of anticipated behaviours by A and/or B will simply
reinforce their respective behaviours. When social interaction is symmetric, cooperative behaviour such as in a Prisoner's Dilemma context will be
reinforced when each individual acts under the assumption that the other
individual will act cooperatively to achieve the highest payoff; thus both
individuals receive the reward for jointly cooperative behaviour and
thereby reinforce their respective assessments. But continuing with symmetric social interaction is not necessary and one or the other of the
interacting individuals may revert to action/reaction as a post behaviour.

Symmetric social interaction

Social interaction as a learned behaviour depends both on (1) a cognitive
learning system that is sufficiently evolved so as to be able to estimate the
parameter values for the likelihood of post behaviour b_B by individual B
when individual A engages in prior behaviour b_A (i.e. $\varphi_{A,B} = \Pr(b_B \mid b_A)$)
and (2) sufficiently stable encounter outcomes between individuals that
individual A can track the response of individual B in situations where A
has engaged in behaviour b_A in the presence of individual B and vice versa.

The non-human primate taxa most closely related to *Homo sapiens*
include an increasingly evolved cognitive learning system, hence we might
expect social interaction to be introduced with the more closely related
non-human primates. However, acting against this is the trend towards
increased individualization of behaviour (Read 2004). This makes learned
behaviour as a basis for interaction of individuals in the same group
problematic, thus reducing the likelihood of conditions under which
learned social interaction would arise even with an evolved cognitive
learning system.

Interference between these two trends occurs with the common chimpanzees (*Pan troglodytes*). Their form of social organization has evolved

from a cohesive troop form of social organization based on learned interaction, into communities. Though a community can be as large as, or larger than a troop, its internal dynamics are more complex and less cohesive. Briefly, a chimpanzee community is characterized by:

- dispersal of females at time of puberty (Wrangham 1979);
- significantly more frequent and longer rates of grooming with more time spent in social dyads by males in comparison to females (Lehmann & Boesch 2008 and references therein);
- variation in sociality of females: asocial females in East Africa (Arnold & Whiten 2003; Goodall 1986; Wrangham et al. 1992), more social females in West Africa (Lehmann & Boesch 2008);
- temporary, fission-fusion subgroups in larger communities composed primarily of males (Gagneux et al. 1999);
- unstable male dominance hierarchies (Muller & Mitani 2005);
- extensive grooming of adult males (Spruijt et al. 1992), especially upon subgroup reformation (Bauer 1979), in contrast with extensive biological mother/daughter and sister/sister grooming among female philopatric (females remain in natal troop) Cercopithecoids (Gouzoules & Gouzoules 1987);
- high levels of conflict within communities: female–female conflict over access to food and defence of offspring, male–male conflict over dominance rank and male–female conflict over sexual access (Nishida 1979); and
- highly aggressive and violent community territorial defence by males that can lead to inter-community killings (Nishida & Hiraiwa-Hasegawa 1987).

Rather than a cohesive, well-integrated social system as is found with the Cercopithecoids, a chimpanzee community is characterized by instability at virtually all levels except aggressive maintenance of its boundaries.

Embedded within this pattern of instability are several examples of learned social interaction. First, males form 'short-term coalitions in which two individuals join forces to direct aggression toward third parties' (Muller & Mitani 2005, 278). These dyads are not based on kin-relatedness (Mitani et al. 2002). Instead, '[i]ndividuals belonging to the same age cohort may be particularly attractive social partners because they grow up together, are generally familiar with each other, and share similar social interests and power throughout their lives' (Mitani et al. 2002, 14); that is, the two males forming the dyad have had sufficient encounters with each other for each to learn the parameter values for the other for social interaction (i.e. $\varphi_{A,B} = \Pr(b_B \mid b_A)$ and $\varphi_{B,A} = \Pr(b_A \mid b_B)$). Second, although the reasons why male chimpanzees may share meat after killing a prey are not fully known, one 'hypothesis proposed to explain meat sharing implicates the use of meat as a political tool' via 'male chimpanzees shar[ing] meat strategically with others in order to curry their favor and support' (Mitani et al. 2002, 18). Third, when patrolling community boundaries 'males who patrol together also groom and form coalitions with each other frequently' (Muller & Mitani 2005, 308), and patrol 'with partners with whom they have strong social bonds and on whom they can rely to take risks' (Mitani et al. 2002, 19). And fourth, grooming by males is not along biological kin lines. Instead 'Male chimpanzees use grooming to cultivate and reinforce social bonds with others upon whom they rely for coalitionary support' (Muller & Mitani 2005, 306).

In sum, the non-human primates present us with a phylogenetic evolutionary trend of individuals incorporating more precise information about the behaviour of other group members while collective social behaviour increases in complexity with increased individuation. When symmetric social interaction takes place, each individual acts in the manner anticipated by the other individual, thereby reinforcing coordinated behaviour, but asymmetric social interaction behaviour may arise through the well-known problem of cheaters. Either party to symmetric social interaction can cheat and revert to a post behaviour action/reaction strategy that may be more beneficial, at least in the short term, than social interaction behaviour.

Symmetric social interaction is also costly to learn and must be maintained constantly—'Given the importance of coalitions, *male chimpanzees work hard* to obtain this valuable social service' (Muller & Mitani 2005, 314, emphasis added)—and is hence a constraint on learned symmetric social interaction becoming the behavioural basis for social groups. The solution to forming large, cohesive groups based on symmetric social interaction that was found during the evolution of *Homo sapiens* involved a shift to a constructed cultural kinship relation basis for symmetric social interaction, rather than learned, experiential interaction.

FROM EMERGENT TO CONSTRUCTED SYSTEMS OF SYMMETRIC SOCIAL INTERACTION

The evolutionary pathway undertaken by our hominin ancestors from experientially to relationally based social interaction builds on two cognitive capacities; the first of these appears to be present in the chimpanzees while evidence for the second is more equivocal: (1) a concept of self and (2) a 'theory of mind'.

Unique to the evolution of *Homo sapiens* is the introduction of two other cognitive capacities critical to the shift from experiential- to relational-based social interaction: (3) categorizations based on the concept of a relation between individuals, and (4) formation of new social categories/units through recursive composition of relations. We begin this section by briefly describing the first two of these four capacities. Then we consider in more detail how (3) and (4) gave rise to an internally coherent, stable system of socially interacting individuals through a conceptually formulated, logically consistent, computational system of relations—the precursor to a kinship terminology system—that defines the cohort of socially interacting individuals comprising what we refer to as a society. A cultural transmission process that cultural anthropologists refer to as enculturation enabled the faithful transmission (both vertically and horizontally) of this conceptual basis, a necessary condition for a group of individuals to form a society based on kin relations (Read et al. in press).

Four cognitive capacities

Concept of self

By the 'concept of self' we mean the cognitive awareness of one's existence, or identity, in contrast to the existence of others. Experimental evidence for a concept of self, at least as measured through recognition of oneself in a mirror image, is substantial for the chimpanzees (Schilhab 2004), so we may assume that a concept of self was already present in a primate ancestor common to the chimpanzees and the hominins.

Theory of mind

By a theory of mind we mean not only that one has awareness of one's own basis for action and one's own mental representations, but that one is able to appreciate that other conspecifics may also have their own action and/or mental representations. Experimental work on the presence of a theory of mind in chimpanzees is equivocal (Heyes 1998; Povinelli & Vonk 2004), though there is general agreement that while chimpanzees do not have a theory of mind comparable to humans (Call & Tomasello 2008), they are capable of reasoning about behaviour. Less clear is whether they are able to attribute and reason about mental states in others (Focquaert et al. 2008). We will assume that if a cognitive capacity for theory of mind was not already present in a common ancestor, it arose early during hominin evolution.

Categorization based on relations

By categorization based on relations, we mean a shift to categorization based on a conceptual relation linking pairs of individuals rather than on the properties of individuals themselves. The extent to which categorization based on relations occurs among the non-human primates is unknown except for one experiment with long-tailed macaques (Dasser 1988a, 1988b). Though categorization based on relations may be rare among the non-human primates, the capacity for this kind of categorization did arise among our hominin ancestors. Categorization based on a conceptual relation linking pairs of individuals contrasts with the more common categorization based on attributes of objects, and the shift from attribute- to relation-based modes of categorization was a critical evolutionary development, as it makes possible the formation of new relations from pre-existing ones through recursion-based conceptual products of relations, rather than purely through experience. Categorization based on attributes of objects depends on experience with those objects and new, non-hierarchical, attribute categories cannot be inferred from existing attribute categories. In contrast, relation categories coupled with recursive reasoning makes possible the formation of new relations and relation categories directly from currently identified relations. However, the power of recursive reasoning is not available to non-human primates, including chimpanzees (Hauser et al. 2002; Spinozzi et al. 1999), probably due to insufficient working memory (Read 2008).

Recursive reasoning and relation formation

We can illustrate the way in which a new relation may be formed from an already identified relation through recursion by considering the construction of a family tree. Assume we already know that a 'mother' relation assigns to a given person that person's mother. We can now form a new relation, 'mother's mother', by defining it recursively from just the 'mother' relation. To do so, start with ego—the focal person for the family tree—apply the 'mother' relation to ego, and trace to ego's mother. Now take ego's mother as ego, apply the 'mother' relation to this new ego and trace to (ego's mother's) mother; that is, to ego's 'mother's mother'. We now define the 'mother's mother' relation to be the female determined in this manner; that is, the 'mother's mother' relation applied to ego traces from ego to ego's mother's mother. Other relations such as 'mother's father', 'father's mother' or 'father's father' may be defined recursively in a similar manner if the 'father' relation is already known. Or the recursion may be continued further to define the relation 'mother's mother's mother', and so on. Thus, unlike the situation with attribute categorization, recursive reasoning makes possible the formation of new relation categories based on ones already identified.

Next, we want to sketch out how a system of recursively defined relations might arise from an evolutionary viewpoint, and the implications this had for social organization and structure. We will begin by assuming a single relation, the M ('mother') relation—based on categorization of actual biological mother/offspring relations—is already part of the cognitive repertoire of individuals; note that the argument will apply equally to any conceptual relation expressed in the form of dyads and not just the mother relation. Now assume that we have a set of individuals, I, each having the four cognitive properties discussed above as part of their cognitive repertoire. In Figure 10.3 (1), female A, the biological daughter of female B, conceptualizes the relation between herself and her biological mother as an instantiation of the M relation. By virtue of theory of mind, she believes her mother, B, also instantiates the same M relation between herself (B) and a female C believed by A to be the biological mother of B. Thus the (B, C) dyad is believed by A to be an instantiation of the M relation perceived by her mother, B (see Figure 10.3 (2)). The instantiation is a belief from the perspective of A since A projects onto her mother A's belief that her mother also perceives an M relation. The thought cloud in Figure 10.3 (2) is in grey for female B to indicate that this is the relation that A *believes* is held by her mother, which may or may not correspond to what is actually conceptualized by her mother.

By recursion, individual A can now construct the MM relation through which individual A perceives that she and female C form an instantiation of the constructed MM relation (see Figure 10.3 (3); for details, see also Box 10.2). The relation MM differs in a crucial way from the M relation. The MM relation is constructed from the M relation through recursive reasoning and not from categorization of actual 'biological grandmother/ biological granddaughter' dyads. Though the M relation may arise from a categorization of biological relations, recursive reasoning leads to the construction of a new relation, MM, without depending upon prior categorization of dyads based on biological relations. Instead, categorization now becomes a *consequence* of the new relation formed via recursive reasoning

Box 10.2. Recursive relation construction

To illustrate the recursive construction of relations, let the two place predicate $M(\_, \_)$ represent the biological mother/biological daughter relation for a set of individuals, B, so that, for all A, B in I, $M(A, B)$ is true when, and only when, B is the biological mother of A. We can recursively form a new relation, $MM(\_, \_)$, where $MM(A, C)$ is true if, and only if, there is a B in I with $M(A, B)$ and $M(B, C)$ both true, as follows. Since there is a single B for which $M(A, B)$ is true, let $B = M(A,\_)$, hence we can think of B as the unique outcome of applying the single-place predicate $M(A, \_)$ to the set I. Similarly, we can let $C = MM(A, \_)$ when $MM(A,C)$ is true. Note that there is a single C for which $MM(A, C)$ is true. Then $C = MM(A,\_) = M(B,\_) = M(M(A, \_),\_)$, hence MM can be constructed recursively by applying the M relation to the outcome of the M relation.

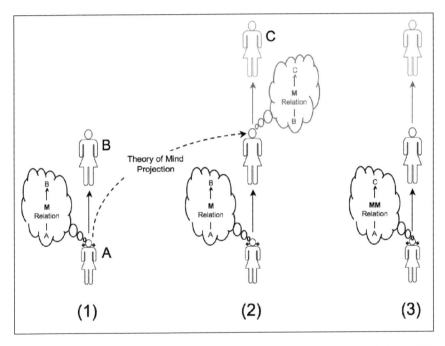

Figure 10.3. (1) Individual A, biological daughter of B, conceptualizes a mother relation and (2) projects, via the theory of mind, the same relation concept to her biological mother B. (3) By composition of relations, individual A constructs a relation linking her to individual C, the female A believes to be the target of the mother relation she has attributed to B.

and would encompass all those instances where, by virtue of theory of mind, individual A projects onto another individual the relation MM. Hence, once constructed, the MM relation gives rise to a category of dyads that are the perceived instantiation of the MM relation. In other words, one of the consequences of constructing a new relation such as

MM using recursion is that the newly constructed relation does not depend on the biological facts of who is related genetically to whom, but on beliefs held by individuals about what—allegedly—the biological facts are. *Recursion of relations leads to decoupling of constructed relations from the biological basis for conceptualizing the relations involved in forming the constructed relations.*

Reciprocal relations

If we consider the relation between *B* and *A* from the perspective of *B*, then *A* will be in a biological daughter relation ***D*** with respect to *B*. Now

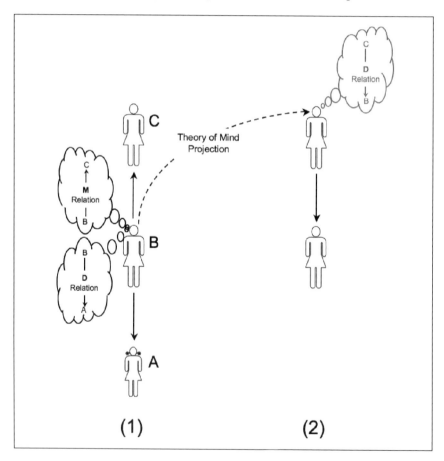

Figure 10.4. (1) Individual *B* conceptualizes an ***M*** (mother) relation to *C* and a ***D*** (daughter) relation to *A*. (2) Individual *B* attributes the ***D*** relation to *C*, hence *B* believes that *C* has *B* as a target for the ***D*** relation, a precursor for a reciprocal social relationship from *B*'s perspective.

consider that individual B perceives both an M relation with C and a D relation with A (see Figure 10.4 (1)) and projects the D relation onto individual C (see Figure 10.4 (2)). An instantiation of the projected D relation will be individual B: hence from the perspective of B, B perceives that individual C will have a daughter relation for which individual B is the instantiation from C's perspective. In other words, B will perceive not only that B has an M relation to C, but B will believe that C perceives a D relation from C to B. Consequently, B will believe that B and C are conceptually linked to each other. Hence the precursor for reciprocal social interaction from B's perspective, namely that B not only perceives a relation with C, but B believes C also perceives a reciprocal relation with B, is in place.

Though illustrated with the M and D relation, the pattern can arise with any relation R that B has with C where there is a corresponding reciprocal relation S that B may be believed to have with A. The projection of the relation S onto C will have B as an instantiation of the S relation from B's perspective and so B will perceive that B has a relation R with C and will believe that C perceives a relation S between C and B.

Functionality of the projected relation: symmetric social interaction

The importance of perceiving a relation R lies not in the relation *per se*, but in behaviours and/or motivation for behaviours that can be associated with the relation and thereby lead not just to interaction, but to social interaction. A behaviour such as altruism, which is introduced through selection based on biological kinship, is not part of social interaction when there is no anticipation on the part of the actor that the behaviour will be reciprocated in some manner. In contrast, a behaviour based on a cultural kinship relation satisfies the conditions for social interaction since the conceptual system that structures cultural kinship (namely a kinship terminology) forms a system of reciprocal relations with expected, reciprocal behaviour. If A recognizes B as a cultural kin, that is, A has a kin term used to refer to B and A knows that B shares with A the same kinship terminology, then A also knows that B has a kin term for A, hence B recognizes A as a cultural kin. Therefore A has expectations about reciprocal behaviour on the part of B by virtue of the fact that A is a cultural kin of B and A and B share the same knowledge about the particular cultural kin relation that A has towards B from B's perspective.

To initiate social interaction, each of *A* and *B* needs to recognize that the one is conceptually linked to the other.[1] Otherwise, there is no reason for expecting reciprocal behaviour. In kin-based societies, typically there cannot be social interaction between individuals *A* and *B* without *A* and *B* first establishing that they are (cultural) kin—which means that *B* is already in the conceptual domain of *A*'s cultural kin and *A* is in the conceptual domain of *B*'s cultural kin and both know that this is true of the other person. Absent a cultural kin relation, an encounter between two individuals who are strangers to each other may be conceived of as a dangerous state of affairs and in some cases may lead to one person killing the other. Among the traditional Waorani of South America, for example, if person *B* comes to *A*'s village and *B* does not have a cultural kin relation with *A*, then whether social interaction could occur between them was resolved in the negative by *A* killing *B* (Davis & Yost 2001). Nor is this extreme example of fear of non-kin an isolated case: on Anuta in the South Pacific '[a]nyone not incorporated into the kinship system is an outsider . . . an open enemy' (Feinberg 1981, 133).

We can include under the theory of mind projection a behaviour (or kind of behaviour) that one individual might engage in vis-à-vis another individual when the behaviour is viewed as being part of a relation *R* linking this pair of individuals. More precisely, suppose that individual *B* has an *R* relation with individual *C* and a reciprocal *S* relation with individual *A*, where the biological relations among *A*, *B* and *C* may be indeterminate. Suppose that individual *B* associates directing behaviour *b* (or the kind of behaviour represented by *b*) towards an individual when that individual is a target of the *S* relation conceptualized by *B* (see Figure 10.5 (1)); for example, *B* may be engaging (even non-socially) in behaviour *b* with *A* as a consequence of *A* being a target of the *S* relation conceptualized by *B*. By theory of mind, individual *B* projects the relation *S* and the conceptually associated behaviour *b* to individual *C* (see Figure 10.5 (2)). Via theory of mind projection, individual *B* believes that individual *C* will engage in the behaviour *b* towards oneself since individual *B* is a target of the *S* relation that *B* believes to be a relation concept held by *C*. Now if individual *B* believes that individual *C* will engage in the behaviour *b* (or *b*-like behaviour) with respect to oneself, then individual *B* can engage in the behaviour *b* directed towards *C* in the belief that

---

[1] A conceptual linkage between individuals is not universally a necessary prerequisite for social interaction as shown by the eusocial insects.

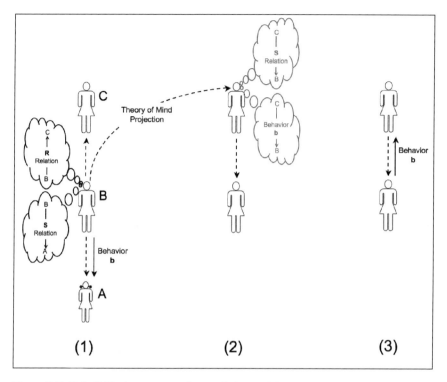

Figure 10.5. (1) Individual *B* conceptualizes a relation **R** with *C* and a reciprocal relation **S** with *A*. In addition, *B* directs behaviour *b* towards individual *A* when *A* is the target of the **S** relation conceptualized by *B*. (2) Individual *B* projects the relation **S** to individual *C* and *B* is the target of the relation **S** believed by *B* to be a relation conceptualized by *C*. (3) Individual *B* directs behaviour *b* towards *C* due to *B*'s belief that *B* is a target of the **S** relation held by *C*. That is, *B* believes *C* will direct behaviour *b* towards *B* since *B* directs behaviour *b* towards *A* due to *B*'s relation with *A*, hence *B* expects *C* to direct behaviour *b* towards *B*.

individual *C* will reciprocate with behaviour *b* directed towards *B* (see Figure 10.5 (3)). *We now have a basis for interaction to become social interaction: one individual acts towards another individual under the belief that the other individual will act in a reciprocal manner. Further, and critically, this basis for social interaction is decoupled from any requirement of biological linkages among the individuals in question.*

Reciprocal relations as a basis for symmetric social interaction

While the projection of a behaviour linked to a relation may lead to the belief that this or a comparable behaviour will be engaged in by the other

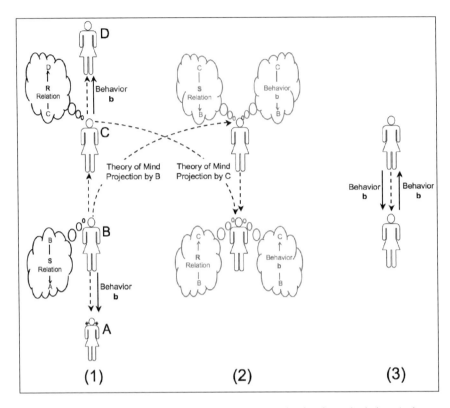

Figure 10.6. (1) Individuals *B* and *C* each share the same pair of reciprocal relations (only one relation from each pair shown for clarity) and each associates behaviour *b* with a relation, with individual *C* directing behaviour *b* to individual *D* and individual *B* directing behaviour *b* to individual *A*. (2) Each of *B* and *C* projects their conceptual relations onto the other individual. (3) Each of *B* and *C* directs behaviour *b* towards the other individual on the basis of one's belief that the other individual will reciprocate with *b* or *b*-like behaviour. The beliefs of both *B* and *C* are reinforced by the behaviour of the other individual.

individual, the reciprocal behaviour need not actually occur unless the other individual has both constructed a complementary belief system about the behaviour of the initiating individual, and reciprocates with a behaviour directed towards the initiating individual. Cheating—defined here to include the situation where reciprocal behaviour is not initiated despite individuals sharing a complementary belief system—is always possible, and if *B* acts towards *C* just under the *belief* that *C* will reciprocate, then *B* has also initiated conditions that favour cheating by *C*.

Symmetric social interaction depends upon each individual actually engaging in reciprocal behaviour. If each person believes that the other will reciprocate the behaviour in question, then the basis for continued, reciprocal behaviours will have been established. For individuals B and C to each have the belief that the other individual will reciprocate with behaviour b, it suffices for individual C to associate behaviour b with the relation R in addition to individual B associating the same behaviour with relation S, where R and S are reciprocal relations, as shown in Figure 10.6 (the reciprocal relations have not been drawn for each individual B and C for clarity of the figure). Under these conditions, individual B will construct the belief that individual C will reciprocate with the behaviour b, and that individual C will independently construct the belief that individual B will reciprocate with the behaviour b. When each individual engages in behaviour b directed towards the other individual based on one's beliefs, one's beliefs are reinforced through confirmation of that belief by the actual behaviour of the other individual.

Coordination through computational conceptual systems

For the functional benefit of reciprocal behaviours to be realized, it is necessary that the individuals in the population recognize in a comparable manner the kind of relation with which a behaviour or complex of behaviours is associated. The relation becomes a marker for individuals who will reciprocate a behaviour b, and agreement between actor and recipient with respect to enactment of the behaviour will occur when both the actor and the recipient happen to associate the behaviour b with the same relation R and its reciprocal relation S. Consequently, the likelihood of the functional benefit potentially accruing from behaviour b actually being realized through reciprocal behaviours is determined by the degree of coordination/agreement among group members with regard to the relations that are recognized and the behaviours associated with those relations. The latter is a precursor to institutionalized social action/role systems (Nadel 1957) that 'are clothed in cultural meaning systems so that institutions cannot be properly represented without . . . reference to shared meanings' (Fararo 1997, 76).

The coordination problem was solved with the construction of cultural kin relations transmitted through enculturation by virtue of the fact that the system of cultural kin relations we find expressed through a kinship terminology in a human society is (1) a computational system through which kin relations may be calculated in a simple manner, (2) a generative computational system which facilitates faithful transmission of the conceptual system and (3) a system of reciprocal kin relations. By a computational system, we mean that two individuals A and B can compute the kin relation they have to each other just by reference to a third individual *C*, for whom each of *A* and *B* knows his or her kin term relation:

> [Maori kin] terms permit *comparative strangers* to fix kinship rapidly . . . With mutual relationship terms all that is required is the discovery of one common relative. Thus, if A is related to B as child to mother, veitanani, whereas C is related to B as veitacini, sibling of the same sex, then it follows that A is related to C as child to mother, although they never before met or knew it. *Kin terms are predictable. If two people are each related to a third, then they are related to each other*. (Sahlins 1962, 155, emphasis added)

This permits defining a binary product, denoted by o, of kin terms as follows. If K is the kin term A (properly) uses to refer to B and L is the kin term B (properly) uses to refer to C, then L o K is the kin term (if any) that A (properly) uses to refer to C. The computational system of kin terms is generative in the algebraic sense, in that there is a subset of the set of kin terms from which all other kin terms can be generated through use of the binary product for the generating kin terms in conjunction with a set of structural equations that determines the structure for the kinship terminology (Read 1984, 2001, 2007b).

It follows that when person A and person B share the same kin term computational system, then they can compute whether they are kin to each other through a third individual as outlined by Sahlins above. Once A knows that A has a kin term relation to B, A also knows that B has a kin term relation to A and that the relation A has to B (from A's perspective) is the reciprocal (in A's computational system) of the relation that B has to A.

Further, A also knows that from B's perspective, the relation B has to A is the reciprocal (in B's computational system) of the relation A has to B. Consequently, once A knows that B is in the domain of individuals with whom A has a kin relation, then the belief that A constructs regarding B (i.e. that B is a person towards whom behaviours associated with kin relations may be directed) should be reciprocated in the behaviour of B, by virtue of B also forming a reciprocal belief about A from B's perspective, as indicated in Figure 10.6. Hence the conditions necessary for symmetric social interaction are satisfied.

The set of persons who mutually recognize each other as cultural kin (or who can compute that they are cultural kin) can form a bounded social system based on symmetric social interaction that does not depend on extensive prior face-to-face interaction for predicting what behaviour will likely be reciprocated. The fact that individuals can compute whether they have a cultural kin relation implies that the size of the group of socially interacting individuals is limited only by the connectedness of individuals through mating/marriage networks, and the latter relates to the likelihood that when individuals A and B encounter one another they can identify a third individual, C, for whom each already has a known cultural kin relation. Empirically, this limit appears to be around 500–800 persons, the modal size for hunter-gatherer societies when social organization is based primarily on a kinship system expressed through a kinship terminology and society-specific marriage rules (either negative in the form of proscription or positive in the form of prescription; Leaf and Read n.d., Appendix).

The modal size of hunter-gatherer societies relates to structural/organizational properties of the kinship terminology conceptual system whose implementation enables symmetric social interaction. Evolutionary change at the conceptual level can restructure social and environmental relationships in a system of interacting individuals through their organization into a structured system of social groupings, such as families and residence groups. Connection is made through cultural instantiation of the units of the conceptual system as individuals, or groups of individuals, rather than the conceptual system emerging out of behavioural processes. A kinship terminology—a system of concepts with a generative structure—does not emerge *from* behaviour, but instead provides a model *for* behaviour and constructs the boundaries for the individuals among whom social interaction may take place.

CONCLUSIONS

Evolution among the higher primates and hominins shows two parallel trends—evolution in the degree to which information regarding other individuals can be taken into account and evolution in the form of social organization. Although symmetric male–male social interactions do occur among the common chimpanzees (and in the form of female–female dyads among the pygmy chimpanzees), the dyads are not stable and depend on extensive interaction. These two trends appear to reach a biological limit among the chimpanzees, due to a third trend of increasing individualization of behaviour. Individualization of behaviour increases the 'cognitive load' when behaviour is modified according to the range of behaviours encountered, including alliances and coalitions. During evolution of the hominins, another trend also came to the fore, namely the cognitive capacity to conceptually categorize on the basis of the relation of one individual to another.

The evolutionary importance of this innovation in categorization, away from features of individuals to relations between individuals, lies in the manner in which new relations may be constructed from current relations through the recursive composition of relations. Through relation composition, new categories of relations can be constructed without the relations requiring prior identification through patterns of behaviour. In addition, a relation that is part of the cognitive repertoire of one individual can become a reciprocal relation when others who are the target of the relation share the same cognitive repertoire and mutually include one another in the range of instantiation for relations. Reciprocal relations provide a basis for symmetric social interaction. The functionality associated with symmetric social interaction will be realized in a community of individuals sharing the same conceptual system of relations: hence the boundary for the community will be determined by those individuals who are mutually enculturated. With social organization based on cultural instantiation of conceptual systems transmitted through enculturation, evolution at the organizational level comes to the fore. This process is driven internally by both the cohesiveness of a conceptual system and its culturally instantiated form, which provides the social context for behaviour (van der Leeuw et al. 2009), and externally by the functionality provided by a system of social organization in competition with the functionality of other systems of social organization.

REFERENCES

Arnold, K. & Whiten, A. (2003). Grooming interactions among the chimpanzees of the Budongo forest, Uganda: tests of five explanatory models. *Behaviour* 140: 519–552.

Baldwin, J. (1896). A new factor in evolution. *American Naturalist* 30: 441–451.

Bauer, H. R. (1979). Agonistic and grooming behaviour in the reunion contexts of Gombe Stream chimpanzees. In: D. A. Hamburg & E. R. McCown (eds) *The great apes*, pp. 395–404. Menlo Park, CA: Benjamin/Cummings Publishing Co.

Call, J. & Tomasello, M. (2008). Does the chimpanzee have a theory of mind? 30 years later. *Trends in Cognitive Science* 12: 187–192.

Crumley, C. (1995). Heterarchy and the analysis of complex societies. In: R. M. Ehrenreich, C. L. Crumley & J. E. Levy (eds) *Heterarchy and the analysis of complex societies*, pp. 1–5. Archaeological Papers of the American Anthropological Association No. 6. Washington, DC: American Anthropological Association.

Dasser, V. (1988a). A social concept in Java monkeys. *Animal Behaviour* 36: 225–230.
Dasser, V. (1988b). Mapping social concepts in monkeys. In: R. W. Byrne & A. Whiten (eds) *Machiavellian intelligence: social expertise and the evolution of intellect in monkeys, apes, and humans*, pp. 85–93. New York: Oxford University Press.
Davis, E. W. & Yost, J. A. (2001). The creation of social hierarchy. In: R. B. Morrison & C. R. Wilson (eds) *Ethnographic essays in cultural anthropology*, pp. 82–120. Belmont, CA: Thomson Publishers.
de Waal, F. B. M. (1992). Coalitions as part of reciprocal relations in the Arnhem chimpanzee colony. In: A. H. Harcourt & F. B. M. de Waal (eds) *Coalitions and alliances in humans and other animals*, pp. 233–257. Oxford: Oxford Science Publications.
di Fiore, A. & Rendall, D. (1994). Evolution of social organization: a reappraisal for primates by using phylogenetic methods. *Proceedings of the National Academy of Sciences, USA* 91: 9941–9945.
Fararo, T. J. (1997). Reflections on mathematical sociology. *Sociological Forum* 12: 73–101.
Feinberg, R. (1981). The meaning of 'sibling' on Anuta. In: M. Marshall (ed.) *Siblingship in Oceania*, pp. 105–148. Ann Arbor: University of Michigan Press.
Focquaert, F., Braeckman, J. & Platek, S. M. (2008). An evolutionary cognitive neuroscience perspective on human self-awareness and theory of mind. *Philosophical Psychology* 21: 47–68.
Gagneux, P., Boesch, C. & Woodruff, D. S. (1999). Female reproductive strategies, paternity and community structure in wild West African chimpanzees. *Animal Behaviour* 57:19–32.
Goodall, J. (1986). *The chimpanzees of Gombe: patterns of behaviour*. Cambridge, MA: Harvard University Press.
Gouzoules, S. & Gouzoules, H. (1987). Kinship. In: B. B. Smuts, D. L. Cheney, R. M. Seyfarth, R. W. Wrangham & T. T. Struhsaker (eds) *Primate societies*, pp. 299–305. Chicago: University of Chicago Press.
Hankins, F. H. (1925). Individual freedom with some sociological implications of determinism. *Journal of Philosophy* 22: 617–634.
Hass, J. (1998). A brief consideration of cultural evolution: stages, agents, and tinkering. *Complexity* 3: 12–21.
Hauser, M. D., Chomsky, N. & Fitch, W. T. (2002). The faculty of language: what is it, who has it and how did it evolve? *Science* 298: 1569–1579.
Heyes, C. (1998). Theory of mind in nonhuman primates. *Behavioural and Brain Sciences* 21: 101–134.
Leaf, M. (2006). Experimental analysis of kinship. *Ethnology* 45: 305–330.
Leaf, M. & Read, D. (n.d.). Empirical formal analysis in anthropology: the new science (manuscript).University of Texas, Dallas.
Lehmann, J. & Boesch, C. (2008). Sexual differences in chimpanzee sociality. *International Journal of Primatology* 29: 65–81.
Lévi-Strauss, C. (1969 [1967]) *The elementary structures of kinship*, revised edn, trans. H. Bell, J. R. von Sturmer & R. Needham. Boston, MA: Beacon Press.
Misztal, B. (2000). *Informality: social theory and contemporary practice*. New York: Routledge.

Mitani, J. C., Watts, D. P. & Muller, M. N. (2002). Recent developments in the study of wild chimpanzee behaviour. *Evolutionary Anthropology* 9: 9–26.

Muller, M. N. & Mitani, J. C. (2005). Conflict and cooperation in wild chimpanzees. *Advances in the Study of Behaviour* 35: 275–331.

Nadel, S. F. (1957). *The theory of social structure*. London: Cohen & West.

Nishida, T. (1979). The social structure of chimpanzees of the Mahale Mountains. In: D. A. Hamburg & E. R. McCown (eds) *The great apes*, pp. 73–122. Menlo Park, CA: Benjamin/Cummings Publishing Co.

Nishida, T. & Hiraiwa-Hasegawa, M. (1987). Chimpanzees and bonobos: cooperative relationships among males. In: B. B. Smuts, D. L. Cheney, R. M. Seyfarth, R. W. Wrangham & T. T. Struhsaker (eds) *Primate societies*, pp. 165–178. Chicago: University of Chicago Press.

Parsons, T. (1964). *The social system*. New York: Free Press of Glencoe.

Povinelli, D. J. & Vonk, J. (2004). We don't need a microscope to explore the chimpanzee mind. *Mind and Language* 19: 1–28.

Read, D. W. (1984). An algebraic account of the American kinship terminology. *Current Anthropology* 25: 417–440.

Read, D. W. (2001). What is kinship? In: R. Feinberg and M. Ottenheimer (eds) *The cultural analysis of kinship: the legacy of David Schneider and its implications for anthropological relativism*, pp. 78–117. Urbana: University of Illinois Press.

Read, D. W. (2004). The emergence of order from disorder as a form of self organization. *Computational & Mathematical Organization Theory* 9: 195–225.

Read, D. W. (2005). Change in the form of evolution: transition from primate to hominid forms of social organization. *Journal of Mathematical Sociology* 29: 91–114.

Read, D. W. (2007a). Culture: the challenge for computational modeling. Paper presented at the 'Computational Models in Anthropology: What Are They Good For? Why Should You Care?' Symposium, Annual Meeting, American Anthropological Association, 2007.

Read, D. W. (2007b). Kinship theory: a paradigm shift. *Ethnology* 46: 329–364.

Read, D. W. (2008). Working memory: a cognitive limit to non-human primate recursive thinking prior to hominid evolution. *Evolutionary Psychology* 6: 676–714.

Read, D. & Behrens, C. (1990). KAES: an expert system for the algebraic analysis of kinship terminologies. *Journal of Quantitative Anthropology* 2: 353–393. Postprint available at: http://repositories.cdlib.org/postprints/2647.

Read, D., Lane, D. & van der Leeuw, S. (2009). The innovation innovation. In: D. Lane, S. van der Leeuw, D. Pumain and G. West (eds) *Complexity perspectives on innovation and social change*, pp. 43–84. Berlin: Springer Verlag.

Sahlins, M. (1962). *Moala: culture and nature on a Fijian island*. Englewood Cliffs, NJ: Prentice Hall.

Schilhab, T. S. S. (2004). What mirror self-recognition in nonhumans can tell us about aspects of self. *Biology and Philosophy* 19: 111–126.

Service, E. (1962). *Primitive social organization: an evolutionary perspective*. New York: Random House.

Simpson, G. G. (1953). The Baldwin effect. *Evolution* 7: 110–117.

Spinozzi, G., Natale, F., Langer, J. & Brakke, K. E. (1999). Spontaneous class grouping behaviour by bonobos (*Pan paniscus*) and common chimpanzees (*P. troglodytes*). *Animal Cognition* 2: 157–170.

Spruijt, B. M., van Hooff, J. A. R. A. M. & Gispen, W. H. (1992). Ethology and neurobiology of grooming behaviour. *Physiological Reviews* 72: 825–852.

van der Leeuw, S., Lane, D., Read, D. & White, D. (2009). The long-term evolution of social organization. In: D. Lane, D. Pumain, S. van der Leeuw & G. West (eds) *Complexity perspectives on innovation and social change*, pp. 85–116. Berlin: Springer Verlag.

Wrangham, R. W. (1979). Sex differences in chimpanzee dispersion. In: D. A. Hamburg & E. R. McCown (eds) *The great apes*, pp. 481–489. Menlo Park, CA: Benjamin/Cummings Publishing Co.

Wrangham, R. W., Clark, A. P. & Isabirye-Basuta, G. (1992). Female social relationships and social organisation of the Kibale Forest chimpanzees. In: T. Nishida, W. C. McGrew, P. Marler, M. Pickford & F. B. M. de Waal (eds) *Topics in primatology, human origins*, vol. 1, pp. 81–98. Tokyo: University of Tokyo Press.

11

Networks and the Evolution of Socio-material Differentiation

CARL KNAPPETT

THE TITLE OF THIS SYMPOSIUM—'Social Brains and Distributed Minds: Inter-disciplinary and Evolutionary Perspectives'—is a good place to begin. We see four terms that are loosely juxtaposed: 'social brains', 'distributed minds', 'inter-disciplinary' and 'evolutionary'. But how are they interconnected? In other chapters in this volume the idea of the 'social brain' is strongly associated with evolutionary perspectives; likewise, the 'distributed mind' is arguably an inter-disciplinary perspective. While there are overlaps, the distributed mind perspective has not been especially evolutionary in outlook, and likewise the social brain hypothesis has not looked across the cognitive sciences in the ways that it might. Hence the aim of this symposium: to encourage articulations between these two domains in the hope of forging stronger understandings of the human past and present.

A further distinction is at work here too, essentially that between the distant and recent pasts. Much of the evolutionary perspective of the social brain concerns the distant past, that is to say, the Palaeolithic, while the intersection of the distributed mind perspective with archaeology has tended to involve the more recent past, that is to say the Bronze Age and onwards (e.g. Knappett 2005; Malafouris 2008a, 2008b). Some of those working primarily on Palaeolithic archaeology have sought to extend their approach down in time beyond the Holocene (Gamble 2007; Mithen 2004); and similarly the distributed mind, or 'material engagement' approach, has been driven back in time by those more habitually working in later periods (Renfrew 2004). The treatment of earlier periods by those engaged with the recent past is a line taken also in this volume by Chapman (ch. 20), with fascinating implications. What I seek to do in this chapter, however, is to remain in the recent past, tackling predominantly

Proceedings of the British Academy **158**, 231–246. © The British Academy 2010.

the Bronze Age using a distributed mind perspective but with my ear to the ground for the rumblings from much earlier periods.

Why the Bronze Age? Evidently this needs qualification as the Bronze Age means rather different things in social terms across Eurasia; here I shall be focusing on the East Mediterranean and Aegean. The Bronze Age in these areas is generally associated with the growth of social complexity, or 'the emergence of civilisation' (Renfrew 1972). This transformation has been characterized in a variety of ways, and has also been glossed as the 'urban revolution' (Childe 1942). But what it can perhaps be boiled down to is a marked increase in social differentiation, both vertical (stratification) and horizontal (specialization). These features are sought in particular material markers (monuments, public works, rich burials, specialized crafts), which are seen to reflect changing socio-political structure and economic organization.

Yet at the same time a parallel observation might be made: that the material culture of the Near East and east Mediterranean in later prehistory is so abundant and diverse—particularly in pottery, stone vases, metalwork and wall paintings—that specialists spend most of their time processing and classifying this mass of material. The interpretative process of seeking to explain social change is almost an afterthought, a luxury, so engrossing is this classificatory project.[1] It might seem that there is little point in stepping back to reflect on *why* and *how* such material culture diversity appears at this time in the archaeological record.[2] It is at worst unconnected with ideas of social complexity, and at best viewed as reflective of or secondary to social complexity.

SOCIO-MATERIAL DIFFERENTIATION

What I argue here, however, is that we should stop simply describing the material world while interpreting the social, and instead seek to describe *and* explain both. These two phenomena are not hierarchically related; rather, each enacts the other, and thus we should really talk of the emergence of *socio-material* differentiation. Theoretical support for this programmatic statement may be sought in a number of domains, not least

---

[1] For example, many Bronze Age sites on Crete can easily measure their finds in ceramics by the ton, though this kind of quantification is rare.

[2] In a sense, one might see it as the birth of the modernist obsession with objects (the excess of supermodernity, even; see Augé 1995).

the 'symmetrical anthropology' espoused by Latour and others in Actor-Network Theory. Here we can find all kinds of examples of the 'symmetrical' role of both artefacts and agents in practices ranging from firing a gun (Latour 2005) to accessing an apartment block (Latour 2000).

But do such accounts really succeed in accounting for why the social co-opts the material? Actor-Network Theory is not cognitive in its outlook, but a cognitive approach is required, I would argue, to get to the heart of the matter. The role that artefacts play in scaffolding cognitive processes has been ably demonstrated in the 'distributed mind' literature by the likes of Hutchins (1995), Clark (1997), Kirsh (1995) and Goodwin (1994), and this has been taken on board in archaeology, if only in a limited way, as signalled by a recent Cambridge conference entitled 'The Cognitive Life of Things' (Malafouris & Renfrew in press). In this chapter, I argue for a distinction between objects and things, inspired by the work of Brown (2001), Mitchell (2005) and Gosden (2004), suggesting that this separation helps us to understand the human cognitive processes that make use of artefacts to establish categorical relationships that can transcend proximate experiential interactions with artefacts.

THINGS AND OBJECTS; NEAR AND FAR

Anchoring and scaffolding processes demand a particular understanding of the artefact: as *object* rather than *thing*. We tend to use these two terms interchangeably, though recent scholarship has sought to differentiate between the two. Gosden (2004, 38–39), for example, suggests that *things* are embedded in assemblages, and are inalienable and unquantifiable, whereas *objects* are disembedded, alienable and quantifiable. This move is echoed in a growing literature in art history, literary criticism and cultural theory, in the shape of what Brown calls 'thing theory' (2001, 2003; Mitchell 2005; Schwenger 2006). Things are ambiguous and undefined; when someone says 'pass me that green thing over there', the thing is unintelligible in some way.

Objects, on the other hand, are named, understood and transparent. Objects might be pulled out of the miasma of thingness (through naming, for example). It is important to note that objecthood and thingness are relational registers, in that the status of the material entity is partly contingent upon the perceiver: a thing to one onlooker might be an object to another. On a journey, for example, looking out of the car window as a passenger, everything may just pass by in a blur, one unnamed thing merging into another: alternatively, particular landmarks and features may be recognized, named, isolated from the flow. *Aides mémoires* provide another example: imagine placing keys by the door of the apartment to remember them upon leaving; or knotting a handkerchief to remember that there is something to remember. While the keys and the handkerchief may very often be experienced as *things*, in the background and embedded, in their function as *aides mémoires*, knotted or placed on a table near the door, they come to the fore as *objects*. And insofar as such artefactual scaffolds mediate action sequences unfolding in other times and places, they allow for the distribution of cognition beyond the proximate (Hutchins 2005; Knappett in press a, in press b; Sinha 2005).

Artefacts can thus act at different scales. In their role as things they are caught up in everyday proximate experience; but in their role as objects they can transcend the proximate and speak to other times and places. When we consider the growth of artefact quantities and diversity in the Bronze Age in these terms, then we might imagine that more and more artefacts create increasing opportunities for cognitive scaffolding and the extension of human practice beyond the confines of the everyday. This might be true if artefacts could be constantly 'controlled' as objects; however, there is an ineluctable pressure that brings objects back into thingness. Large numbers of artefacts might hold cognitive potential, but at the same time they threaten to be excessive and overwhelming. As more and more artefacts accrue, some spill out beyond the proximate, so that not all of them can be present. Only those things that have been cognized as objects can be rendered cognitively present while physically absent.[3]

CREATING OBJECTS FROM THINGS

How, then, are things transformed into objects? Let us for now consider three possibilities. The first is 'naming': naming a thing objectifies it and, if one follows Peter Schwenger (2006), is a 'murder' of the thing, denying its thingness. Things are of course named in language, but also in script; this too can be an effective means of objectifying the thing, as seen in

---

[3] This demands at some level a semiotic perspective, as within Actor-Network Theory (e.g. Latour 2005), though the semiotic dimension is generally implicit. A more explicit semiotic approach is offered in some quarters, particularly in the work of those following the semiotic of Charles Sanders Peirce (e.g. Keane 1997; Preucel 2006). This field has much potential, but I wish here to follow a different tack.

many early administrative systems in the Near East and Aegean for controlling the flow of commodities. In scripts there is also an imagistic aspect, particularly in pictographic scripts, like the Cretan Hieroglyphic of the Cretan Middle Bronze Age (Knappett 2008). Making an image of the thing is indeed a second means of objectifying it. This can occur in scripts, in pictorial depictions and even in display, which is effectively a process of image-making: in a museum or gallery setting, for example, the things of everyday life are converted into objects and engaged with as objects (Gosden 2004). Changing the scale of an artefact is also a form of imaging, through either monumentalization or miniaturization (Knappett in press a). Moreover, making skeuomorphic versions of artefacts can create iconic images too. A third means is fragmentation (Chapman 2000; Chapman & Gaydarska 2007): the complete, indissoluble thing is deliberately or accidentally fragmented and in some sense objectified in the process. This relates at some level to the change of status that occurs when an artefact works smoothly, such as a hammer in the hands of a skilled builder; it is in this moment a thing, barely cognized as something separate from the user. But as soon as it breaks it very quickly reverts to objecthood, its qualities (or lack of) quickly revealed. This distinction is one made by Heidegger, distinguishing between readiness-to-hand and presence-at-hand respectively (Harman 2005; Wheeler 2005).

Now it is time to work through some of the above theoretical statements using examples from the later prehistory of the Aegean and east Mediterranean. First we will consider the role of material culture in scaffolding and anchoring social practices and ideas, demonstrating the co-enactment of the social and the material. The example is the development of containers from the late Mesolithic into the early Neolithic. Second, we will look at the more systematic objectification of artefact assemblages in the Bronze Age, through processes of imaging and fragmenting; this is tackled via the example of rhyta.

CONTAINERS[4]

Containers were first made c. 12,000 to 9,000 BP, in a range of materials but arguably most emblematically in clay. This innovation may be

---

[4] This section draws on a co-authored paper with Lambros Malafouris and Peter Tomkins (Knappett et al. in press); many of the insights are theirs and I thank them for allowing me to draw on this paper here.

understood as 'the introduction of a different topology—*a surface around a void*' (Read & van der Leeuw 2008, 1965; see also van der Leeuw 2000; van der Leeuw et al. 2009). We might assume that this innovation took place through a metaphorical transfer from the source domain of the human body: it is hard to escape from the basic metaphor of body as container, and evidently the body takes precedence over the relatively late innovation of ceramic and other containers. Yet perhaps we should resist this easy formulation whereby the material world is a reflection of human-derived concepts. After all, 'body as container' is a strongly Western conception rather than some universal metaphor. Furthermore, it is quite conceivable that the very idea of containing evolved through the enactment of various practices in which both human body and materials were entwined; in the practice of various gestures, working on surfaces, media and substances in specific ways, some sense of 'containment' may have emerged jointly in relation to both bodies and material culture (Ingold 2007; Warnier 2006).[5] This moves us away from the idea of the pot as container, as some static entity, and towards a more dynamic conception of 'containing' as a set of gestures and practices that engenders particular relationships among surfaces, substances and media. When we think of this in terms of the meshes of everyday activities, some of these activities have scale-traversing metaphorical properties enabling the idea of containment to extend from an individual across different scales, even to the extent of a whole kingdom (see Warnier 2007; see also Knappett et al. in press).

Clay vessels in particular have the potential to transcend scale, as more and more are produced, going far beyond the level of the household in terms of their distribution and consumption (cf. Gamble 2007, 272). The relative ubiquity of clay as a resource, and its almost endless plasticity, make it a particularly flexible means of creating a surface around a void. In later prehistory, c. 2500 BC (in the Aegean at least), we see the manufacture of containers in a new material, also with considerable malleability: metal. Bronze in particular is used to create containers that intersect substantially with existing shapes in clay and stone; nonetheless this new material creates what has been dubbed 'Metallschock' (see Nakou 2007), as it brings radical new properties, such as the potential for melting down and recycling, and hence new possibilities for socio-material expression.

---

[5] See also van der Leeuw (2000), who suggests that leather-working, whereby skin, one kind of 'container', can be transformed into another kind of container, may have been the key craft through which containing was 'discovered'.

Furthermore, metals differ profoundly from clay in the extremely uneven distribution of their ores. Whereas clay is more or less ubiquitous in the east Mediterranean, metal ores are very restricted: Crete, famously, has no metal resources to speak of. This implies that any metal vessel (or instrument, for that matter) in use is much more likely to have an impressive 'back story' to it in terms of its production and circulation. Callon and Law, in their discussion of the role of technologies in the commingling of people and things over space and time, cite the following maxim: 'invisible but present beside the ploughman is the blacksmith who made his ploughshare' (2004: 6). The 'back story' of metal vessels means that they too cross different spatial and temporal scales, albeit in different ways from ceramics.

BRONZE AGE OBJECTS: RHYTA

The use of metals to manufacture containers of various kinds from the Early Bronze Age onwards is a significant development, not least because of the cross-referencing that occurs between metals and other materials. Ceramics begin to imitate new metal forms, while stone vessels are also made in imitation of different media. One particular kind of container that serves as a useful point of discussion for cross-referencing and the creation of object assemblages is the 'rhyton' (see Koehl 2006). This is a particular kind of vessel designed to release as much as to contain: it has a small secondary hole c. 0.5 cm in diameter through which any liquids poured into the primary opening soon escape. Rhyton means 'flow' in Greek. The earliest rhyta occur in the Early Bronze Age on Crete, c. 2500 BC, and are exclusively zoomorphic, most often in the shape of bulls (Koehl 2006). The metaphorical connection with bodies as containers is thus quite explicit. This association continues over many centuries, as seen in the famous bull's head rhyta of the Neopalatial period (c. 1700–1500 BC), though by then we also see more and more non-zoomorphic types that are conical or ovoid in profile (Koehl 2006). Neopalatial rhyta are varied not only in shape but also in material, with specimens in metal, stone, ceramic and faience. The creation of rhyta in very similar shapes but different media could be seen as a means of stabilizing the concept of the rhyton, or at least the practices it invokes, through a kind of diversification. But these multiple connections go further still.

Rhyta are not only metaphorically associated with animal and human bodies as containers; they are also linked to another form of container, the house. There are numerous instances documented ethnographically of houses being treated as bodily containers of a kind (Blier 1987; Tilley 1999; Warnier 2007). Rhyta are connected to houses through their frequent deposition in foundation deposits; such deposits are found frequently in Minoan Crete, often in the form of small structured depositions in wall niches or beneath floors, consisting often of just a single whole vessel, usually a cup or jug (Herva 2005; MacGillivray et al. 1999). These foundation deposits also include rhyta on occasion, such as the example of the bull's head rhyton from the Little Palace at Knossos (Herva 2005, 217).

A further aspect of rhyta that may also speak to their multiple connections is their possible use in deliberate acts of fragmentation. Chapman (2000) has developed a fascinating body of work theorizing the role of the deliberate fragmentation of objects in creating social relations among individuals and groups through what he calls 'enchainment'. Most of his examples are from the later prehistory of the Balkans, though the sense is that this is a much wider phenomenon. Independently of Chapman's analysis, Rehak (1995) has identified what he sees as the deliberate fragmentation of Minoan stone bull's head rhyta. He hypothesizes that this kind of rhyton acted as a simulacrum of the sacrificed bull, with a ritual smashing of the stone muzzle signifying the bull's sacrifice (Rehak 1995, 451). Though there is nothing to suggest that the fragments from this ritual destruction were then distributed among participants to form enchained relations that endure beyond the event, as Chapman argues in his fragmentation theory, we might nonetheless observe that this process of fragmentation is a very material means for establishing metaphorical connections across domains.[6]

Rehak (1995, 450) observes that stone bull's head rhyta 'seem to be part of a much larger iconographic network'. To this I would add that the

---

[6] Fragmentation may well be a more widespread practice in Minoan Crete than has currently been recognized. One of the most dramatic and well-documented examples of deliberate fragmentation comes from the site of Palaikastro, where recent excavations uncovered evidence for a remarkable event in and around 'Building 5'. This construction suffered a fire destruction at the close of the Late Minoan IB period, and found within its ruins were a number of pieces of a fine chryselephantine statue, a male figure which came to be dubbed the kouros (MacGillivray et al. 2000). However, many other pieces of it were found outside the building's entrance, in a small courtyard. Piecing together the various fragments the excavators surmised that the kouros must have been deliberately smashed in the courtyard, with its face particularly badly disfigured, and then the legs thrown into the building, which then burnt to the ground. Arguably what we are seeing here is the harnessing of the metaphorical power of release and fragmentation, in the conjoined acts of desecration of the statue, possibly a cult figure, and the burning of the building.

network is not solely iconographic but is actually much more broadly cultural. While in prehistory we might struggle with the specifics, rhyta do seem to enact a series of practices and concepts concerning ideas of containing and releasing, ideas that cross-cut humans, animals, houses and artefacts. The existence of intertwining material metaphors has been documented ethnographically, for example in the Andes where metaphors of grinding and pounding as productive of life are seen to run across all kinds of bodily practices and gestures, from grinding corn, to pounding clay into a workable powder and even crushing enemies in battle (Sillar 1996).

Thus, on the one hand, rhyta are intimately connected with bodily gestures and metaphors that underlie all kinds of daily practices. On the other hand, their multiple interconnections, their cross-media referencing and their objectification through fragmentation make them rather more than just sets of things that are experienced on no more than a day-to-day level. All these connections lend rhyta a kind of iconic status that allows them to exist across time and space as objects and not just as things. What I will argue next is that these connections take the form of a network of objects; and that this network topology is a crucial development in the long-term evolution of human artefact assemblages.

NETWORKS

At the level of everyday lived experience the idea of the network may not seem particularly relevant. As one interacts seamlessly with the artefacts that make up one's daily space there is perhaps a feeling of flow and of continuous experience, rather than of a series of interconnected nodes (as the network implies). Perhaps here we might co-opt a term recently suggested by Ingold (2007), the idea of 'meshwork'. Everyday experience is more like a set of criss-crossing lines, trajectories along which we move, and which at certain intersections may take the character of place. But these places of intersection are not nodes as in a network, because the lines are continuous and overlapping. In these meshworks we experience artefacts as things, in the sense defined earlier. They are encountered experientially as groups at the micro-scale. Objects, on the other hand, exist in networked assemblages, more in the domain of ideas than phenomena (van der Leeuw 2008), and can transcend the proximate.[7]

---

[7] This is essentially the difference between grouping and classification, the former concerning things, the latter objects; archaeologists have, arguably, often mistaken their grouping as classification (van der Leeuw 1976, and pers. comm.).

Let me give an example of this difference between the experience of things and the conception of objects. It comes in fact from the domain of graph theory and is often cited in connection with the birth of graph theory in the mid-18th century. The citizens of Königsberg would go for walks around their town, which had seven bridges across different stretches of river. At some point they began to wonder whether it would be possible to walk around the town crossing each bridge only once and returning to the same starting point; but the answer to this problem eluded them. That was, until a Swiss mathematician Leonhard Euler took on the problem by treating each segment of land as a node and each bridge as a link. By analysing the problem as a graph of nodes and links, he was able to come up with a solution to the Seven Bridges of Königsberg question—and indeed no such path around the town crossing each bridge only once was possible.

What this story tells us is that in the midst of lived experience we follow paths and these intersect and overlap in complex meshes, i.e. mesh-works (Ingold 2007). This experiential understanding is important; but it does not necessarily provide the basis for an analysis of some properties of those meshes. Even if not experienced explicitly as 'networks' by the inhabitants, nonetheless by converting the meshwork into a network, composed of defined nodes and links (or vertices and edges), Euler was able to grasp some other, systematic characteristics of that same experience. Meshwork and network are two topologies, and not necessarily the only two. In this example we see that different topologies may coexist, as may different registers: that is to say objecthood and thingness may be simultaneous. However, it is networks of objects that facilitate relational thinking across scales. And, I would argue, it is by conceiving of the world in terms of networks of objects that socio-material differentiation, expansion and innovation is (and was) enabled.

A PRIORI/A POSTERIORI, INVENTION/INNOVATION

Let us consider briefly this notion that object networks facilitate socio-material differentiation and the ever-increasing expansion of material culture that has grown exponentially from the Neolithic to the present day, with its overwhelming material excess (Read & van der Leeuw 2008; Read et al. 2009). Observations made recently by van der Leeuw (2008) connecting things and objects with invention and innovation are partic-ularly pertinent here. In the course of everyday experience, as we interact with artefacts as things, we may come across some new way of doing something; a creative process of invention. This invariably happens 'in the moment', moving forward in the action a priori, such that one does not necessarily have a clear sense of exactly what transpired to create something new (van der Leeuw 2008). It might be a slight shift of the hands to create a new shape on the wheel, or a slightly higher temperature in kiln firing that gave the fired clay new and unexpected properties. But this process of 'invention' is far removed from the process of innovation; such inventive moments occur all the time, but only rarely do they come to be transmitted more widely across society as innovations. The need to treat invention as just one small part of innovation was stated 20 years ago in the archaeological literature (e.g. van der Leeuw & Torrence 1989), but innovation has not been much of an explicit concern in archaeology, for various reasons (Knappett & van der Leeuw in preparation). Van der Leeuw goes on to state that innovation, on the other hand, in contrast to invention, requires an a posteriori handling of what just happened, stepping back into the networked object world, and trying to attribute functionality in a rather more detached fashion. Experientially both these perspectives are required in invention and innovation; however, in analysis of invention and innovation the a priori and a posteriori perspectives become detached, and we tend to pursue a solely a posteriori approach, meaning that the creative, inventive dimension is under-analysed and misunderstood. We need to think both 'backwards' and 'forwards' to really get to grips with all aspects of the process, rather than just assigning invention to 'personal creativity' and as such somehow beyond the bounds of rigorous social science. By the same token we should not tackle socio-material differentiation solely from the perspective of objects, as there is an inherent tension between objecthood and thingness that reproduces that between a posteriori and a priori thinking respectively.

When considered in terms of containers broadly, or rhyta more specifically, we may begin to understand that a single category—a ceramic bowl, for example—is somewhat isolated and prone to being treated just as a thing. But if that bowl occurs in exactly the same shape in wood, and indeed in stone; and if that bowl is also made in miniature form for use in particular rituals; and if that bowl is also used as a hieroglyphic sign, and depicted in wall paintings; then we can see how a network of sorts is formed which holds that bowl in a conceptual place that transcends its particular everyday instantiation. When this networking process becomes more complex still—as is surely the case with rhyta, with more and more elaborate material used, with connections to houses and bodies, and with intricate metaphorical processes of fragmentation—then one can perhaps imagine how any single moment of invention might more readily be transmitted across time and space, in part thanks to this objectified network. And the more categories that are established in a network, the more connections are made possible.

CONCLUSIONS

So what allows for the evolution of socio-material differentiation? As artefacts proliferate and spill out beyond the proximate, a significant problem arises. They accentuate the problem that not everything that is known is immediately present. More and more things, more and more tangled agent–artefact webs, create problems of cognitive load for the human mind. Yet with the problem comes a solution. By specifying the properties/qualities of a particular artefact, by blending material structure with conceptual structure, these overspilling artefacts can actually be harnessed and used to occupy and control these non-proximate times and spaces. As *things*, artefacts occupy the world of phenomena, embedded in the meshworks of everyday life; but as *objects*, with specific properties in networks of relations, they can also occupy the world of ideas (van der Leeuw 2008). Things are understood relationally with respect to individual and group lived experience, while objects exist in more structured relations independent of experience (see Read ch. 10 this volume). A shift from things to objects also implies a capacity to evoke assemblages of interrelated objects that transcend the proximate: this is what we might dub 'network thinking'. Furthermore, it seems possible that network thinking might have facilitated yet further artefactual innovation, which does seem to increase exponentially in later prehistory (Read et al. 2009) since (unlike invention) it demands a clear attribution of functionality and in some sense an objectification in the world of ideas. The continuing expansion of agent–artefact space (and of spatial and temporal scales) is arguably only possible through a conceptual framework that specifies nodes and links, i.e. the network; and it is perhaps the expansion of arte-factual assemblages in later prehistory that kickstarts network thinking. It is objecthood, with its network qualities, that allows agents to fit an invention into a system of innovations a posteriori and effect a system-wide change. This, I argue, is what underlies 'the innovation innovation'

(Read et al. 2009)[8]—a shift in action-perception-thought such that the world is treated as a network of objects in tension with a meshwork of things.

But of course these networks do not just emerge in later prehistory of their own accord. They are not just materials enacting themselves. Human agents are entangled in these networks too. And some agents are better placed in these dynamic networks than others. Assemblages of objects have a political dimension, in that some agents are always acting at the expense of others; and political inequalities are as much enacted by objects as by humans in these networks. Moreover, because of the constant pull of things on objects, these networks can become naturalized, pulled back into everyday experience. Things are thus almost impossible to challenge politically. If we bring ourselves full circle back to the issues of social and material differentiation with which we started this chapter, then perhaps we begin to see a clearer path for studying the explosion of typological diversity and artefactual abundance in later prehistory as a deeply political process. Stratification and specialization have to be understood as entangled parts of these networked assemblages, rather than behind or above them.

REFERENCES

Augé, M. (1995). *Non-places: introduction to an anthropology of supermodernity*, trans. J. Howe. London: Verso.

Blier, S. P. (1987). *The anatomy of architecture: ontology and metaphor in Batammaliba architectural expression.* Cambridge: Cambridge University Press.

Brown, B. (2001). Thing theory. *Critical Inquiry* 28(1): 1–22.

Brown, B. (2003). *A sense of things: the object matter of American literature.* Chicago: University of Chicago Press.

Callon, M. & Law, J. (2004). Guest editorial. *Society and Space* 22: 3–11.

Chapman, J. (2000). *Fragmentation in archaeology: people, places and broken objects in the prehistory of southeastern Europe.* London: Routledge.

Chapman, J. & Gaydarska, B. (2007). *Parts and wholes: fragmentation in prehistoric context.* Oxford: Oxbow Books.

Childe, V. G. (1942). *What happened in history.* Harmondsworth: Penguin.

Clark, A. (1997). *Being there: putting brain, body and world together again.* Cambridge, MA: MIT Press.

---

[8] Note also Read (ch. 10 this volume) on the important shift to relational thinking as expressed through kinship terminology—and that it allows social organization that can transcend individual behaviour and experience: relations can be understood structurally rather than purely through experience.

Gamble, C. (2007). *Origins and revolutions: human identity in earliest prehistory.* Cambridge: Cambridge University Press.

Goodwin, C. (1994). Professional vision. *American Anthropologist* 96(3): 606–633.

Gosden, C. (2004). Making and display: our aesthetic appreciation of things and objects. In: C. Renfrew, C. Gosden & E. DeMarrais (eds) *Substance, memory, display: archaeology and art,* pp. 35–45. Cambridge: McDonald Institute for Archaeological Research Monographs.

Harman, G. (2005). Heidegger on objects and things. In: B. Latour & P. Weibel (eds) *Making things public: atmospheres of democracy,* pp. 268–271. Cambridge, MA: MIT Press.

Herva, V.-P. (2005). The life of buildings: Minoan building deposits in an ecological perspective. *Oxford Journal of Archaeology* 24(3): 215–227.

Hutchins, E. (1995). *Cognition in the wild.* Cambridge, MA: MIT Press.

Hutchins, E. (2005). Material anchors for conceptual blends. *Journal of Pragmatics* 37: 1555–1577.

Ingold, T. (2007). Materials against materiality. *Archaeological Dialogues* 14: 1–16.

Keane, W. (1997). *Signs of recognition: powers and hazards of representation in an Indonesian society.* Berkeley, CA: University of California Press.

Kirsh, D. (1995). The intelligent use of space. *Artificial Intelligence* 73: 31–68.

Knappett, C. (2005). *Thinking through material culture: an interdisciplinary perspective.* Philadelphia, PA: University of Pennsylvania Press.

Knappett, C. (2008). The neglected networks of material agency: artefacts, pictures and texts. In: C. Knappett & L. Malafouris (eds) *Material agency: towards a non-anthropocentric approach,* pp. 139–56. New York: Springer.

Knappett, C. (in press a). Meaning in miniature: semiotic networks in material culture. In: M. Jensen, N. Johanssen & H. J. Jensen (eds) *Excavating the mind: cross-sections through culture, cognition and materiality.* Aarhus: Aarhus University Press.

Knappett, C. (in press b). Communities of things and objects: a spatial perspective. In: L. Malafouris & C. Renfrew (eds) *The cognitive life of things: recasting the boundaries of the mind.* Cambridge: McDonald Institute.

Knappett, C. & van der Leeuw, S. E. (in preparation). The space of innovation: cognitive, social and physical considerations.

Knappett, C., Malafouris, L. & Tomkins, P. (in press). Ceramics as containers. In: D. Hicks & M. Beaudry (eds) *The Oxford handbook of material culture studies.* Oxford: Oxford University Press.

Koehl, R. (2006). *Aegean Bronze Age rhyta.* Philadelphia, PA: INSTAP Academic Press.

Latour, B. (2000). The Berlin key or how to do words with things. In: P. M. Graves-Brown (ed.) *Matter, materiality and modern culture,* pp. 10–21. London: Routledge.

Latour, B. (2005). *Reassembling the social: an introduction to Actor-Network-Theory.* Oxford: Oxford University Press.

MacGillivray, J. A., Sackett, L. H. & Driessen, J. (1999). 'Aspro Pato': a lasting liquid toast from the master-builders of Palaikastro to their patron. In: P. P. Betancourt, V. Karageorghis, R. Laffineur & W.-D. Niemeier (eds) *Meletemata: studies in Aegean archaeology presented to Malcolm H. Wiener as he enters his 65th year,* pp. 465–568. Liège: Aegaeum 20.

MacGillivray, J. A., Sackett, L. H. & Driessen, J. M. (2000). *The Palaikastro kouros*. London: BSA Studies 6.

Malafouris, L. (2008a). Between brains, bodies and things: tectonoetic awareness and the extended self. *Philosophical Transactions of the Royal Society B* 363: 1993–2002.

Malafouris, L. (2008b). Is it 'me' or is it 'mine'? The Mycenaean sword as a body-part. In: J. Robb & D. Boric (eds) *Past bodies: body-centred research in archaeology*. Oxford: Oxbow Books.

Malafouris, L. & Renfrew, C. (eds) (in press). *The cognitive life of things: recasting the boundaries of the mind*. Cambridge: McDonald Institute.

Mitchell, W. J. T. (2005). *What do pictures want? The lives and loves of images*. Chicago: University of Chicago Press.

Mithen, S. (2004). *After the ice: a global human history 20,000–5000 BC*. Cambridge, MA: Harvard University Press.

Nakou, G. (2007). Absent presences: metal vessels in the Aegean at the end of the third millennium. In: P. M. Day & R. C. P. Doonan (eds) *Metallurgy in the Early Bronze Age*, pp. 224–244. Sheffield Studies in Aegean Archaeology, 7. Oxford: Oxbow Books.

Preucel, R. (2006). *Archaeological semiotics*. Oxford: Blackwell.

Read, D. & van der Leeuw, S. E. (2008). Biology is only part of the story . . . *Philosophical Transactions of the Royal Society B* 363: 1959–1968.

Read, D., Lane, D. & van der Leeuw, S. E. (2009). The innovation innovation. In: D. Lane, S. E. van der Leeuw, D. Pumain & G. West (eds) *Complexity perspectives in innovation and social change*, pp. 43–84. Berlin: Springer.

Rehak, P. (1995). The use and destruction of Minoan stone bull's head rhyta. In: R. Laffineur and W.-D. Niemeier (eds) *Politeia: society and state in the Aegean Bronze Age*, pp. 435–460. Liège: Aegaeum 12.

Renfrew, C. (1972). *The emergence of civilisation: the Cyclades and the Aegean in the third millennium BC*. London: Methuen.

Renfrew, C. (2004). Towards a theory of material engagement. In: E. DeMarrais, C. Gosden & C. Renfrew (eds) *Rethinking materiality: the engagement of mind with the material world,* pp. 23–31. Cambridge: McDonald Institute for Archaeological Research.

Schwenger, P. (2006). *The tears of things: melancholy and physical objects*. Minneapolis: University of Minnesota Press.

Sillar, B. (1996). The dead and the drying: techniques for transforming people and things in the Andes. *Journal of Material Culture* 1(3): 259–289.

Sinha, C. (2005). Blending out of the background: play, props and staging in the material world. *Journal of Pragmatics* 37: 1537–1554.

Tilley, C. (1999). *Metaphor and material culture*. Oxford: Blackwell.

van der Leeuw, S. E. (1976). *Studies in the technology of ancient pottery*, 2 vols. Amsterdam: University Printing Office.

van der Leeuw, S. E. (2000). Making tools from stone and clay. In: T. Murray & A. Anderson (eds) *Australian archaeologist. Collected papers in honour of J. Allen*, pp. 69–88. Canberra: ANU Press.

van der Leeuw, S. E. (2008). Agency, networks, past and future. In: C. Knappett & L. Malafouris (eds) *Material agency: towards a non-anthropocentric approach*, pp. 217–247. New York: Springer.

van der Leeuw, S. E. & Torrence, R. (eds) (1989). *What's new? A closer look at the process of innovation.* London: Routledge.

van der Leeuw, S. E., Lane, D. & Read, D. W. (2009). The long-term evolution of social organization. In: D. Lane, S. E. van der Leeuw, D. Pumain & G. West (eds) *Complexity perspectives in innovation and social change*, pp. 85–116. Berlin: Springer.

Warnier, J.-P. (2006). Inside and outside: surfaces and containers. In: C. Tilley, W. Keane, S. Küchler, M. Rowlands & P. Spyer (eds) *Handbook of material culture*, pp. 186–195. London: SAGE.

Warnier, J.-P. (2007). *The pot-king: the body, material culture and technologies of power.* Leiden: Brill.

Wheeler, M. (2005). *Reconstructing the cognitive world: the next step.* Cambridge, MA: MIT Press.

PART IV

THE REACH OF THE BRAIN: MODERN HUMANS AND DISTRIBUTED MINDS

12

When Individuals Do Not
Stop at the Skin

'WHEN INDIVIDUALS DO NOT STOP AT THE SKIN' has become a common notion in psychology, in sociology, in anthropology and even in archaeology: for example, Clive Gamble and Martin Porr have discussed the idea of an individual in an environment which includes both material objects and other individuals. They have argued for the definition of the individual as 'a social actor constituted by his/her relation to these other individuals' (Gamble & Porr 2005, 10). This notion of the individual, rather than individual as *agent*, is the one I want to explore in this article.

I will examine this idea in ways that I think can throw light on human evolution, especially with regard to its relation to concepts like culture, community, kinship and communication. My examples are drawn mainly from my own experience of field research among southern African hunter-gatherers and semi-hunter-gatherers and their neighbours. I also want to look at what I see as an unacknowledged background to the distributed mind hypothesis, which lies in social theory. I will bring this together with aspects of Robin Dunbar's extended brain hypothesis (e.g. Dunbar 1998), which forms one of the two bases of my own recent theory of the co-evolution of language and kinship.

THE COHERENCE OF CULTURE-BEARING
SOCIAL FORMATIONS

Boyd and Richerson on 'culture'

In *The origin and evolution of cultures*, Robert Boyd and Peter Richerson (2005) have collected a wonderful set of their own papers, written over a 30-year period but all arguing a single thesis. For Boyd and Richerson, culture is part of human biology, but operates not only directly through

Proceedings of the British Academy **158**, 249–267. © The British Academy 2010.

biological mechanisms but also by analogy with them. Let me mention two of the papers in the volume.

In the first, they consider 'Why culture is common, but cultural evolution is rare' (Boyd & Richerson 2005, 52–65). They point out that cultural variation and cultural learning occur in a number of animal species, from chimpanzees to pigeons, but that only in humans does accumulated cultural change regularly lead to the evolution of behaviour beyond that which could be invented by an individual. Their argument is short, but it is complex. If I may change their terminology slightly, they suggest that some form of socially conscious learning, through observation, imitation and the deliberate transmission of ideas, is necessary to build culture. All this requires that individuals possess a *theory of mind*: the capacity to understand that others may have different ideas in their heads from oneself. From this, cultural evolution follows: the abilities to make a better tool, tell a story or elaborate on one, draw a picture or see a picture and understand it. I agree with Boyd and Richerson, and would go further than they do. Because of the integrated nature of cultural domains (kinship, religion and so on), after a certain stage of cultural sophistication, cultural accumulation makes cultural evolution virtually inevitable. What that stage of cultural accumulation is, must remain debateable. Presumably too, change may occur either gradually or in revolutionary transformations.

In the second paper, written with colleagues Monique Borgerhoff-Mulder and William Durham, Boyd and Richerson (2005, 310–336) pose the question: 'Are cultural phylogenies possible?' Through analogies with biology, they propose four hypotheses relating to the possible reconstruction of such cultural phylogenies. (1) Cultures are 'species', either isolated from each other or so structurally coherent that the borrowing of traits is limited. (2) Cultures are integrated but hierarchical systems, with peripheral elements that may be borrowed and core elements that will not be. (3) Cultures are assemblages, each coherent, but none easily definable as a core domain or a peripheral one. (4) Cultures are collections of things, operating without the functional coherence of a hierarchy of domains (Boyd & Richerson 2005, 317–319).

My own vision of culture, which I argued in *Hunters and herders of southern Africa* (Barnard 1992), is similar to the second of these, with core and peripheral elements, and in my view with core elements shared with related cultures. In other words, although I now question the degree to which it is useful to think of 'cultures' as countable units, I believe that entities such as Khoisan culture, Australian Aboriginal culture, Lowland

South American culture, or even Western culture, each has within them not only core elements but also underlying structural principles. These underlying structural principles, not random sets of traits, are what distinguish one culture complex, culture area or ethnographic region, from another. Usually, there will be a point of common cultural origin, but convergence, with new shared core features, is also possible—as in what some linguists call a *Sprachbund* or linguistic area (e.g. Güldemann 1998).

Cultural structures in kinship

Two Khoisan individuals may live in different countries, thousands of miles apart, speak different languages, and practise different subsistence activities, but they may share the same understandings of how to classify and behave towards one another through shared kinship ideology and its principles, such as the joking/avoidance dichotomy, the alternation of generations, the principle of universal kin classification and the rule, 'When in doubt, treat a friend as a "grandrelative".' Among Khoe-speaking Central Bushmen or San, these are derived in part from common principles of Khoe kinship, but shared elements also figure typically in other hunter-gatherer societies and are found among non-Khoe Khoisan like Ju/'hoansi and !Xóõ. (Khoe is a subset of Khoisan, and includes both Khoekhoe herders and Central Bushmen or San hunter-gatherers.)

More subtly, structural convergence and the accumulation of peripheral features may alter the ways in which underlying principles are played out. I have argued, for example, that when some hundreds of years ago a Khoe system known as Naro (Nharo) borrowed Ju/'hoan (!Kung) personal naming practices, the relevant kinship term was slotted into the structurally different Naro system to replace two previous Khoe terms (Barnard 1988). The naming practice, through which Ju/'hoansi and Naro receive the names of senior grandrelatives (grandparents or, loosely, uncles/aunts) and trace kinship through names as if namesake equals 'self', renders the previous senior/junior distinction, still found in all other Khoe systems, irrelevant. I did fieldwork with Naro, and my Naro name is !A/e (in Nguni-based Naro orthography, spelled Qace). If I meet another !A/e, I call him 'grandfather' or 'grandchild'. It is immaterial whether he is simply a namesake, or (if I were a Naro) my real grandfather, cross-uncle, cross-cousin, cross-nephew or grandchild. These genealogical positions are terminologically all the same—the Naro category I refer to in English as 'grandrelative'.

At least one cultural domain apart from language, namely kinship, is so structured that it always forms a whole (cf. Bickerton 1998). You will never find, anywhere among *Homo sapiens*, half a kinship system. You will of course find systems in transition, but they always seek stabilization. Partly, this is due to the principle of uniform reciprocals. In any system, if I call someone, say, 'nephew' or 'niece', they will call me 'uncle' or 'aunt'. 'Father', 'brother' or 'son' (or their female equivalents) are not options. We are born into kinship structures, and these more than any other cultural realm both constrain our behaviour and define us as individuals.

This principle is even more true in hunter-gatherer societies than in others, because almost invariably such societies possess universal kin classification: every member of society stands in a precise kin relationship to every other (Barnard 1978). The mechanisms will vary from place to place: egocentrically through friendship or name relationships in Africa, or socio-centrically through moiety and genealogical level in South America, or through moiety, section or subsection membership in Australia. But in such systems, there is no such thing as non-kin. The real test of universality is classification of outsiders. I am not Naro and therefore have no Naro genealogy, but through my name and my namesakes in their genealogies, every one of the 15,000 Naro can, and must, classify me individually as belonging to some category in relation to themselves. Particularly for opposite-sex people, this determines whether to behave in a formal way (e.g. parent/child or brother/sister), or informal way (e.g. grandrelative or husband/wife)—how close to sit, whether to tell rude jokes or not, and so on. If, for example, someone's father-in-law is called !A/e, the fact that I happen to bear that name, even though I am not really a Naro, means that they will classify me and treat me as if I were their father-in-law. (If I were actually a Naro and therefore had a Naro genealogy, and I were the older, I would do the classifying and they would reciprocate appropriately.)

Finally, it is worth recalling that where everyone is kin, possibly no-one is structurally privileged (in terms of social category) for the kind of sharing that we might think of as characterizing kin relations in other kinds of society. Of course, Khoisan hunter-gatherers, like anyone else, recognize the difference between close kin and distant, but they also have other mechanisms to enable the redistribution of resources. The best known, though not the only one, is the relationship of delayed balanced reciprocity known as *hxaro* (Wiessner 1982) which transcends kin category. It is, in a sense, quasi-kinship by choice. Ironically, *hxaro* (or *//aĩ*, as some groups call it) is not quite unique to hunter-gatherers, and not found among the majority of Bushman groups. Yet for those groups that practise it, it is a highly effective social and economic tool. Individuals choose their partners and define their place in the world according to their partnerships, which in turn allow access to the resources which their partners own.

CULTURE, COMMUNITY AND LOCAL GROUPS

Ernest Gellner once defined 'culture', and defined it in two quite different ways. In its more abstract sense, he argued, culture is 'a system of constraints' analogous to language, which in turn is itself 'a system of prohibitions' (Gellner 1989, 515–519). In both cases, language and culture, our predisposition for acquiring and adhering to such limiting behaviours is part of what makes us human. In its more specific sense, Geller reasoned, culture is 'what a population shares and what turns it into a community', while a community is simply 'a population which shares a culture' (1989, 515).

Locality and community

The group that Robert Layton and Sean O'Hara (ch. 5 this volume) call the 'community' is possibly the most socially important unit for hunter-gatherers—in the present or in prehistoric times. Essentially, this is the unit which is often in the southern African literature called the 'nexus', or what I have called the 'band cluster'. If it aggregates seasonally, it is what North Americanists sometimes call the 'maximal band' or 'macro-band'. It is larger than the 'band', 'camp' or what Australianists used to call the 'horde', but smaller than the grouping considered in traditional Australianist terminology a 'tribe', or elsewhere for hunter-gatherers a 'society' or 'speech community'. The latter, larger unit is more akin to Gellner's idea of a 'community'. In my primary fieldwork area in central-western Botswana, the speech community is the people who speak Naro. The band cluster, or community I worked in, is N//oa//xai, and the camp or band location I lived in for most of my early fieldwork was called ≠Aã. During my one-year stay at ≠Aã in 1974–1975, the population varied from about 20 to 25. On return visits I found population size down to zero in 1979, and then up to about 25 again in 1982. None of the people of ≠Aã in 1975 had returned in 1982, although I caught up with several of them in nearby locations. When I visited the area in 1995, ≠Aã had again been abandoned, but individuals who had lived there in the 1970s were located nearby.

In fact, ≠Aã was, and is, a specific location—more permanent in residence than what we might usually want to label a 'camp' but much more fluid in composition than what we tend to think of as a 'band'. Meyer Fortes' (1958) idea of the 'developmental cycle of domestic groups' comes to mind. Working with Ghanaian agriculturalists, Fortes deduced the temporal patterns that must lie behind what the fieldworker sees. The duration of the cycle, from nuclear family compound, to extended family compound, to death and division, and so on, might take 40 or 60 years. The ethnographer, though, might be there for just two years, and must recognize that the different observed social units in fact represent different points in a temporal sequence: that one over there will become like this one over here in 15 years, and then split to become two units like those over the hill. In other words, the dynamics of group structure in, say, a 60-year cycle cannot be observed in one or two years in the field, but must be inferred. Through deduction, then, the seemingly random movement of individuals on the ground becomes the temporal pattern in the ethnographer's mind.

One thing that interests me here is whether hunter-gatherers conceptualize their social units in terms of such temporal patterns. The evidence of ethnography, for example on the Ju/'hoansi (Lee 1979, 333–369; Marshall 1976, 156–200), suggests that they do. They know the history of their own individual movements between locations, and of others, and they explain their residence and use of resources in terms of returning to where they lived, their parents lived, or their grandparents lived, and therefore where they retain rights in band territory and band membership.

Are hunter-gatherers different?

Are hunter-gatherers different from non-hunter-gatherers? Recent perspectives in archaeology suggest that there was no Neolithic Revolution. Clive Gamble (2007), for example, in *Origins and revolutions* argues that human cultural evolution is gradual and marked by an uneven gradient of development from instruments to containers. Its timescale covers the period before symbolic culture up until the Neolithic and the times after. In his view, there was no Neolithic Revolution and no Human or Symbolic Revolution either. Yet widely accepted notions in social anthropology distinguish between hunter-gatherer and non-hunter-gatherer ways of life. The most influential of these is James Woodburn's (e.g. 1980) distinction between immediate and delayed-return economies. Woodburn argues that once a people have made this economic transition, their way of thinking is

altered. Immediate-return peoples do not plan for the future in their economic activities and are reluctant to invest time in making complex hunting equipment, let alone spending the time required to grow crops or look
after livestock. Even Australian Aborigines, in Woodburn's words, 'farm
out' their women through complex kinship arrangements, thus denying
themselves the status of an immediate-return economic ideology.

However, in my view both Gamble and Woodburn go too far in making their respective points. There was a 'Neolithic Revolution'—in the
sense that the transition from food-gathering and hunting to food production was, ultimately, revolutionary. There is no doubt that it was slow
and gradual, taking perhaps about 1,500 years according to estimates for
both Europe and southern Africa (see Barnard 2007, 17). The revolutionary point, if it can be dated, occurred not at the beginning (as
Woodburn's distinction would imply), but rather at the end of the long
Neolithic transition. I have suggested this indirectly in several papers on
what I have called the foraging or hunting-and-gathering mode of
thought (e.g. Barnard 2002, 2007). Neolithic and post-Neolithic thinking
involve permanent settlement and planning for the future. For example, a
number of things change with the acquisition of livestock: the need for
herding skills; the search for grazing; the possession of a guaranteed supply of meat; the practice of trading it as opposed to just sharing it; the
longer work hours required for herding over hunting and gathering; the
possibility of increasing the number of possessions through sale or trade
of livestock; greater worries over the supply of water; and above all the
necessity to plan for the future of the herd and the human social group.
A similar set of attributes is applicable to the acquisition of cultivating
practices (Barnard 2007, 16–17).

Figure 12.1 shows an example from my paper on modes of thought
through the Neolithic transition. It illustrates just one of several changes
in perception required when one moves from hunting and gathering, to
herding or horticulture. An individual's relations with the group change
with regard to the contrast between accumulation and immediate consumption. Accumulation, which was in hunter-gatherer times anti-social,
becomes social through the ability to pass possessions, including livestock, through the generations. This is contrasted with immediate consumption, which is not a purely individual act for hunter-gatherers, but a
social one, as it is equated with sharing. One can think of the model as
'hunter-gatherers consume' or 'hunter-gatherers share', but I find it more
meaningful to think of it as 'non-hunter-gatherers accumulate (but manage
to do this in a socially acceptable way)'.

MESOLITHIC MODE OF THOUGHT

Accumulation   Anti-social (equated with not
                                            sharing)

Immediate consumption   Social (equated with sharing with
                                            family and community)

NEOLITHIC MODE OF THOUGHT

Accumulation   Social (equated with saving for self
                                            and dependants)

Immediate consumption   Anti-social (equated with not saving)

Figure 12.1. Sharing (immediate consumption) and accumulation (from Barnard 2007, 10)

THE DISTRIBUTED MIND IN SOCIAL THEORY

The distributed mind hypothesis suggests mind beyond the self, broadly in the sense that an individual's mind is located in his or her environment as much as it is within his or her brain. Particularly in archaeology, this is generally taken to imply that the material world, especially material culture, shapes the thinking of individuals just as much as an individual shapes the artefacts of that culture (see also Gamble ch. 2 this volume). Yet environments can be social as well as natural, and immaterial as well as material. In this sense, earlier ideas in the social sciences, as well as in the biological sciences (cf. Wilson 2005), can also imply a distributed mind. Examples from the social sciences might include Durkheim's *conscience collective* (or 'collective consciousness'), Bateson's version of the early 20th-century idea of a cultural 'configuration', and Lévi-Strauss's *esprit humaine* (often translated as 'collective unconscious').

Durkheim's 'collective consciousness' is a social mind exerting its collective will on individuals. In his statistical study of suicide in France, Durkheim (1951 [1897]) showed that even this seemingly ultimate individual act is in part socially determined. There is a correlation between religion and the incidence of suicide. Protestants and Jews in 19th-century France were more prone to kill themselves than were Catholics. Similarly, Gregory Bateson (1980 [1936], 30–31) described the 'configuration' of a culture as a combination of its 'ethos', or emotional emphases, and its 'eidos', or system of cognitive processes. Lévi-Strauss's 'human spirit' or 'collective unconscious' is a mind distributed not among members of a single culture or society, but one distributed throughout humankind as a whole. This is most obvious to me in Lévi-Strauss's early work on kinship (1969 [1949]), in which he suggests that every kinship system in the world can be defined according to the way it utilizes the generating principles that underlie all human kinship structures. Other anthropologists, no doubt, would point to Lévi-Strauss's writings on the savage mind, totemism or mythology, in all of which the seemingly culturally specific is explained as part of deeper and universal cultural determinants.

A somewhat more mystical and much more extreme version is found too in anthropology, in A. L. Kroeber's theory of 'the superorganic' (1917). In Kroeber's 1917 article of that title, the individual was pushed to the side in favour of cultural forces which drive human invention. Kroeber points to the fact that the telescope, the telephone, photography, the phonograph and so on were each simultaneously invented by two or more people; and oxygen, Neptune and the North and South Poles similarly discovered almost simultaneously by more than one individual. His article brought immediate criticism though, from Edward Sapir (1917), who attacked Kroeber for overemphasizing material aspects of culture. Sapir attributed invention in philosophical, religious and aesthetic activities to autonomous individual activity, albeit activity by culture-bearing individuals in social contexts.

Let me sum up this brief excursion into social theory with three points. First, notions resembling the present-day concepts of 'distributed mind' are not all recent. They have been around in sociological and anthropological thought for some time, and I know that psychologists can cite examples from their discipline as well. Second, as the earlier ideas suggest, there are different levels of collective consciousness or mind distribution. They need not be confined to countable 'cultures', but may be present at any level: from family, community or society to a deeper configuration comprising 'culture' as a whole, in the abstract. Third, there have been serious disagreements, even among close colleagues of the same intellectual school, about fundamental things like the locus of culture, the relation between biological, psychological and social phenomena, and whether or not to see individuals as embodying culture to such a degree that they cease to be able to act as individuals at all.

The evolutionary question that comes to mind is less how 'deep' cultural universals may be, but how old. Let me again set aside our current knowledge and examine this question of time-depth with reference to a debate from a few decades ago. At the 'Man the Hunter' conference in 1966, there was a heated exchange between Claude Lévi-Strauss and L. R. Hiatt, over the historical and evolutionary interpretation of Gidjingali marriage arrangements and of Australian kinship structures more broadly (see Hiatt 1968; Hiatt & Lévi-Strauss 1968; Lévi-Strauss 1968). Let me quote from the post-conference, edited version of Lévi-Strauss's paper.

Lévi-Strauss (1968: 351) writes: 'Hiatt has suggested two possible explanations for the discrepancy between model and reality in Australian society . . .' Lévi-Strauss refers here to Hiatt's comment that, in order to salvage Lévi-Strauss's idealist interpretation of present-day Australian systems, we might envisage the imperfect systems that we see today either as survivals from a time when behaviour did conform to reality, or as 'a chronologically unrealized unconscious model' (Hiatt 1968: 172). 'However', Lévi-Strauss continues, alongside these possibilities:

> . . . there is also a third worth considering—that at one time, all this completed theory was clearly conceived and invented by native sociologists or philosophers. Thus, what we are doing is not building a theory with which to interpret the facts, but rather trying to get back to the older native theory at the origin of the facts we are trying to explain. After all, we know that mankind is about one or two million years old, but while we are ready to grant man this great antiquity, we are not ready to grant man a continuous thinking capacity during this enormous length of time. I see no reason why mankind should have waited until recent times to produce minds of the caliber of a Plato or an Einstein. Already, over two or three hundred thousand years ago, there were probably men of a similar capacity, who were probably not applying their intelligence to the solution of the same problems as these more recent thinkers; instead, they were probably more interested in kinship! (1968, 351)

It is worth recalling too Richard Lee and Irven DeVore's words in the preface to *Man the hunter*:

> We cannot avoid the suspicion that many of us were led to live and work among hunters [or hunter-gatherers] because of a feeling that the human condition was likely to be more clearly drawn here than among other kinds of societies. (1968, ix)

In other words, through the study of contemporary hunter-gatherers we can hope to uncover something of an earlier time, when perhaps, if Lévi-

Strauss is right, we might have seen kinship coming to be debated, or practices being modelled and models being practised.

Exactly when this was of course we do not know, but elsewhere I have suggested a trajectory, based in fact on the social brain hypothesis—to which I shall now turn.

THE SOCIAL BRAIN HYPOTHESIS, LANGUAGE AND KINSHIP

The social brain hypothesis suggests that the anthropoid primate brain evolved along with social complexity. In the brain, this involved the expansion of the neocortex, and in society it involved, among other things, a parallel expansion in group size and consequent selection for language over grooming as basis of communication around the time of *Homo erectus* (e.g. Dunbar 2001, 190–191).

In recent papers, I have coupled this hypothesis with (a) a rough and not strictly essential trajectory in relation to fossil hominins, from *Homo habilis* or *Homo erectus* to *Homo heidelbergensis* to *Homo sapiens*; (b) Calvin and Bickerton's three-phase model of the evolution of language (2000): from proto-language (words and symbolic communication) to rudimentary language (simple and ambiguous sentences) to true language (with full syntax); and (c) a parallel model of the evolution of kinship. The last involves a proto-kinship phase of inclusive kinship and sharing, which is different from pre-linguistic kin patterns among chimpanzees, bonobos or (I speculate) australopithecines; building on that, a rudimentary kinship phase of us/them kinship, incest avoidance and exchange of all kinds; and then a full kinship phase with universal kin categorization and explicit rules of sharing, exchange and kin behaviour. This third phase, which entails loosely Lévi-Straussian elementary structures (Lévi-Strauss 1969), eventually breaks down after Neolithization and the transition from universal to non-universal classification systems and the re-emergence of genealogical distance over category as the basis of kin relationships (Barnard 2008, 2009).

This theory is expressed in Figure 12.2. There is more to it, of course, but the relevance of it here is to suggest that the dawn of *Homo*, which is traditionally regarded as the dawn of tool-making (although this may now be in dispute), also marks the beginnings of linguistic communication, which is in turn coupled with the evolution of kinship structures. Leslie Aiello and Peter Wheeler (1995) have also argued a relation

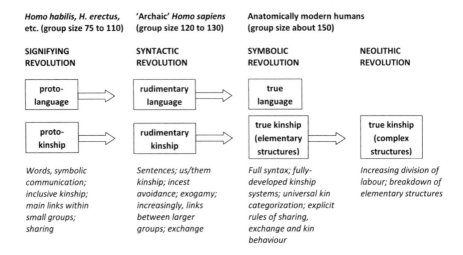

Figure 12.2. The co-evolution of language and kinship

between brain size, gut size and a transition to intensive meat-eating, which in turn suggests larger group sizes and increasing intellectual abilities, which are required not only to make tools but also to teach tool-making skills. The evolution of kinship structures through the phases which I call 'signifying', 'syntactic' and 'symbolic' involve an ever-increasing concern with classification as the basis of identity—until the destabilizing Neolithic. An individual in human society is never isolated. In a universal system, he or she is also never without specific relationship to everyone else, for kinship does not stop at the family but at the very end of social interaction. No individual is non-kin, but always my joking partner (e.g. wife or grandmother) or my avoidance partner (e.g. usually a man's sister, or mother).

HUMAN NATURE?

Distributed mind and extended brain

The distributed mind hypothesis implies that humans are naturally cultural, and possibly that we are naturally cultural to an unlimited degree. Furthermore, culture has no bounds, in that at least certain aspects of culture are cumulative and can be amplified by the storage capacity of language, and, beyond that, by the unnatural means of writing or computers. A further comparison with language may be relevant here. Marc Hauser et al. (2002, 1570) note that there is a difference between language as 'a culturally specific communication system' and language as 'an internal component of the mind/brain'. The notion of culture, it seems to me, could similarly be divided into two forms, with analogous meanings. Hauser et al. further discuss the distinction between the 'faculty of language in the broad sense' (FLB) and the 'faculty of language in the narrow sense' (FLN). The former includes sensory-motor and conceptual-intentional systems, whereas the latter includes specifically recursion— the embedding of a sentence within a sentence. And they argue that although other animals have FLB, only humans have FLN. Recursion, for them, is the single defining property of human, as opposed to animal, communication. But the most relevant point they make for our discussion here is that to find the mechanism required for the evolution of language to include recursion, we probably have to look beyond language itself: they suggest to numerical ability, navigation and (unspecified) social relations.

The extended brain hypothesis implies that humans are naturally social, but only to a certain degree. More specifically, humans achieve maximal sociality at roughly 150 individuals per group (or per 'community', which may be larger or smaller), according to predictions by neocortex ratio. While there is no limit to culture, this seems to be the natural limit to sociality for humans (see Aiello & Dunbar 1993, 189). However, I question these limits on both counts. It is not that culture has no natural bounds or that sociality is impassably bounded, but rather, that we in our post-natural age have broken the constraints of nature on the first count and found cultural solutions to social boundaries on the second count. Let me explain. In a sense, the cultural limits of human nature lie at the end of hunter-gatherer society. And by 'hunter-gatherer society' I mean those societies which function primarily (if not exclusively) by hunting and gathering and possess a foraging mode of thought. Arguably, the production and processing of vegetables and grain, and the possession of edible and milk-, yoghurt- and cheese-giving animals, does not lie within the 'natural' confines of a human way of life. It lies easily within human capability, of course, but beyond normal human nature.

Likewise, group sizes of thousands and millions of humans per social entity lie clearly within human capability, but well beyond the predictions for humans based on neocortex size alone. Dunbar (e.g. 1993) has explained this with ingenious examples of maximal units among anarchical intentional communities such as Hutterites. They themselves explain the limit of 150 as the largest community which they can sustain without a police force or other hierarchical mechanisms to maintain order. Beyond that, we do seem to need such *unnatural*, and therefore arguably un-human, hierarchical mechanisms of social constraint. As it happens, I live in a fairly self-regulating hamlet (in the Scottish Borders) of almost exactly 150 individuals. It is not an intentional community, but an accidental and indeed very diverse one. The vast majority of humanity, though, live in villages, towns or cities that are considerably larger. They do this by extending not their brains, but their unnatural, *cultural* elaboration of social segmentation and social order.

African or Australian?

In an earlier paper (Barnard 1999) I raised the question of which represented the better model of early symbolic cultural humanity: contemporary African hunter-gatherers, or contemporary Australian ones. I suggested that there are six ways in which Australian hunter-gatherers differ from southern African hunter-gatherers, and that these are mainly also ways in which the former differ from all other hunter-gatherers. These include: belief in the Rainbow Serpent, spiritual relations to land, the possession of elaborate forms of totemism, complex rights and obligations to kin through clan membership, elaborate marriage rules governed by sociocentric categories, and the application of the same classification principles in a larger world order which is unified through such principles. All these, it seems to me, are reasons for looking elsewhere. African hunter-gatherers, whose social and cosmological structures are simpler and more like those of other hunter-gatherers, are more likely to represent the earlier form.

Let me now add a seventh reason. In a recent paper, Doron Behar et al. (2008) show that the genetic distance between different branches of humanity is greatest in Africa, and within Africa greatest in southern Africa, and within southern Africa greatest among Khoisan peoples. The rest of the world really represents a small subset of human genetic diversity (at least in female lines). According to Behar and his colleagues, the matrilineal divergence of the Khoisan population was between 150,000 and 90,000 years ago, and the Out of Africa dispersal between 70,000 and 60,000 years ago. I shall return to that point in a moment.

There are several specific forms of kinship classification among southern African hunter-gatherers, but broadly these can be collapsed into two basic forms. These basic forms are the same the world over (see Barnard 2008, 238–239). One emphasizes genealogical distance and the other emphasizes egocentric cross/parallel and alternating-generation categories. As among other hunter-gatherers, both forms are universal, in that everyone is categorized as kin. But, unlike most Australian or South American systems, these operate entirely without sociocentric categories. If such categories were embedded within human nature, I would expect to find at least one system in Africa too with remnants of them. The parallel/cross- and alternating-generation categories are not vestiges of these, but rather the building blocks of both such egocentric systems and the sociocentric ones of Australia and South America.

On a worldwide scale, my view seems to go against Clark Wissler's age–area hypothesis (e.g. Wissler 1923, 58–61), which for smaller regional units like 'culture areas', often does work. Wissler's age–area hypothesis is indeed sustained if we look to eastern and southern Africa, and not the whole world, as the relevant unit. In the early 20th century, Wissler hypothesized that typically within a culture area the oldest items of culture will be those found on the periphery, not those in the centre. That is because the centre is the seat of change, and things diffuse outwards (from centre to periphery). One might ask why this is of any relevance today, in our era of absolute dating with radioactive isotopes. As Sapir pointed out in his argument against Kroeber, it is relevant because not all culture is material culture. We might indeed want to know which kinship structures, social practices or cosmologies came first among modern humans in general, or in a subcontinent or region. In a monumental book called *Configurations of culture growth*, Kroeber (1944) did eventually try his hand at explaining the things Sapir had criticized him for leaving out. Indeed, it is not the accumulated specifics, material or ethereal, which define what is in essence a relation between culture and individual. It is the configuration, or to borrow the Chomskyan phrase, the 'faculty of *culture* in the narrow sense', which allows the description of specific social relations to be embedded in abstractions such as a 'kinship system'. In my own work (e.g. Barnard 1992), such configurations are as often as not definable as structural elements held in common across a culture area or region like Khoisan southern Africa or Aboriginal Australia—in other words, larger than specific 'cultures'. The fact that both Aborigines and Bushmen can not only classify strangers but also make connections between systems when describing them hints at cognitive configurations that lie between a 'culture' and the universe of cultures.

CONCLUSION

Let me conclude with a brief return to Behar et al.'s paper (2008) in light of the social brain and extended mind hypotheses. Humanity is descended in the common matriline from a small group of people living between 210,000 and 140,000 years ago. There are more than 40 mtDNA lineages in the African population, but only two such lineages in the Out of Africa migration. This, according to Behar, suggests that humanity at the point of dispersal was divided into small, isolated groups, and, further, that matrilineal organization was likely. I would say that uxorilocality would be a better description, but the details of that matter little in terms of the wider social organization of the groups. These people of the African Middle Stone Age no doubt possessed all the attributes shared by humanity today. They also, I believe, possessed specifically those elements of culture and social life common to all or nearly all human hunter-gatherers today or in ethnographic memory. These would include at least the following: a low population density compared to non-hunter-gatherers; a band level of social organization; an egalitarian social organization; gender differentiation in subsistence and in ritual; customs governing the distribution of the products of hunting and gathering activities; universal kin classification; belief in communication with animals or a symbolic association between animals and humans (Barnard 1999). They probably had a world-view based on twos or fours (not threes), and their religion was one of animism or monotheism (not polytheism and probably not totemism, which is dependent on more complex relations to land or among groups). And above all, their social order was characterized by flexibility, even if their cosmological order was more rigid.

This society of natural, but fully cultural, humanity spread across the globe and became all of us. Those who went south have kept most closely the knowledge and social ways of all our ancestors. Those who went elsewhere have all lost elements of social structure that are adaptive for southern and eastern African hunter-gatherer life and which still characterize many fully modern hunter-gatherer communities in southern and eastern Africa and—though to a lesser extent—elsewhere in the world. Such attributes include the individual ability to classify as 'kin' everyone with whom one normally associates, but nevertheless without the formal assignment of individuals to sociocentric categories such as moieties or sections. The classification of kin in such a way would be coincident with formally restricting but nevertheless empirically flexible rules of marriage.

Other attributes would include the ability to form groups, aggregate and disperse according to seasonal and other environmental circumstances, and, importantly, the recognition of common cultural configurations across physical group boundaries.

   Human nature is within us all, but more precisely embedded within some forms of social structure than others. This is not the same thing as hominin nature, because in humans language and the consequent development of kinship structures replace other forms of social bonding. Human nature is more embedded in the social structures of African hunter-gatherer populations than elsewhere because such populations, at least until very recently, have been able to maintain relations to land, to resources, and to people through symbolic and socio-environmental ideologies undoubtedly reminiscent of those once shared by all humanity. It is not that these peoples are in any sense primitive, but rather that the rest of us are, through our social condition, in a sense deviant: we have lost part of that aspect of human nature that defines post-symbolic but pre-political sociality.

REFERENCES

Aiello, L. C. & Dunbar, R. I. M. (1993). Neocortex size, group size and the evolution of language. *Current Anthropology* 34: 184–193.

Aiello, L. C. & Wheeler, P. (1995). The expensive tissue hypothesis: the brain and the digestive system in human and primate evolution. *Current Anthropology* 36: 199–221.

Barnard, A. (1978). Universal systems of kin categorization. *African Studies* 37: 69–81.

Barnard, A. (1988). Kinship, language and production: a conjectural history of Khoisan social structure. *Africa* 58: 29–50.

Barnard, A. (1992). *Hunters and herders of southern Africa: a comparative ethnography of the Khoisan peoples*. Cambridge: Cambridge University Press.

Barnard, A. (1999). Modern hunter-gatherers and early symbolic culture. In: R. Dunbar, C. Knight & C. Power (eds) *The evolution of culture: an interdisciplinary view*, pp. 50–68. Edinburgh: Edinburgh University Press.

Barnard, A. (2002). The foraging mode of thought. In: H. Stewart, A. Barnard & K. Omura (eds) *Self- and other images of hunter-gatherers*, pp. 5–24, Senri Ethnological Studies 60. Osaka: National Museum of Ethnology.

Barnard, A. (2007). From Mesolithic to Neolithic modes of thought. In: A. Whittle & V. Cummings (eds) *Going over: the Mesolithic–Neolithic transition in north-west Europe*, pp. 5–19, Proceedings of the British Academy 144. London: Oxford University Press for the British Academy.

Barnard, A. (2008). The co-evolution of language and kinship. In: N. J. Allen, H. Callan, R. Dunbar & W. James (eds) *Early human kinship: from sex to social reproduction*, pp. 232–243. Oxford: Blackwell Publishing.

Barnard, A. (2009). Social origins: sharing, exchange, kinship. In: R. Botha & C. Knight (eds) *The cradle of language*, pp. 356–381. Oxford: Oxford University Press.

Bateson, G. (1980 [1936]). *Naven: a survey of the problems suggested by a composite picture of the culture of a New Guinea tribe drawn from three points of view*, 2nd edn. London: Wildwood House.

Behar, D. M., Villems, R., Soodyall, H., Blue-Smith, J., Pereira, L., Metspalu, E. et al. (2008). The dawn of human matrilineal diversity. *American Journal of Human Genetics* 82: 1–11.

Bickerton, D. (1998). Catastrophic evolution: the case for a single step from proto-language to full human language. In: J. R. Hurford, M. Studdert-Kennedy & C. Knight (eds) *Approaches to the evolution of language: social and cognitive bases*, pp. 341–358. Cambridge: Cambridge University Press.

Boyd, R. & Richerson, P. J. (2005). *The origin and evolution of cultures*. Oxford: Oxford University Press.

Calvin, W. H. & Bickerton, D. (2000). *Lingua ex machina: reconciling Darwin and Chomsky with the human brain*. Cambridge, MA: MIT Press.

Dunbar, R. I. M. (1993). Coevolution of neocortical size, group size and language in humans. *Behavioral and Brain Sciences* 16(4): 681–735.

Dunbar, R. I. M. (1998). The social brain hypothesis. *Evolutionary Anthropology* 7: 178–190.

Dunbar, R. I. M. (2001). Brains on two legs: group size and the evolution of intelligence. In: F. B. M. de Waal (ed.) *Tree of origin: what primate behavior can tell us about human social evolution*, pp. 173–192. Cambridge, MA: Harvard University Press.

Durkheim, E. (1951 [1897]). *Suicide: a study in sociology*, trans. J. A. Spaulding & G. Simpson. New York: Free Press of Glencoe.

Fortes, M. (1958). Introduction. In: J. Goody (ed.) *The developmental cycle in domestic groups*, pp. 1–15. Cambridge: Cambridge University Press.

Gamble, C. (2007). *Origins and revolutions: human identity in earliest prehistory*. Cambridge: Cambridge University Press.

Gamble, C. & Porr, M. (2005). From empty spaces to lived lives: exploring the individual in the Palaeolithic. In: C. Gamble & M. Porr (eds) *The individual in context: archaeological investigations of Lower and Middle Palaeolithic landscapes, locales and artefacts*, pp. 1–12. London: Routledge.

Gellner, E. (1989). Culture, constraint and community: semantic and coercive compensations for the genetic under-determination of *Homo sapiens sapiens*. In: P. Mellars & C. Stringer (eds) *The Human Revolution: behavioural and biological perspectives in the origins of modern humans*, pp. 514–525. Edinburgh: Edinburgh University Press.

Güldemann, T. (1998). The Kalahari basis as an object of areal typology—a first approach. In: M. Schladt (ed.) *Language, identity, and conceptualization among the Khoisan*, pp. 137–169, Research in Khoisan Studies 15. Cologne: Rüdiger Köppe Verlag.

Hauser, M. D., Chomsky, N. & Fitch, T. (2002). The faculty of language: what is it, who has it, and how did it evolve? *Science* 298: 1569–1579.

Hiatt, L. R. (1968). Gidjingali marriage arrangements. In: R. B. Lee & I. DeVore (eds) *Man the hunter*, pp. 165–175. Chicago: Aldine.

Hiatt, L. R. & Lévi-Strauss, C. (1968). Gidjingali marriage arrangements: comments and rejoinder. In: R. B. Lee & I. DeVore (eds) *Man the hunter*, pp. 210–212. Chicago: Aldine.

Kroeber, A. L. (1917). The superorganic. *American Anthropologist* 19: 163–213.

Kroeber, A.L. (1944). *Configurations of culture growth*. Berkeley: University of California Press.

Lee, R. B. (1979). *The !Kung San: men, women, and work in a foraging society*. Cambridge: Cambridge University Press.

Lee, R. B. & I. DeVore, I. (1968). Preface. In: R. B. Lee & I. DeVore (eds) *Man the hunter*, pp. vii–ix. Chicago: Aldine.

Lévi-Strauss, C. (1968). The concept of primitiveness. In: R. B. Lee & I. DeVore (eds) *Man the hunter*, pp. 349–352. Chicago: Aldine.

Lévi-Strauss, C. (1969 [1949]). *The elementary structures of kinship*, revised edn, trans. J. H. Bell, J. R. von Sturmer & R. Needham. London: Eyre & Spottiswoode.

Marshall, L. (1976). *The !Kung of Nyae Nyae*. Cambridge, MA: Harvard University Press.

Sapir, E. (1917). Do we need a 'superorganic'? *American Anthropologist* 19: 441–447.

Wiessner, P. (1982). Risk, reciprocity and social influences on !Kung San economics. In: E. Leacock & R. Lee (eds) *Politics and history in band societies*, pp. 61–84. Cambridge: Cambridge University Press.

Wilson, R. A. (2005). Collective memory, group minds, and the extended mind thesis. *Cognitive Process* 6(4): 227–236.

Wissler, C. (1923). *Man and culture*. New York: Thomas Y. Crowell Co.

Woodburn, J. (1980). Hunters and gatherers today and reconstruction of the past. In: E. Gellner (ed.) *Soviet and Western anthropology*, pp. 95–117. London: Duckworth.

13

Cliques, Coalitions, Comrades and Colleagues: Sources of Cohesion in Groups

HOLLY ARROW

THE SOCIAL BRAIN HYPOTHESIS proposes that a major factor driving the evolution of large brain size and enhanced cognitive capacity in primates is social complexity, for which the maximum size of organized groups is used as a proxy (Dunbar 1993). In line with our fission-fusion pattern of social organization (see Layton & O'Hara ch. 5 this volume; Lehmann et al. ch. 4 this volume), human groups occur in a variety of characteristic sizes rather than being smoothly distributed along a continuum from small to large (Caporael & Baron 1997; Dunbar 1998; Zhou et al. 2005). Attention to the different sorts of 'adhesives' that hold groups together can provide insight into why the apparently strong constraints limiting the size of some kinds of groups do not apply to groups held together with different sorts of ties. Freed of many of the environmental constraints that limit community size for hunter-gatherer societies living in harsh environments (see Layton & O'Hara ch. 5 this volume), some groups can grow to huge sizes, while others stay small. The architecture of cohesion helps explain why.

Social psychologists distinguish between the dyadic ties that connect two individuals (interpersonal relationships), and the connection between an individual and a group (group identification or social identity). They also distinguish between the strong bonds of socio-emotional cohesion and the more flexible adhesives of exchange or task cohesion (Evans & Dion 1991; Stokes 1983). Combining these two variables yields four adhesives for forming groups: strong and weak dyadic ties and primary and secondary group identification. After explaining in more detail the multiple sources of cohesion as understood by social psychologists, I will provide a fuller picture of the group prototypes these give rise to. The mix of strong and weak adhesives and the greater scalability offered by the

Proceedings of the British Academy **158**, 269–281. © The British Academy 2010.

member–group bond in particular has facilitated the assembly of large-scale societies that are orders of magnitude larger than ancestral human groups, without creating unmanageably large demands on the social brain.

The focus of this chapter is on how groups of three or more people who are not necessarily close kin are structured and held together. In small-scale hunter-gatherer societies and in ancestral bands and tribes, most members of a band are kin, whether close or more distant. Family members also form an important part of the personal networks of modern humans (see Roberts ch. 6 this volume), as do the pair bonds (see Dunbar ch. 8 this volume) that are embedded in and generative of families. The family ties of kin relations and mates are clearly fundamental to human communities.

Social psychologists studying groups, however, have largely ignored kin groups and kin relations, and mating and marriage are not generally studied in relation to larger groups. Research into groups has either composed groups from scratch in order to manipulate variables such as task, group size or leadership structure, or it has focused on the existing non-kin groups that are ubiquitous in communities, the workplace, sports, social networks and the military. While social network studies reveal more of the private social sphere (Roberts ch. 6 this volume; Wallette ch. 7 this volume), studies of existing groups in modern industrial societies tend to 'find' groups in more public and accessible settings.

It is abundantly clear that genetic relatedness promotes cooperative relations and—in many mammalian species—acts of altruism that benefit both direct offspring and other kin (e.g. Mateo & Holmes 1997). However, genetic relatedness falls off sharply as one moves from siblings to first cousins to more distant relations, and thus the glue of inclusive fitness is not by itself sufficient to construct massively large and complex societies. Read (ch. 10 this volume) notes a limit of around 500–800 individuals for social organizations based on an extended kinship system. A next step for categorization beyond relatedness is universal kin classification (see Barnard ch. 12 this volume) by which pairs of people are classified as related based on, for example, sharing the same name. This generalization falls into the realm of non-kin-based social adhesives that is the focus of the present chapter.

Briefly sketched, the four group prototypes chosen to illustrate different architectures of cohesion are cliques, coalitions, comrades and colleagues. Cliques are dense clusters of individuals linked by strong, interconnected dyadic bonds. Coalitions, which also depend on dyadic ties, are strategic alignments that improve the relative power positions of the individuals involved (de Waal & Harcourt 1992). Comrades and colleagues are examples of groups that do not depend on dyadic ties. Comrades are united by collective action, joint membership and shared commitment to the group. Groups of colleagues are drawn together by common interests and shared social identity (for example, academics interested in the social brain). Dyadic relationships that develop among comrades and colleagues can be strong and enduring, but they are not fundamental building blocks for such groups.

These four prototypes should not be considered an exhaustive list of non-kin-based groups. Rather they constitute an informal typology designed to illuminate structural differences in cohesion that affect the cognitive loads on group members and the consequent group size limits. In other words, it is a typology created for the niche defined by this book. Existing typologies and category systems in group and organizational studies (e.g. Arrow & McGrath 1995; Hackman 1990) are less useful for this purpose as they tend to distinguish groups based either on the specific task they perform (e.g. top management groups or customer service teams) or on the different models used by managers and supervisors in creating work groups.

The rest of the chapter is organized as follows. First I discuss some different aspects of self and identity, social attraction and group cohesion. The relative importance of different forms of attraction and cohesion in different groups helps explain how they can be cohesive without having close interpersonal bonds among members. After establishing this groundwork, I consider the four exemplar group types in more depth, and discuss how the last two types in particular provide a mechanism for cohesion in very large organizations and societies.

THE MANY ASPECTS OF SELF AND IDENTITY

The self has been broadly defined by social psychologists as including the totality of thoughts about one's self (Trafimow et al. 1991). It is generally understood to be a complex psychological structure that includes a multiplicity of 'selves', some of which are more explicitly social than others. Distinctions are made between the private, public and collective self (Triandis 1989); the independent and interdependent self (Markus & Kitayama 1991); and the personal, relational and collective self (Brewer & Gardner 1996). As Barnard (ch. 12 this volume) might put it, some of our selves stop at the skin, and some do not. One approach to studying the self is to have people complete the sentence 'I am' multiple times and then classify the statements as belonging to different aspects of self. Statements such as 'I am tall' reference the personal or independent self; 'I am Susie's mom' refers to the relational self, and 'I am American', 'I am a Methodist' or 'I am a wide receiver for the Broncos' are aspects of the collective self. As these examples suggest, the relational self is most relevant to dyadic interpersonal relationships, while the collective self involves membership in and identification with a larger group.

Beyond these distinctions, research on self-concepts and self-esteem provides abundant evidence that the self is a special and privileged psychological structure that we are prone to enhance and that evokes strong favouritism. For example, even fleeting connection with the self makes objects more special and valued. A host of experiments have demonstrated a robust 'endowment' effect: the tendency to value 'my cup' more highly than other cups, even if has only been 'my' cup briefly, and to demand a higher price to sell it than to purchase an otherwise identical cup (Kahneman et al. 1991). This effect has clear implications for any relationship or group that is incorporated into the relational and collective self. The 'stickiness' of the self and our corresponding attachment to anything connected with the self provides a powerful adhesive that helps relationships and groups stay together.

Social identity theory focuses primarily on the collective self in the context of inter-group relations (Hogg et al. 2004). Social identity is a person's knowledge of belonging to a social group, including demographic categories such as European or women; it is enhanced by contrast with 'outgroups', whether these comprise a general category (e.g. men) or a more specific group (e.g. a rival football club). When people think of themselves as group members their feelings and actions are biased in favour of the group in the same way that the self is generally accorded special privilege in our thoughts, feelings and actions.

FORMS OF SOCIAL ATTRACTION

Attraction among fellow members of a group has long been recognized as a source of cohesion. It can take several forms. *Interpersonal attraction* is positive feeling between individuals independent of whether they are in a relationship or a group. It is promoted by inter-individual similarity (Hogg & Hardie 1991) and other bases of interpersonal attraction, such as physical attractiveness. *Depersonalized attraction* (Hogg & Hains 1996) describes attraction between individuals based on shared category membership. It is similar to the much older notion of solidarity among people who feel they are in similar circumstances. Hogg and colleagues (Hogg & Hains 1996; Hogg & Hardie 1991) have demonstrated that depersonalized attraction may be distinguished from interpersonal attraction both in cause and effects. It is also stronger the more a person is seen as prototypical of the category or group, as depersonalized attraction is derivative: the primary attraction is to the group, and the more prototypical a member is, the stronger the association between that person and the attractive group.

Group members may feel and act upon loyalty to one another based on depersonalized attraction regardless of whether they particularly like one another personally. Whereas dyadic bonds are promoted and cemented by interpersonal attraction, groups based on membership rely instead on depersonalized attraction.

A third form of social attraction, *inter-member attraction*, denotes positive feelings based on satisfying role relations within a group context (Brewer & Gardner 1996). It is grounded in interaction.

GROUP COHESION

A broad and often ambiguous concept (Hogg 1987; Mudrack 1989), 'cohesion' originally referred both to a quality of group structure such as compactness (Festinger et al. 1950) and to the totality of forces that act on members to keep them in the group (Festinger 1950). This confusing use of the term as both an attribute and a process continues to resist resolution (Brawley et al. 1987; Drescher et al. 1985; Keyton & Springston 1990; Stokes 1983). However, despite the lack of a consensus definition and it has become clear that cohesion has many sources and is also a multidimensional construct. For our purposes the most important distinction is that between socio-emotional cohesion and task cohesion (Tziner 1982).

Socio-emotional cohesion is typically measured by asking group members how much they like one another, enjoy socializing and are friends. It has obvious connections with interpersonal attraction, and addresses needs for intimacy and belonging (Baumeister & Leary 1995). Task cohesion refers instead to attraction to the group's activity and effective integration of members in pursuing the group task (Carron et al. 1985). A third type of cohesion rarely mentioned in the literature is exchange-based cohesion (Thibaut & Kelley 1959), which is based on satisfaction with an exchange relation.

CLIQUES: CLUSTERS OF CLOSE INTERPERSONAL TIES

Drawing on these distinctions, cliques evoke the relational self and are held together by dyadic bonds, interpersonal attraction, and socio-emotional cohesion. Knowing what keeps a group together also reveals what will threaten the group's integrity. In a friendship clique, disruptions of dyadic ties are traumatic not just for the two people involved, but for the whole group. Heider's balance theory applies strongly in cliques: if two friends embedded in the same cluster become openly hostile this can be a signifi-cant problem for the group (Cartwright & Harary 1956). The need for close monitoring of any disruption in the network of dyadic ties and the rippling effect of troubles in any one dyad or triad make the maintenance of cliques socially demanding, even beyond the direct costs of maintain-ing the dyadic bonds in which one is directly involved. The proliferation of dyads and triads that must be monitored and managed means that costs escalate as the clique gets larger. Small group size (4–5 members) helps keep these social cognitive costs reasonable and also makes it easier for the group to coordinate joint activities.

In the literature on prototypical human group sizes, the size of the smallest core of human personal networks—the support clique—typi-cally ranges from 3 to 7, with the mean varying in part based on how data is gathered (McPherson & Smith-Lovin 1987; Marsden 1987; Stiller & Dunbar 2007). However, such 'cliques' are not necessarily cliques in the network or group sense, as an individual may have others in their support clique who have no relationship with one another. In the network sense, the support clique is an ego-centric star, and need not be a fully connected cluster. When two dyads are not tied together into a triad, the challenge of maintaining balance in all three of the dyads is less significant. Instead, stresses created by increased demands from one dyadic partner may reduce time available to attend to the other relationships. When the dyads are fully clustered, a crisis for one member can be handled cooperatively by the group and the support load flexibly distributed. This reduces the cumulative risk posed by multiple dyadic obligations and protects against the damage to a bond that might otherwise result when one cannot respond effectively to a sudden need by a partner.

COALITIONS: EXCHANGE-BASED
STRATEGIC ALIGNMENTS

The ethological literature on coalition formation in primates (e.g. Harcourt & de Waal 1992) distinguishes between momentary coalitions that emerge for a single interaction and more enduring alliances among partners who routinely come to each other's aid or defence. Studies of coalitions in the social sciences (e.g. Komorita & Kravitz 1983; Mannix 1993; Murnighan 1985) typically do not make this distinction, and use the term 'coalition' to refer to strategic groupings regardless of stability.

Coalitions rely on exchange-based cohesion and, for those that endure over time, on dyadic obligations of reciprocal favours. Structurally, a coalition is based on the perception of shared advantages to grouping together, and to persist all members must remain convinced that the coalition benefits them more than some alternate political grouping. The emphasis on the individual self (and not the relationship or the collective) makes this a weak adhesive. In contrast to inwardly focused cliques, coalitions are focused on the external political context. Individuals solicit support from others to help counteract the power of some other individual or group. They need not like one another or feel depersonalized attraction based on shared category membership, for coalitions can bring together 'strange bedfellows' who otherwise have little in common.

Group theories based on social exchange (e.g. Moreland & Levine 1982; Thibaut & Kelley 1959) fit the coalition model. They assume that members are regularly scanning the environment and assessing other potential groups that might offer a better deal. If they find one, they will leave or threaten to leave to get a better deal from the group. In an ecology of shifting coalitions (e.g. the US Congress or a parliament), any membership change has political consequences, especially when allies who abandon one coalition join another. In this case dyadic ties of obligation can exacerbate the threat to the group rather than keep it together. A departing member may actively recruit others to leave with them, especially if he or she has a few strong allies within the coalition. Maintaining a positive power position thus requires constant monitoring not only of one's own dyadic alliances within the coalition but also the strength of political alignment of all other members with one another. For advanced players, monitoring the ties of coalition members with others outside the current group is also wise, as the value of any particular coalition is always relative. The social cognitive challenges of this Machiavellian monitoring are very high.

Despite these challenges, coalitions can be relatively large if the behavioural demands on members are modest ('vote with me on this; let others know by your presence that you support me'). Members can minimize the demands of monitoring the political situation by keeping track of a small subset of partners within their shifting coalitions, and by delegating comprehensive monitoring to dedicated roles such as the 'whips' of US congressional politics who keep track of the commitments and intentions of all relevant players. A coalition of hundreds in a deliberative body, however, is a more fragile grouping than a coalition among just a few people who can more easily monitor one another.

COMRADES: BONDED COLLECTIVE ACTION GROUPS

The defining characteristics of comrades are collective action and strong bonding to a group. The prototype of comrades is a war party, in which all members are bonded collectively (rather than dyadically) to one another in service of a joint goal. This bond with the group is essential to ensure loyalty and commitment in trying circumstances, as in military action the small group and not the individual soldier is the fundamental unit of effectiveness (Marshall 1947). Although powerful dyadic relationships can and do form among comrades, they are not essential as the primary attraction is depersonalized, the primary form of cohesion task cohesion, and the primary identity the collective self. A Marine feels a bond with another Marine and can immediately coordinate with him or her in joint action even if they are working together for the first time.

Comrades illustrate the difference between an acting group and a standing group or pool from which acting units are assembled or recruited. This is similar to the distinction between the interacting bands of a hunter-gatherer society and the larger communities of members from which the bands are composed (see Layton & O'Hara ch. 5 this volume). For comrades, the standing group can be very large (as with the Marines) even though the effective acting unit of soldiers for a particular mission is small. Among ancestral humans, the pool of comrades would probably be a sex- and age-stratified group of male adults eligible for missions such as hunting large dangerous game or conducting raids against other groups.

The norms that govern bands of comrades are strong and rigorously instilled through training and initiation. In contrast to coalitions, members do not come and go according to shifting political winds; instead, membership in the pool is permanent and defection a serious violation. The psychological machinery of induction helps to ensure loyalty via a powerful collective identity and attachment to the group, and hence the need for constant monitoring of intentions is minimized.

The size of a pool of comrades can be scaled up through a stratified structure of nested groups of different size. In the military, a squad is nested within a platoon, platoons are collected into companies, which is turn make up battalions, and so on up to an army composed of tens of thousands. In day-to-day action an individual's strongest attachment is to their smaller unit, in which interpersonal bonds can help the unit cohere. The strength of socio-emotional connection should also be especially strong with the cohort with which one was initiated. However, the ultimate loyalty is to the larger-scale unit to which each cohort belongs.

In the organization of comrades with cells and larger units, a new layer of social is complexity is evident. Belonging is generalized so that smaller groups in turn 'belong' to larger units. In this way groups are themselves linked and subordinated in a hierarchical structure. While inter-group rivalries can still be a source of tension and prove problem-atic in joint actions, awareness of shared membership in a larger unit to which both units belong can temper inter-group conflicts. In the social psychology literature, this phenomenon is studied under the rubric of categorization and re-categorization (Gaertner et al. 2000).

COLLEAGUES: SHARED INTERESTS AND SOCIAL DISTINCTIVENESS

Colleagues, like comrades, are connected via a shared social identity and depersonalized attraction. However, groups of colleagues differ from comrades as collectives and in the form of social organization in two important ways. First, colleagues with specialized skills or training are often dispersed across many primary action groups in which they play a specialized role. Thus what colleagues share is not membership in fully nested groups but boundary-spanning ties based on common training and similar roles. For example, accountants share a common training and interests, and may get together regularly at seminars and talk together on listserves, but many will be the only accountant in their immediate work group or organization.

Clustering of specialized colleagues in primary work groups (like comrades) is a phenomenon that probably developed gradually as the scale of human societies increased. Small bands of hunter-gatherers might each have a shaman, for example, and each shaman might have one or two apprentices. Gatherings of shamans, however, would occur only at seasonal gatherings of the larger tribe, when shamans could get together and share information and techniques, and perform ceremonies together. In towns and cities, however, people with the same specialized occupation can cluster together in guilds and live and work concentrated in the same district.

In the transition from smaller units to larger societies, the 'invisible colleges' of colleagues can provide connections across bands and also across tribes, as specialists can recognize one another's common distinctiveness even when there is a language barrier to overcome. Shared training and identity can also help to promote the development of norms and rules that transcend tribal boundaries. For example, European armies observed common rules of protocol regarding the surrender and ransoming of officers. During the battle of Waterloo British infantry who took temporary cover among freshly wounded Frenchmen engaged in what amounted to shop talk, exchanging professional opinions about how the battle might end (Keegan 1976, 204). The mutual recognition of colleagues made cordial exchanges possible even between official enemies.

GROUPS AND SOCIAL COMPLEXITY

A full account of social complexity needs to incorporate the ways in which groups can bind people together and coordinate their actions on a large scale without overwhelming their social and cognitive capacities. Groups such as bands and colleagues rely on the cross-level ties of membership as a source of cohesion beyond dyadic relationships, which are costly to maintain and monitor. The generalization of attachments beyond dyads to larger units provides a more flexible array of building blocks for creating large complex societies. In such societies, all four of the group types described here (plus others not detailed) operate, serving different functions. The ability of people to simultaneously belong to cliques, coalitions, and groups of comrades and colleagues adds social complexity. At the same time, group norms and roles—including the special role of leadership—can simplify the social demands of everyday life. One of the essential insights in the study of complexity is that complex structures are not necessarily generated by highly complicated processes

(Holland 1995). A small number of building blocks can generate highly complex architecture. And a large number of agents, following simple rules that make their actions dependent on the actions of others, can generate patterns of action and structure that are staggeringly complex.

REFERENCES

Arrow, H. & McGrath, J. E. (1995). Membership dynamics in groups at work: a theoretical framework. *Research in Organizational Behavior* 17: 373–411.

Baumeister, R. F. & Leary, M. R. (1995). The need to belong: desire for interpersonal attachments as a fundamental human motivation. *Psychological Bulletin* 117(3): 497–529.

Brawley, L. R., Carron, A. V. & Widmeyer, W. (1987). Assessing the cohesion of teams: validity of the Group Environment Questionnaire. *Journal of Sport Psychology* 9(3): 275–294.

Brewer, M. B. & Gardner, W. (1996). Who is this 'we'? Levels of collective identity and self-representations. *Journal of Personality and Social Psychology* 71: 83–93.

Caporael, L. R. & Baron, R. M. (1997). Groups as the mind's natural environment. In: J. A. Simpson & D. T. Kenrick (eds) *Evolutionary social psychology*, pp. 317–344. Hillsdale, NJ: Lawrence Erlbaum Associates.

Carron, A. V., Widmeyer, W. N. & Brawley, L. R. (1985). The development of an instrument to assess cohesion in sport teams: the Group Environment Questionnaire. *Journal of Sport Psychology* 7(3): 244–266.

Cartwright, D. & Harary, F. (1956). Structural balance: a generalization of Heider's theory. *Psychological Review* 63: 277–293.

de Waal, F. & Harcourt, A. H. (1992). Coalitions and alliances: a history of etho-logical research. In: F. de Waal & A. H. Harcourt (eds) *Coalitions and alliances in humans and other animals*, pp. 1–9. Oxford: Oxford University Press.

Drescher, S., Burlingame, G. & Fuhriman, A. (1985). Cohesion: an odyssey in empirical understanding. *Small Group Behavior* 16(1): 3–30.

Dunbar, R. I. M. (1993). Coevolution of neocortical size, group size and language in humans. *Behavioral & Brain Sciences* 16(4): 681–735.

Dunbar, R. I. M. (1998). The social brain hypothesis. *Evolutionary Anthropology* 6(5): 178–190.

Evans, C. R. & Dion, K. L. (1991). Group cohesion and performance: a meta-analysis. *Small Group Research* 22(2): 175–186.

Festinger, L. (1950). Informal social communication. *Psychological Review* 57(5): 271–282.

Festinger, L., Schachter, S. & Back, K. (1950). *Social pressures in informal groups*. Stanford, CA: Stanford University Press.

Gaertner, S. L., Dovidio, J. F., Banker, B. S., Houlette, M., Johnson, K. M. & MacGlynn, E. A. (2000). Reducing intergroup conflict: from superordinate goals to decategorization, recategorization, and mutual differentiation. *Group Dynamics* 4(1): 98–114.

Hackman, J. R. (ed.) (1990). *Groups that work (and those that don't)*. San Francisco: Jossey Bass.

Harcourt, A. H. & de Waal, F. (eds) (1992). *Coalitions and alliances in humans and other animals*. New York: Oxford University Press.

Hogg, M. A. (1987). Social identity and group cohesiveness. In: M. A. Turner, O. P. J. Hogg, S. D. Reicher & M. S. Wetherell (eds) *Rediscovering the social group: a self-categorization theory*, pp. 89–116. Oxford: Basil Blackwell.

Hogg, M. A. & Hains, S. C. (1996). Intergroup relations and group solidarity: effects of group identification and social beliefs on depersonalized attraction. *Journal of Personality & Social Psychology* 70(2): 295–309.

Hogg, M. A. & Hardie, E. A. (1991). Social attraction, personal attraction, and self-categorization—a field study. *Personality and Social Psychology Bulletin* 17(2): 175.

Hogg, M. A., Abrams, D., Otten, S. & Hinckle, S. (2004). The social identity perspective: intergroup relations, self-conception, and small groups. *Small Group Research* 35(3): 246.

Holland, J. H. (1995). *Hidden order: how adaptation builds complexity*. Reading, MA: Addison-Wesley.

Kahneman, D., Knetsch, J. L. & Thaler, R. H. (1991). The endowment effect, loss aversion, and status quo bias. *Journal of Economic Perspectives* 5(1): 193–206.

Keegan, J. (1976). *The face of battle*. New York: Penguin.

Keyton, J. & Springston, J. (1990). Redefining cohesiveness in groups. *Small Group Research* 21(2): 234–254.

Komorita, S. S. & Kravitz, D. A. (1983). *Coalition formation: a social psychological approach*. In: P. B. Paulus (ed.) *Basic group processes*, pp. 179–203. Hillsdale, NJ: Erlbaum.

McPherson, J. & Smith-Lovin, L. (1987). Homophily in voluntary organizations: status distance and the composition of face-to-face groups. *American Sociological Review* 52(3): 370–379.

Mannix, E. A. (1993). Organizations as resource dilemmas: the effects of power balance on coalition formation in small groups. *Organizational Behavior & Human Decision Processes* 55(1): 1–22.

Markus, H. R. & Kitayama, S. (1991). Culture and the self: implications for cognition, emotion, and motivation. *Psychological Review* 98(2): 224–253.

Marsden, P. V. (1987). Core discussion networks of Americans. *American Sociological Review* 52(1): 122–131.

Marshall, S. L. A. (1947). *Men against fire: the problem of battle command in future war*. Oxford: The Infantry Journal Press.

Mateo, J. M. & Holmes, W. G. (1997). Development of alarm-call responses in Belding's ground squirrels: the role of dams. *Animal Behaviour* 54(3): 509–524.

Moreland, R. & Levine, J. M. (1982). Socialization in small groups: temporal changes in individual–group relations. In: L. Berkowitz (ed.) *Advances in experimental social psychology* 15, pp. 137–192. New York: Academic Press.

Mudrack, P. E. (1989). Defining group cohesiveness: a legacy of confusion? *Small Group Behavior* 20(1): 37–49.

Murnighan, J. (1985). Coalitions in decision-making groups: organizational analogs. *Organizational Behavior & Human Decision Processes* 35(1): 1–26.

Stiller, J. & Dunbar, R. (2007). Perspective-taking and memory capacity predict social network size. *Social Networks* 29(1): 93–104.

Stokes, J. P. (1983). Components of group cohesion: intermember attraction, instrumental value, and risk taking. *Small Group Behavior* 14(2): 163–173.

Thibaut, J. W. & Kelley, H. H. (1959). *The social psychology of groups*. New York: John Wiley & Sons, Inc.

Trafimow, D., Triandis, H. C. & Goto, S. G. (1991). Some tests of the distinction between the private self and the collective self. *Journal of Personality & Social Psychology* 60(5): 649–655.

Triandis, H. C. (1989). The self and social behavior in differing cultural contexts. *Psychological Review* 96(3): 506–520.

Tziner, A. (1982). Differential effects of group cohesiveness types: a clarifying overview. *Social Behavior & Personality* 10(2): 227–239.

Zhou, W. X., Sornette, D. & Dunbar, R. I. M. (2005). Discrete hierarchical organization of social group sizes. *Proceedings of the Royal Society B: Biological Sciences* 272(1561): 439.

14

The Socio-religious Brain:
A Developmental Model

DANIEL N. FINKEL, PAUL SWARTWOUT & RICHARD SOSIS

> Therefore, a prince must have great care that . . . to see him and hear him,
> he appear all piety, all faith, all integrity, all humaneness, all religion.
> And there is nothing more necessary to seem to have than this last qual-
> ity. And men in general judge more by the eyes than by the hands;
> because to see is for everyone, to feel for a few. (Machiavelli, *The Prince*
> 1997 [1532], 67)

THE SOCIAL BRAIN HYPOTHESIS has made significant progress toward
explaining why humans have such large brains for their body size (Byrne
& Whiten 1988; Dunbar 1998, 2003; Whiten & Byrne 1997). Our large
brains have enhanced our social capacities—particularly the ability to
track multiple interconnecting relationships—and introduced selective
pressures to maintain and heighten these abilities in order to keep pace in
the competitive landscape (Byrne 1998). Here we examine the role of religion in this evolutionary dynamic. Any of the core elements of human
society—political structure, economics, kinship, resource acquisition,
art, religion, etc.—could have independently played an important role in
the development of the social brain. Why distinguish religion among
these core elements? Is religion an important part of the repertoire of
social manoeuvres that are linked to brain size? Or even, as Machiavelli
advises, the most important?

Religion stands out from other aspects of society because it is the
medium through which enculturation and social bonding took place
during the bulk of our evolutionary past. Components of the religious
system, such as ritual participation, supernatural belief, myth recitation
and sacred/taboo distinctions are the language in which human sociality
is transmitted. The specifics of each system vary from culture to culture,
but there are important cross-cultural similarities, including a consistent
pattern of developmental timing that is linked to neural development
and universal life history phases.

Proceedings of the British Academy **158**, 283–307. © The British Academy 2010.

Following brief introductions to the social brain hypothesis and relevant concepts in the evolutionary study of religion, we discuss religion as a medium for enculturation. We argue that human sociality is inextricably linked to religion and offer a developmental account of the socio-religious brain through four phases of the life course—childhood, adolescence, adulthood and post-reproductive adulthood. The developmental account highlights the vital role that religion has played in transmitting and sustaining the cultural information that guides our social lives.

THE SOCIAL BRAIN HYPOTHESIS

There are fitness costs and benefits for individuals living in groups. The most significant costs include increases in pathogen exposure and direct competition for mates and resources (Byrne & Bates 2007). The proposed benefits of group living, which presumably outweigh these costs, include increased access to environmental information, safety from predation and cooperative resource acquisition that yields increased per capita returns. In order for individuals to reap these rewards effectively they must possess a suite of cognitive abilities that allow them to successfully negotiate living among a relatively large number of intricately intertwined relationships. The social brain hypothesis posits that selection favoured increased investment in hominin brain growth, especially the neocortex, to navigate a complex social world (Dunbar & Shultz 2007).

If human brain size is a consequence of selective pressures for increased social cognition, there should be differences between humans and other primates in the number, types, duration and complexity of social relationships. Dunbar (1998) has shown that group size, a measure of social complexity, is significantly correlated with neocortex size for the anthropoid primates. This relationship is robust to changes in metrics for the relevant variables (Dunbar 1995). While total number of individuals is only a proxy for interactions that take place within social groups, other measures of social complexity are also related to brain size, including social clique size (Kudo & Dunbar 2001), frequency of deception (Byrne & Corp 2004) and social play (Lewis 2000). Dunbar and colleagues have shown that the human mind could realistically maintain personal, not solely official, relationships with about 150 individuals (Hill & Dunbar 2003). Beyond this number, the cognitive demands imposed are expected to be too great, and groups of greater size are predicted to either fission or collapse.

A more recent version of the social brain hypothesis emphasizes the role of pair-bonding. In a groundbreaking study, Shultz and Dunbar (2007) found a positive correlation between brain size and long-term pair-bonds among carnivores, artiodactyls, birds and bats, but not anthropoid primates. The authors suggest that perhaps primate sociality is different from sociality in other taxa because primates have extended the qualities of their pair-bonded relationships to other social partners (Dunbar & Shultz 2007).

The benefits of group living are typically achieved through collective action, which creates a tension between individual and group interests. If some individuals are able to put forth less effort in a collective task (e.g. foraging and defence) than others, while still reaping the same benefit (e.g. food and safety), defection should spread. But if too many defect in this manner then eventually cooperation will fail. Presumably, both the ability and the tendency to defect should increase with group size since detecting free-riders is more difficult in larger groups (Olson 1965). However, this is not what we find in human groups. Humans are able to cooperate well in large numbers (Richerson & Boyd 2005) and economic studies in various cultures have shown that we tend to cooperate even when defection is not particularly costly (Fehr & Fischbacher 2003; Roth et al. 1991), though these studies do often find a small minority of participants playing a free-rider strategy. Given the potential benefits of free-riding, why does it seem that cooperation is in fact the dominant strategy?

RELIGION AND COOPERATION

Religion is one possible solution to the free-rider problem posed by evolutionary theorists attempting to understand group cohesion and cooperation, with three primary mechanisms offered as potential explanations. First, as anthropologists have long noted, ritual activity creates an emotional bond among participants which has been variously (and mysteriously) described as collective effervescence (Durkheim 1995 [1912]) and communitas (Turner 1967). Remarkably, this solidarity is achieved through both positive (e.g. dance, chanting) and negative (e.g. scarification, genital mutilation) affect rituals. The underlying physiological mechanisms that create this sense of cohesiveness during ritual activity remain obscure, but several authors have offered possible causal pathways that require further exploration (see Alcorta & Sosis 2005). The second explanation, referred to as the supernatural punishment hypothesis, focuses on cognitive function and posits that pro-social behaviour can be motivated by fear of supernatural sanctions (Johnson 2005; Johnson & Bering 2006). Norenzayan and Shariff (2008) suggest that when people believe in supernatural beings with access to morally relevant information, this can help reduce defection by invoking evolved reputational concerns.

A third explanation of how religion impacts social cohesion involves costly signalling, in which participation in religious activity serves as a costly and therefore hard-to-fake signal of commitment to the group (Bulbulia 2004; Irons 2004; Sosis 2003; Sosis & Alcorta 2003). Religious systems maintain expectations concerning communal activities, often referred to as the four B's: bans (taboos), badges (markers), behaviours (rituals) and beliefs (Sosis 2006). Willingness to fulfil these obligations signals one's commitment to the values of the community, which typically include in-group cooperation. If fulfilling these obligations is more costly for non-believers than believers, then cooperation can emerge and stabilize.

Religion not only increases in-group cooperation (e.g. Sosis & Ruffle 2003), but it also enables individuals to extend their cooperative alliances beyond their immediate community. Religious signals may have less signalling value within small-scale groups where everyone knows each other well, since reputational concerns can often sustain pro-social behaviour. Rather, signals in small-scale groups may be used to build alliances with individuals who share a common religious identity but live in other communities, and thus whose reputations are less accessible (Sosis 2005). Indeed, in a recent computer simulation Dow (2008) has shown that costly religious signals can emerge when those outside of the group increase their trust of in-group members. Hayden (1987) has argued that inter-band cooperation was essential in our evolutionary history to overcome the challenges of resource stress, and that ecstatic ritual was the key mechanism that enabled inter-band alliances to form. The successful cooperative trade networks among Muslim and Jewish co-religionists of distant communities provide a more recent example of religion's ability to extend across community boundaries (Greif 1989; Landa 2008; Sosis 2005). While we think it is unlikely that religion could extend the cognitive limits of community size, religion does seem to increase *functional* group size by extending cooperation across community boundaries.

RELIGION AS MEDIUM FOR SOCIAL PROCESSES

Has religion's ability to promote cooperation and extend collaborative relationships across time and space played a role in the evolution of the social brain? There are two conceptual problems with this question. The first concerns a definition of religion. Countless scholarly definitions of religion have been offered, but religion is an inherently fuzzy category and there is no definition which has been universally accepted. Therefore, rather than define religion, many scholars have concluded that it can best be studied by considering its constituent parts (Alcorta & Sosis 2005; Atran & Norenzayan 2004; Bering 2005; Bulbulia 2005; Sosis n.d.; Whitehouse 2008), and here we continue this trend. Religion consists of recurrent core features including ritual, myth, supernatural agent concepts, symbolic representation and sacred/profane distinctions, which receive varied emphasis across cultures, but they all play important roles in enculturation.

A related second conceptual problem concerns generalizing this category of religion, however it is defined, across time and space. Anthropologists have long warned about the pitfalls of employing contemporary categories, especially religious ones (Bloch 2008; Evans-Pritchard 1965; Klass 1995), to interpret the behaviours and beliefs of traditional populations. Whereas in contemporary Western societies religion is conceived as a distinct and often separate aspect of social life, in most non-stratified societies traditional religions are not separated conceptually from other aspects of life. Belief systems and ritual practices permeate all other aspects of culture, rather than lying near the centre or periphery of individual identities, as they do in Western societies (Rappaport 1999). Given that the vast majority of our evolutionary history was spent in small hunter-gatherer groups, we must look to these societies if we wish to understand the relationship between religion and the social brain.

In small bands, religious rituals and beliefs *are* the language and method of many forms of cultural transmission. The transmission of these beliefs mediates the enculturation of younger members into the identities, roles and commitments necessary for functioning in the group. If selective pressures favouring sociality drove the evolution of larger brains, then the role played by supernatural belief, ritual and the sacred in this process cannot be overestimated.

Supernatural beliefs, rituals, the sacred and other core elements of religion all combine to form a complex of mechanisms that creates distinct group identities. Social cognitive processes contribute to the polarization that mediates bond (in-group relationships) and prejudice (out-group relationships). Just as children acquire language and theory of mind (ToM) according to distinct but typical developmental patterns, they also acquire the significant features of their own cultures (beliefs, behaviours, rituals, etc.) in a predictable progression of maturation (Morgan & Kegl 2006). The process of enculturation could potentially have innate features—perhaps we also have a 'universal grammar' for religion as we do for language (Alcorta 2006; Bloom 2007; Bulbulia 2005). We may be born expecting to receive and internalize a set of beliefs regarding the world that fit within certain cognitive constraints. The primary function of these beliefs would be to provide social rules and direct social interaction.

In band-level societies, abstract symbols and supernatural beliefs are invested with emotional significance through communal ritual participation, which also serves to promote bonding between the participants who are demonstrating their commitment to one another. While this process still occurs in religious communities today, what is novel in the modern setting is that it is now possible to identify millions of people as members of the same religious group, albeit in a more limited sense than if they actually knew each other. This makes it possible for markers of group membership to tap into evolved associations between religious signals and the trustworthiness of those bearing them (or at least their potential as a cooperative partner; see Sosis 2005). For example, consider the Jewish and Muslim merchants mentioned above—two particular individuals in a business relationship might not have participated in any group rituals with each other during childhood, so they likely are not deeply bonded to each other. They are, however, bound with the distinctive symbols, beliefs and behaviours of their shared religion. Cooperation can then flourish even when reputations are largely unknown because religious identity provides a proxy for treating co-religionists as extended members of an in-group. The great advantage of this system is that it can achieve successful collective action among large numbers of people without imposing the impossible cognitive load required to actually keep track of them.

A DEVELOPMENTAL ACCOUNT OF THE
SOCIO-RELIGIOUS BRAIN

As mentioned above, religious social bonding makes use of communal rituals, supernatural belief and sacred symbols. We suggest that these features are used to organize enculturation and in-group bonding, and that ritual participation and the acquisition of supernatural beliefs vary in their expression and impact over the course of human lifetimes in predictable ways. What follows is a description of how religion mediates social bonding and identity formation during four developmental stages: childhood, adolescence, adulthood and post-reproductive adulthood. We focus especially on the stages in which the influence of religion is least understood—childhood and adolescence.

We propose that our susceptibility to the acquisition of new religious beliefs will be higher during childhood and adolescence in order to take advantage of the cognitive and neural flexibility characteristic of these stages. Sense of self, social cognition and linguistic ability develop during these early stages. Culturally acquired knowledge, self-concept and group bonding are all cemented during adolescence via emotionally salient initiations into adulthood. After adolescence the acquisition of new supernatural beliefs, while certainly still possible (as seen in modern societies in religious conversion) is less likely. Concerns in adulthood shift toward demonstrations of commitment to the group with increased ritual engagement in order to maximize the benefits of group living during reproductive years. Ritual engagement persists in post-reproductive adulthood, as older adults become the primary transmitters of beliefs, roles and rituals for younger generations.

CHILDHOOD

Although developmental psychologists have produced a wealth of literature on moral development (Killen & Smetana 2006), the field has a history of conspicuously ignoring religious cognition in children (Harris 2000). Recently, however, developmental psychologists have turned their attention to experimental examinations of religion with results that point to typical developmental stages in the areas of mind-body dualism and supernatural agent concepts (Bering & Parker 2006; Bloom 2007). A growing body of evidence also suggests an innate tendency in young children to include supernatural beliefs in their view of the world. Studies have demonstrated that children are likely to apply teleological reasoning to explain a wide range of phenomena. This tendency occurs regardless of religious upbringing and in spite of parental tendency to use causal rather than teleological explanations (Kelemen et al. 2005), and only begins to decline in Western societies around the age of 9 or 10 (Kelemen 1999).

Religion and childhood are also intimately linked in the forms of early social interaction known as pretence and play. Dunbar (2003) suggests that the ability to infer intentions and beliefs in other agents, which we expect to have been strengthened throughout the evolution of the social brain, may have relevance for understanding religion. The scaffolding of levels of intentionality achieved by humans is underwritten by a theory of mind (ToM). Reasoning about supernatural agents and their concern with societal norms is expected to carry a significant cognitive load, not least because their behaviour is not directly observable. It is clear that ToM must be involved in the process of thinking about the beliefs and desires of supernatural beings, including the possibility that they may be false or different from one's own. Research on how pretend play and fantasy affect the developmental progression of ToM in children demonstrates that these phenomena are tightly bound to one another. We now explore the idea that religion has assumed some of the functions of play and pretence found in other species, similar to the way that language may have taken over the function of social grooming in humans (Dunbar 1996). Religion engages ToM to simulate interaction with supernatural and unfamiliar agents, assisting people in exploring the boundaries of their social relationships, even as they form and maintain these bonds.

Play and the social brain

Social play is among the behavioural indices of social complexity that are hypothesized to have spurred the evolution of large brain sizes in primates (Dunbar & Shultz 2007). Lewis (2000) found a positive relationship between neocortex ratio and social play behaviour in seven primate species. Similarly, Byers (1999) reports a positive correlation between relative brain mass and frequency of social play in Australian marsupials. Iwaniuk et al. (2001), however, found a play–brain size relationship between orders of mammals, but not within lower taxonomic groups, including primates and marsupials. Other research has shown that amygdala size predicts sexual adult–adult play in primates (Pellis & Iwaniuk 2002), and that amygdala and hypothalamus size are both positively related to all kinds of social play in non-human primates (Lewis & Barton 2006). Another compelling finding is that primate species that have more brain growth occurring postnatally play more as adults (Pellis & Iwaniuk 2000). Humans were not included in this analysis, but human rates of postnatal brain growth are significantly higher than for other primates (Kaplan et al. 2000) and we suspect that humans also maintain among the highest levels of adult play, although this has yet to be assessed in comparative studies. This cumulative evidence points to a relationship between cognitive-emotional processing ability and play behaviour, although the direction of causality remains unclear.

Play appears to offer many benefits. In general, it may be seen as a rehearsal of behaviour in which the animal loses partial control of its body, thereby gaining experience in recovering from abnormal and unexpected situations (Spinka et al. 2001). Social play in particular may aid in learning the boundaries of social relationships in a safe environment where there are relatively few penalties for transgressions (Bekoff 2001). In chimpanzees, play rates become elevated in captive populations just before feeding time (Palagi et al. 2004), and therefore may also function in reducing tension and preventing conflict escalation.

On the other hand, play is also energetically expensive and carries opportunity costs. Social play in particular is cognitively demanding in that it requires the player to understand that its partner is acting 'nonseriously', sometimes communicated through play markers (e.g. Bekoff 1995; Waller & Dunbar 2005). In humans, pretence adds another level of cognitive complexity.

Play and theory of mind

Pretend play in children is often richly imaginative and involves substantial departure from real situations and actual identities. There is an apparent contradiction between children's ability to participate in pretend play before the age of 4 years and their inability to pass false-belief tasks during this period (Lillard 2001, 175). How can a child pretend to be (or be with) different people or animals without a developed understanding that others have distinct knowledge and perceptual states? The answer to this question remains controversial. Pretend play emerges by the second year at the latest, and possibly by 15 months (Lillard 2002, 190). Although children younger than 4 years old tend to fail the standard false-belief task, there is some evidence that they can succeed if demands on speech and memory in the task are limited (see Wellman et al. 2001). Despite uncertainty about the timing of onset for ToM capacity, its correlation with pretence is still strongly supported. First, several studies have uncovered a relationship between ToM, as measured by false-belief tasks, and pretend play or certain constituent play behaviours. Four-year olds' scores on a fantasy/pretence factor were shown to predict their performance on ToM tasks (Taylor & Carlson 1997). Children observed performing more social pretence fared better on false-belief tasks seven months later (Youngblade & Dunn 1995). Theory of mind is positively correlated with joint action proposals and explicit role assignments (Astington & Jenkins 1995) or object substitution and role assignment behaviours (Nielsen & Dissanayake 2000). Second, autistic children, who have long been described as having a theory of mind deficit (Baron-Cohen et al. 1985), have difficulty producing spontaneous, creative pretend play (Jarrold 2003). Third, some evidence from neuroimaging suggests that brain areas associated with making mental state judgements are activated when adults watch others engaging in pretend situations (German et al. 2004).

Supernatural agents are no ordinary 'others', but they are assumed to have minds, which raises the question of whether the developmental progression of ToM applies to their cognition as well. Barrett et al. (2001) presented children aged 2–6 years with a false-belief task in which the researchers showed the children a box with a picture of crackers on it, revealed that it had rocks inside instead of crackers, and then showed them a paper bag that actually had crackers inside. When asked where Mom, God and a few other agents would look for crackers, there was a significant correlation with age in assuming that Mom would have the false belief and look in the cracker box, but age was not correlated with responses about God. Children typically assumed that God did not have false beliefs. Similar results have been found for Yucatec Maya (Knight et al. 2004) and Greek Orthodox children (Makris & Pnevmatikos 2007, but see authors' discussion). If these children conceived of God as just another kind of agent, they might attribute false beliefs to God when they understand that their fellow humans have them. Instead, they seem to retain the (culturally specific) 'theologically correct' (Barrett et al. 2001) belief that God is omniscient past the age at which they pass the false-belief task. Either they have a somewhat intuitive understanding that God's mind is different from humans', or they are flexibly reversing their ToM prediction when thinking about God. In either case, children appear well-equipped to reason about supernatural minds.

Play and religion

Similar to the study of religion, the study of play focuses on seemingly 'purposeless' composites of multiple interacting systems, with little consensus about its adaptive value. This is true for both play in animals and for pretend play in children. However, recent attempts to compare possible evolutionary functions across taxa have had success (Burghardt 2005; Mitchell 2002; Power 2000). Here we consider social play in animals as a mechanism for establishing and strengthening social bonds, and pretending in humans as an extension of this function. Imaginative play allows individuals to explore several dimensions of various social situations without actually experiencing them, contributing to a greater understanding of the mental and emotional states of others through simulation.

Religious stories are distinguished from fiction by certain truth values attached to them by those who follow their teachings. But there is no denying that the mythological and literary aspects of religion are spectacularly imaginative and fantastical. Supernatural characters are right at home in the epics and sagas of world literature, such as the Hindu Mahabharata or the Norse Eddas. Creation myths, eschatological scenarios and everything in between get imaginative treatment from religion. For instance, Black Muslims followed this Final Judgment story in the mid 20th century: a half-mile-long spaceship will descend on North America, releasing 'baby planes' that lay waste to civilization with incendiary bombs, while dropping leaflets in Arabic and English to believers in black Islam that direct them away from the flames (Walker 1990, 345–346). Sometimes the most bizarre and cryptic aspects of religious stories are effective at generating commitment, as with David Koresh's obsession with opening the 'seven seals' of Revelation 5.

Individuals engaging in religious cognition past the age of 4 years old are clearly not practising their ToM skills in order to develop the ability to make inferences about mental states, but they are exercising this capacity. If the links between pretend play and ToM are preserved over the life course, religion, in its deployment of both, may conserve some of the functionality of play found phylogenetically and ontogenetically. Psychological approaches have traditionally considered pretence only in the juvenile period, tending to ignore it altogether afterward (Göncü & Perone 2005). This is unfortunate because failing to study pretence among adults has obscured links between juvenile pretence behaviour and its adult manifestations, including art, literature, cinema, sports, comedy

Table 14.1. How pretence can encourage social understanding, and instances of its use in children's play and in Christianity. Pretence behaviors are from Lillard (1998, 15–16); examples are the authors' except where noted.

Pretence behaviour	Children's example	Religious example
Confronting others' beliefs through script negotiation	I'll be Batman and you be the Joker. Oh, alright, you can be Batman and I'll be the Joker	Dialectical engagement of pre-existing religious concepts in new belief introduction (Rappaport 1999)
One entity as two things at once	I'm a kid, but I'm also a dinosaur	Jesus as man and deity at once (John 1: 14)
One entity as representing another	This banana is a telephone (Leslie 1987)	This cracker is the body of Christ—often understood in practice as a representation (Burnham & Giaccherini 2005)
Role-playing, perspective-taking	I'm a fireman, I need to save the kittens from the pet store fire	What would Jesus do? (Fiala 2007)
Acting out conflicts with emotional resonance	I'm the mommy, and I don't like it when you hit my baby!	Story of the binding of Isaac (Genesis 22: 1–19)

and, most notably for our purposes, religion. Lillard (1998, 15–16) suggests five ways by which pretending could encourage social understanding: (1) negotiating topic and script of pretence, thereby confronting the beliefs of others, (2) seeing one entity as two things at once, (3) seeing one entity as representing another, (4) role-playing and assuming the mental representations of others, and (5) acting out conflicts that may have emotionally vivid connotations. Table 1 shows how religion carries over all of the socially salient pretend play behaviours described by Lillard into adulthood for familiar Christian examples. Religious cognition possesses some of the structure and content of pretend play, and is manifest in religious narratives. The allegorical and pedagogical features of religious stories make them a safe arena for exploring social norms and power relationships. This is expected to be especially important in early human groups and contemporary small-scale societies, whose norms are not codified into a system of secular contracts like those found in large-scale societies.

Furthermore, the influence of religious imagination on an individual's ability to signal his or her commitment to the community must be explored (Sosis & Alcorta 2003). Knowledge of religious texts, history and the supernatural realm in general commonly carries a certain amount of prestige in groups across the world. Participation in religious rituals, which entail shared imaginative acceptance of a pretence situation accompanied by physical arousal, can be a potent signal of individual commitment. Religious narratives drive the mental exploration of socially relevant situations, as well as provide relatable characters. As such, they can be powerful aids to the internalization of beliefs, which can alter cost-benefit equations and make costly commitment attractive (Sosis 2003). In this way, signals of religious commitment are lent force by receivers' understanding that the signaller must be exploring the same social landscape and internalizing the norms that they share. This additional dimension for signalling theory will benefit from the input of research on play markers in animals, because they both communicate intent to enter into a specific kind of relationship and to follow the rules implicit in it (Palagi 2008).

ADOLESCENCE

The adolescent stage carries several distinct goals as the bridge between childhood and reproductive adulthood. Adolescents must form and perpetuate friendships and alliances of increasing complexity, conform to societal gender roles, and understand and control their developing sexuality. The stakes in this developmental stage are higher—one's actions and the perceptions of one's character are directly relevant to one's status within the community and affect future reproduction. Consequently, deviations from social expectations become more costly because individuals are assumed to have achieved a grasp of basic social interaction in childhood. They must also learn to forgo short-term benefits for long-term benefits, although the tension between these priorities is characteristic of this stage. Of course, these cost-benefit ratios will be different for boys and girls, and there may be conflicting behavioural and morphological strategies for children and parents at this time (Surbey 1998).

We now know that brain development continues through adolescence in humans. Recent neuroimaging studies show that areas involved in processing social information continue to develop during adolescence, including the medial prefrontal cortex (mPFC), and the superior temporal sulcus (STS) (Blakemore 2007). These areas show increases in grey matter, an indication of synaptogenesis, through childhood up to its peak during adolescence, followed by a decrease in grey matter in adulthood, a sign of neural pruning and the formation of stable connections. Other evidence shows that neural correlates of 'socially integrated self-concept' undergo important development during adolescence (Blakemore 2008). This neural reorganization suggests that adolescence is indeed an important time during the development of social cognition. Adolescence has been characterized as 'experience expectant' (Alcorta 2006), which highlights the idea that this phase is ontogenetically designed to receive environmental information regarding both individual personality differences and socio-cultural features. We examine two major tasks for the developing adolescent brain and how they are aided by religious behaviour: (1) how out-group distinctions are formed while generating strong in-group relationships, and (2) how social structure is utilized to become socially integrated and position oneself for reproduction.

In-group/out-group belonging

During adolescence we are primed to commit ourselves to belonging to certain groups and not belonging to others. Again we can see radical differences in the way this process unfolds in small bands and large societies. In small societies, adolescence is marked by the ceremonial transition to adulthood, usually mediated by an initiation ritual. The extreme costliness of these rituals may contribute to increased group cohesion by signalling commitment and demonstrating that those who participate are not likely to shrink from pain and danger when it counts (Sosis et al. 2007). Whitehouse (1996) has further argued that such emotionally intense rites may be stored as 'flashbulb' memories, making it more likely for them to be retained in long-term memory. Whether these memories are recalled more accurately than others or not (Talarico & Rubin 2007), the events and the ways they transform relationships are highly salient, even for more benign rituals.

In large-scale societies, the content of in-group relationships has been heavily altered by changed ecological demands. For individuals in these societies, religious rituals continue to mark major transitions between life stages (e.g. circumcision—bar mitzvah—marriage—funeral), cementing sense of identity within a particular religion. However, in demographically mobile societies fewer individuals spend their lives within the same religious community. Moreover, secular groups engaged in sustained cooperation like sports teams, fraternities and sororities, and military units (Richerson & Boyd 1999) have co-opted features of religious initiation rites in order to manipulate identity. These organizations follow a standard progression of steps used in initiation rites: separation, liminality and reintegration (Turner 1969). Initiates are removed and given physically, mentally or emotionally challenging tasks to complete according to ritual formulae. They live in a liminal phase for a certain amount of time (sports training camps, fraternity houses during 'hell week', military housing), but once they demonstrate their commitment satisfactorily, they are reintegrated into the group with a new sense of identity. To a lesser extent, we find the same features in summer camps, youth groups, and sometimes even in schools. These institutions aim to educate as well as instil a sense of belonging to a certain group. Concurrently, religion not only supplies rituals that unite cooperative units but also instils beliefs that can help categorize others as members of out-groups. For example, even when tempered by liberal attitudes toward religious pluralism, a significant proportion of American adolescents express exclusivist religious beliefs, claiming that only one religion can be true (Trinitapoli 2007).

Social integration

Before their attention turns to reproduction and sustaining families, interpersonal interaction with peers becomes more prevalent for adolescents (Steinberg & Morris 2001). Religion may act to direct them toward resources for social support in order to encourage healthy development. Results from Western societies indicate that religion has a modest positive influence on the outcomes of several dimensions of adolescent lives, including physical and emotional health, education, volunteerism and political involvement, and family well-being (reviewed in Regnerus 2003). These effects are likely to be stronger in small-scale societies where each dimension is even less readily extricable from each other one.

There is evidence that a solid cultural-religious framework of belief is important for good mental health and positive adjustment (Alcorta 2006). Doubts about the truth or value of one's religious beliefs have been linked to greater susceptibility to depressive symptoms (Krause & Wulff 2004). Religious doubt seems to exert the greatest effect on psychopathology at younger ages, and this influence erodes as individuals age (Galek et al. 2007). We interpret this as support for the idea that religion has played and continues to play an organizing role in the construction of socially informed world-views. When the behavioural guidelines that inform individual decisions and bind together virtually all of one's peers and superiors are called into question, the result is cognitive dissonance and social anxiety.

In the US, as adolescence progresses religiosity tends to decline (Smith et al. 2002). Yet religiosity may prepare adolescents for the challenges of adulthood. Barry and Nelson (2005) found that the most religious 18–20-year-olds in their sample (Mormons) consistently perceived themselves as having achieved the necessary criteria for adulthood to a greater extent than any other group. The underlying cause of this effect is likely the church's mobilization of large social networks, prohibitions on diet and conduct, and extensive ritual engagement.

If religion is an important medium of enculturation and social bonding, then adolescence clearly plays an enormously transformative role in this process. It is during this time that the practice and play of childhood culminate in more serious and costly rituals, which both create and demonstrate commitments among participants. Though rituals and beliefs continue into adulthood, the cessation of neural plasticity in brain areas involved in social cognition at this time suggests that bonds and beliefs acquired in this stage may be fundamentally different from those acquired later in life.

ADULTHOOD

Though ritual and belief play a major role during adolescence in the formation of self-concept, social cognition and in-group identity, ritual and belief certainly continue to be important features of life during young adulthood. This stage of life is characterized (or defined) by reproduction. The first offspring are typically born during the early or mid twenties, with the number of living offspring peaking during the thirties and forties. This stage of life is rarely included in developmental accounts since physical development is complete by its onset. In our account, however, the role of religion in mediating social bonding continues unabated, and the introduction of children makes the cultural education afforded by religion more attractive.

Religion and sociality in young adulthood

In the US, adolescents primarily attend religious services with their parents, and parents are more likely to attend than non-parent adults (Sherkat 2001). Parents expose their children to the beliefs and rituals of their group in order for them to build identity and bond with their cohort. The trend noted above, that religious affiliation and attendance diminish later in adolescence, continues into young adulthood (Uecker et al. 2007).

Religious affiliation and attendance increase with marriage, and increase again with reproduction.

Interestingly, the costs of such attendance are likely higher for parents with young children or adolescents since there can be associated membership fees, time and energy costs are greater, and children may be resistant. However, the benefits of belonging to such a community, such as receiving aid during times of difficulty, may be crucial in order for parents to raise their children successfully, and such attendance is also likely the only way for them to inculcate a sense of religious affiliation or identity.

Religious trends in adulthood

McCullough et al. (2005), in their study on adult religious development, found three independent trends in religiousness throughout the adult life course. One trend showed an initial high level of affiliation that grew slightly during the life course. Another trend showed a low-level religiosity that decreased very slightly (but significantly). The third showed a parabolic trend, beginning in between the other trends (medium religiosity), increasing during peak reproductive years (thirties to fifties), and then decreasing to original medium levels in the seventies. These trends are likely based on the interaction of personality characteristics and situational exigencies, and reflect the ability of individuals in large societies to avoid religion in their daily lives. The major factor associated with the low religiosity trend was remaining unmarried for the duration of one's life. The main factors associated with the high religiousness trend were 'religious upbringing' and 'agreeableness'. Those in the parabolic trend were more likely to be married than either other trend, and also were more likely to be women. We interpret the parabolic trend to depict those who rely on religious communal life to support reproductive costs as described above. Peacock and Poloma (1999) also examined religiosity through the adult life course. They suggest that during the first half of adulthood (18–50) spirituality is associated with 'development of identity . . . mutual relationships with others, and a sense of spiritual transcendence' (Peacock & Poloma 1999, 336), which again supports the developmental perspective proposed above.

POST-REPRODUCTIVE ADULTHOOD

Human life history is characterized by an extended period of juvenile dependence, high rates of male provisioning, a long lifespan and support of reproduction by older, post-reproductive individuals (Hill & Kaplan 1999). With their reproduction finished, their cultural milieu mastered, and their personality characteristics set, older individuals will not benefit directly from the interaction between religion and social cognition we have detailed for earlier developmental stages. Yet religion remains a significant feature past the reproductive years. Now these individuals are on the transmitting end of the flow of enculturation and are able to influence their descendants via religion. In most small-scale societies, those knowledgeable about religion and those who hold important spiritual 'offices' can be respected well beyond their functional abilities. Elderly individuals may be remembered shortly after their deaths as supernatural beings still concerned with the state of affairs in the living world. Maintaining religious involvement ensures that one will remain a compelling paragon of pro-social behaviour from beyond the grave.

In large-scale modern societies, there has been a conceptual shift from viewing older people as venerable to treating them as vulnerable (Davie & Vincent 1998). The function of religion for older individuals in these societies may have followed suit, now treated as a way to restore health and maintain competence or independence. An enormous literature has emerged documenting positive relationships between religion and physical (Koenig et al. 2001), as well as mental (Koenig 1998), health. Especially well-supported is the inverse relationship between frequency of church attendance and mortality rates (Gillum et al. 2008). In terms of mental health, religious individuals tend to rate their well-being and their global satisfaction with life higher than those who are not religious (McFadden 1999). As mentioned above, religious doubt is less troublesome and challenges to belief structures are more easily accommodated. The underlying causal mechanisms are unclear, but one candidate is social integration and support, including social network size (Musick et al. 2000). Religion seems to sustain older individuals as they attempt to sustain their descendants. Some individuals report a shift in the content of their prayers as they age, from self-interest in early adulthood to increased social consciousness and compassion in later years (Ingersoll-Dayton et al. 2002). By participating in the institution that will transmit desirable cultural information to relatives, post-reproductive individuals communicate their continuing endorsement of those beliefs, influence future behaviour, and derive socially mediated health benefits.

CONCLUSION

We begin childhood ready to soak up the particular beliefs of our own group in much the same way we are prepared to learn our own language. We practise these beliefs and begin our experiences with ritual during the childhood processes of pretence and play, which continues into adulthood via religion. We cement our beliefs and relationships with our age cohorts (and the rest of our in-groups) during the initiation rites of adolescence, though modern society has a wide range of options available to fill this role if religion is not present or salient. We continue our ritual engagement into adulthood, further strengthening communal ties based on signals of solidarity and commitment. In post-reproductive adulthood we engage with the younger generation as models, teachers and guides.

Machiavelli noted that religion's influence rests in its ability to represent the underlying qualities of those who participate in it. That is, in fact, the thesis of this chapter. Religion is a way of *packaging information*. The process of development takes an individual through the early stages of first unwrapping this package to the later stages when he or she ties a bow on it and gives it to others. The information contained therein reciprocally informs and is enabled by social cognition. In large-scale modern societies, many of the contents of the religion package have been scattered into a variety of more or less discrete sources. But for nearly all of human evolutionary history, religion united vast amounts of cultural knowledge into frameworks of belief and behaviour that guided the kinds of social manoeuvres described by the social brain hypothesis.

Note. We thank Candace Alcorta, Benjamin Purzycki and John Shaver for very helpful comments on earlier drafts of this manuscript, and the Russell Sage Foundation, US–Israel Binational Science Foundation, and Templeton Foundation for financial support.

REFERENCES

Alcorta, C. S. (2006). Religion and the life course: is adolescence an 'experience expectant' period for religious transmission? In: P. McNamara (ed.) *Where God and man meet: how the brain and evolutionary sciences are revolutionizing our understanding of religion and spirituality*, pp. 55–79. Westport, CT: Praeger.

Alcorta, C. S. & Sosis, R. (2005). Ritual, emotion, and sacred symbols: the evolution of religion as an adaptive complex. *Human Nature* 16: 323–359.

Astington, J. W. & Jenkins, J. M. (1995). Theory of mind development and social understanding. *Cognition and Emotion* 9(2/3): 151–165.

Atran, S. & Norenzayan, A. (2004). The evolutionary landscape of religion. *Behavioral and Brain Sciences* 27: 713–770.

Baron-Cohen, S., Leslie, A.M. & Frith, U. (1985). Does the autistic child have a 'theory of mind'? *Cognition* 21: 37–46.

Barrett, J. L., Richert, R. A. & Driesenga, A. (2001). God's beliefs versus mother's: the development of nonhuman agent concepts. *Child Development* 72(1): 50–65.

Barry, C. M. & Nelson, L. J. (2005). The role of religion in the transition to adulthood for young emerging adults. *Journal of Youth and Adolescence* 34(3): 245–255.

Bekoff, M. (1995). Play signals as punctuation: the structure of social play in canids. *Behavior* 132: 419–429.

Bekoff, M. (2001). Social play behaviour: cooperation, fairness, trust, and the evolution of morality. *Journal of Consciousness Studies* 8(2): 81–90.

Bering, J. M. (2005). The evolutionary history of an illusion: religious causal beliefs in children and adults. In: B. Ellis & D. Bjorklund (ed.) *Origins of the social mind: evolutionary psychology and child development*, pp. 411–437. New York: Guilford Press.

Bering, J. M. & Parker, B. D. (2006). Children's attributions of intentions to an invisible agent. *Developmental Psychology* 42(2): 253–262.

Blakemore, S. J. (2007). The social brain of a teenager. *Psychologist* 20: 600–602.

Blakemore, S. J. (2008). The social brain in adolescence. *Nature Reviews Neuroscience* 9: 267–277.

Bloch, M. (2008). Why religion is nothing special but is central. *Philosophical Transactions of the Royal Society B* 363: 2055–2061.

Bloom, P. (2007). Religion is natural. *Developmental Science* 10: 147–151.

Bulbulia, J. (2004). The cognitive and evolutionary psychology of religion. *Biology & Philosophy* 19: 655–686.

Bulbulia, J. (2005). Are there any religions? *Method and Theory in the Study of Religion* 17: 71–100.

Burghardt, G. M. (2005). *The genesis of animal play: testing the limits*. Cambridge, MA: MIT Press.

Burnham, D. & Giaccherini, E. (eds) (2005). *The poetics of transubstantiation: from theology to metaphor*. Burlington, VT: Ashgate.

Byers, J.A. (1999). The distribution of play behaviour among Australian marsupials. *Journal of the Zoological Society of London* 247: 349–356.

Byrne, R. W. (1998). Machiavellian intelligence. *Evolutionary Anthropology* 5(5): 172–180.

Byrne, R. W. & Bates, L. A. (2007). Sociality, evolution and cognition. *Current Biology* 17: R714–R723.

Byrne, R. W. & Corp, N. (2004). Neocortex size predicts deception rate in primates. *Proceedings of the Royal Society B* 271: 1693–1699.

Byrne, R. W. & Whiten, A. 1988. *Machiavellian intelligence*. Oxford: Clarendon Press.

Davie, G. & Vincent, J. (1998). Religion and old age. *Ageing and Society* 18: 101–110.

Dow, J. (2008). Is religion an evolutionary adaptation? *Journal of Artificial Societies and Social Simulation* 11(2): 2.

Dunbar, R. I. M. (1995). Neocortex size and group size in primates: a test of the hypothesis. *Journal of Human Evolution* 28: 287–296.

Dunbar, R. I. M. (1996). *Grooming, gossip, and the evolution of language*. Cambridge, MA: Harvard University Press.

Dunbar, R. I. M. (1998). The social brain hypothesis. *Evolutionary Anthropology* 6: 178–190.

Dunbar, R. I. M. (2003). The social brain: mind, language, and society in evolutionary perspective. *Annual Review of Anthropology* 32: 163–181.

Dunbar, R. I. M. & Shultz, S. (2007). Evolution in the social brain. *Science* 317: 1344–1347.

Durkheim E. (1995 [1912]). *The elementary forms of religious life*. New York: Free Press.

Evans-Pritchard, E. E. (1965). *Kinship and marriage among the Nuer*. London: Oxford University Press.

Fehr, E. & Fischbacher, U. (2003). The nature of human altruism. *Nature* 425: 785–791.

Fiala, A. (2007). *What would Jesus really do? The power and limits of Jesus' moral teachings*. Lanham, MD: Rowman & Littlefield.

Galek, K., Krause, N., Ellison, C. G., Kudler, T. & Flannelly, K. J. (2007). Religious doubt and mental health across the lifespan. *Journal of Adult Development* 14: 16–25.

German, T. P., Niehaus, J. L., Roarty, M. P., Giesbrecht, B. & Miller, M. B. (2004). Neural correlates of detecting pretense: automatic engagement of the intentional stance under covert conditions. *Journal of Cognitive Neuroscience* 16(10): 1805–1817.

Gillum, R. F., King, D. E., Obisesan, T. O. & Koenig, H. G. (2008). Frequency of attendance at religious services and mortality in a US national cohort. *Annals of Epidemiology* 18(2): 124–129.

Göncü, A. & Perone, A. (2005). Pretend play as a life-span activity. *Topoi: An International Review of Philosophy* 24: 137–147.

Greif, A. (1989). Reputation and coalitions in medieval trade: evidence on the Maghribi traders. *Journal of Economic History* 49: 857–882.

Harris, P. (2000). On not falling down to earth: children's metaphysical questions. In: K. S. Rosengren, C. N. Johnson & P. L. Harris (eds) *Imagining the impossible: magical, scientific, and religious thinking in children*. New York: Cambridge University Press.

Hayden, B. (1987). Alliances and ritual ecstasy: human responses to resource stress. *Journal for the Scientific Study of Religion* 26: 81–91.

Hill, K. & Kaplan, H. (1999). Life history traits in humans: theory and empirical studies. *Annual Review of Anthropology* 28: 397–430.

Hill, R. & Dunbar, R. I. M. (2003). Social network size in humans. *Human Nature* 14(1): 53–72.

Ingersoll-Dayton, B., Krause, N. & Morgan, D. (2002). Religious trajectories and transitions over the life course. *International Journal of Aging and Human Development* 55(1): 51–70.

Irons, W. (2004). An evolutionary critique of the created co-creator concept. *Zygon: Journal of Religion and Science* 39: 773–790.

Iwaniuk, A. N., Nelson, J. E. & Pellis, S. M. (2001). Do big-brained animals play more? Comparative analyses of play and relative brain size in mammals. *Journal of Comparative Psychology* 115(1): 29–41.

Jarrold, C. (2003). A review of research into pretend play in autism. *Autism* 7(4): 379–90.

Johnson, D. D. P. (2005). God's punishment and public goods: a test of the super-natural punishment hypothesis in 186 world cultures. *Human Nature* 16(4): 410–446.

Johnson, D. D. P. & Bering, J. M. (2006). Hand of God, mind of man: punishment and cognition in the evolution of cooperation. *Evolutionary Psychology* 4: 219–233.

Kaplan, H., Hill, K., Lancaster, J. & Hurtado, A. M. (2000). A theory of human life history evolution: diet, intelligence, and longevity. *Evolutionary Anthropology* 9: 156–184.

Kelemen, D. (1999). Why are rocks pointy? Children's preference for teleological explanations of the natural world. *Developmental Psychology* 35: 1440–1452.

Kelemen, D., Callanan, M. A., Casler, K. & Perez-Granados, D. R. (2005). Why things happen: teleological explanation in parent–child conversations. *Developmental Psychology* 41: 251–264.

Killen, M. & Smetana, J. (2006). *Handbook of moral development*, 1st edn. Mahwah, NJ: Lawrence Erlbaum Associates.

Klass, M. (1995). *Ordered universes: approaches to the anthropology of religion.* Boulder, CO: Westview Press.

Knight, N., Sousa, P., Barrett, J. L. & Atran, S. (2004). Children's attributions of beliefs to humans and God: cross-cultural evidence. *Cognitive Science* 28: 117–126.

Koenig, H. G. (ed.) (1998). *Handbook of religion and mental health.* San Diego, CA: Academic Press.

Koenig, H. G., McCullough, M. E. & Larson, D. B. (eds) (2001). *Handbook of religion and health.* New York: Oxford University Press.

Krause, N. & Wulff, K. M. (2004). Religious doubt and health: exploring the potential dark side of religion. *Sociology of Religion* 65(1): 35–56.

Kudo, H. & Dunbar, R. (2001). Neocortex size and social network size in primates. *Animal Behaviour* 62: 711–722.

Landa, J. (2008). The bioeconomics of homogeneous middleman groups as adaptive units: theory and empirical evidence viewed from a group selection framework. *Journal of Bioeconomics* 10(3): 259–278.

Leslie, A. M. (1987). Pretense and representation: the origins of 'theory of mind'. *Psychological Review* 94(4): 412–426.

Lewis, K. P. (2000). A comparative study of primate play behaviour: implications for the study of cognition. *Folia Primatologica* 71: 417–421.

Lewis, K. P. & Barton, R. A. (2006). Amygdala size and hypothalamus size predict social play frequency in nonhuman primates: a comparative analysis using independent contrasts. *Journal of Comparative Psychology* 120(1): 31–37.

Lillard, A. S. (1998). Playing with a theory of mind. In: O. N. Saracho & B. Spodek (eds) *Multiple perspectives on play in early childhood education*, pp. 11–33. New York: SUNY Press.

Lillard, A. S. (2001). Explaining the connection: pretend play and theory of mind. In: S. Reifel (ed.) *Theory in context and out*, vol. 3: *Play and culture studies*, pp. 173–178. Westport, CT: Ablex.

Lillard, A. S. (2002). Pretend play and cognitive development. In: U. Goswami (ed.) *Handbook of cognitive development*, pp. 188–205. London: Blackwell.

Machiavelli, N. (1997 [1532]). *The Prince*, trans. A. M. Codevilla. New Haven, CT: Yale University Press.

Makris, N. & Pnevmatikos, D. (2007). Children's understanding of human and supernatural mind. *Cognitive Development* 22: 365–375.

McCullough, M. E., Enders, C. K., Brion, S. L. and Jain, A. R. (2005). The varieties of religious development in adulthood: a longitudinal investigation of religion and rational choice. *Journal of Personality and Social Psychology* 89(1): 78–89.

McFadden, S. H. (1999). Religion, personality, and aging: a life span perspective. *Journal of Personality* 67(6): 1081–1104.

Mitchell, R. W. (ed.) (2002). *Pretending and imagination in animals and children*. New York: Cambridge University Press.

Morgan, G. & Kegl, J. (2006). Nicaraguan sign language and theory of mind: the issue of critical periods and abilities. *Journal of Child Psychology and Psychiatry* 47: 811–819.

Musick, M. A., Traphagan, J. W., Koenig, H. G. & Larson, D. B. (2000). Spirituality in physical health and aging. *Journal of Adult Development* 7(2): 73–86.

Nielsen, M. & Dissanayake, C. (2000). An investigation of pretend play, mental state terms and false belief understanding: in search of a metarepresentational link. *British Journal of Developmental Psychology* 18: 609–624.

Norenzayan, A. & Shariff, A. F. (2008). The origin and evolution of religious prosociality. *Science* 322: 58–62.

Olson, M. (1965). *The logic of collective action: public goods and the theory of groups*. Cambridge, MA: Harvard University Press.

Palagi, E. (2008). Sharing the motivation to play: the use of signals in adult bonobos. *Animal Behaviour* 75: 887–896.

Palagi, E., Cordoni, G. & Borgognini Tarli, S. M. (2004). Immediate and delayed benefits of play behaviour: new evidence from chimpanzees (*Pan trogolodytes*). *Ethology* 110: 949–962.

Peacock, J. R. & Poloma, M. M. (1999). Religiosity and life satisfaction across the life course. *Social Indicators Research* 48: 321–345.

Pellis, S. M. & Iwaniuk, A. N. (2000). Comparative analyses of the role of postnatal development on the expression of play fighting. *Developmental Psychobiology* 36: 136–147.

Pellis, S. M. & Iwaniuk, A. N. (2002). Brain system size and adult–adult play in primates: a comparative analysis of the roles of the non-visual neocortex and the amygdala. *Behavioural Brain Research* 134: 31–39.

Power, T. G. (2000). *Play and exploration in children and animals*. Mahwah, NJ: Lawrence Erlbaum Associates.

Rappaport, R. A. (1999). *Ritual and religion in the making of humanity*. London: Cambridge University Press.

Regnerus, M. D. (2003). Religion and positive adolescent outcomes: a review of research and theory. *Review of Religious Research* 44(4): 394–413.

Richerson, P. J. & Boyd, R. (1999). Complex societies—the evolutionary origins of a crude superorganism. *Human Nature—An Interdisciplinary Biosocial Perspective* 10: 253–289.

Richerson, P. J. & Boyd, R. (2005). *Not by genes alone: how culture transformed human evolution*. Chicago: University of Chicago Press.

Roth, A. E., Prasnikar, V., Okuno-Fujiwara, M. & Zamir, S. (1991). Bargaining and market behavior in Jerusalem, Ljubljana, Pittsburgh, and Tokyo: an experimental study. *American Economic Review* 81: 1068–1095.

Sherkat, D. E. (2001). Tracking the restructuring of American religion: religious affiliation and patterns of mobility, 1973–1998. *Social Forces* 79: 1459–1492.

Shultz, S. & Dunbar, R. I. M. (2007). The evolution of the social brain: anthropoid primates contrast with other vertebrates. *Proceedings of the Royal Society B– Biological Sciences* 274: 2429–2436.

Smith, C., Denton, M. L., Faris, R. & Regnerus, M. (2002). Mapping American adolescent religious participation. *Journal for the Scientific Study of Religion* 41(4): 597–612.

Sosis, R. (2003). Why aren't we all Hutterites? Costly signaling theory and religious behavior. *Human Nature* 14(2): 91–127.

Sosis, R. (2005). Does religion promote trust? The role of signaling, reputation, and punishment. *Interdisciplinary Journal of Research on Religion* 1: 1–30.

Sosis, R. (2006). Religious behaviors, badges, and bans: signaling theory and the evolution of religion. In: P. McNamara (ed.) *Where God and science meet: how brain and evolutionary studies alter our understanding of religion*, vol. 1: *Evolution, genes, and the religious brain*, pp. 61–86. Westport, CT: Praeger.

Sosis, R. (n.d.) The adaptationist-byproduct debate on the evolution of religion: five misunderstandings of the adaptationist program.

Sosis, R. & Alcorta, C. (2003). Signaling, solidarity, and the sacred: the evolution of religious behavior. *Evolutionary Anthropology* 12: 264–274.

Sosis, R. & Ruffle, B. (2003). Religious ritual and cooperation: testing for a relationship on Israeli religious and secular kibbutzim. *Current Anthropology* 44: 713–722.

Sosis, R., Kress, H. C. & Boster, J. S. (2007). Scars for war: evaluating alternative signaling explanations for cross-cultural variance in ritual costs. *Evolution and Human Behavior* 28: 234–247.

Spinka, M., Newberry, R. C. & Bekoff, M. (2001). Mammalian play: training for the unexpected. *Quarterly Review of Biology* 76(2): 141–168.

Steinberg, L. & Morris, A. S. (2001). Adolescent development. *Annual Review of Psychology* 52: 83–110.

Surbey, M. K. (1998). Parent and offspring strategies in the transition at adolescence. *Human Nature* 9(1): 67–94.

Talarico, J. M. & Rubin, D. C. (2007). Flashbulb memories are special after all; in phenomenology, not accuracy. *Applied Cognitive Psychology* 21: 557–578.

Taylor, M. & Carlson, S. M. (1997). The relation between individual differences in fantasy and theory of mind. *Child Development* 68(3): 436–455.

Trinitapoli, J. (2007). 'I know this isn't PC, but . . .': religious exclusivism among US adolescents. *Sociological Quarterly* 48: 451–483.

Turner, V. W. (1967). *The forest of symbols: aspects of Ndembu ritual*. Ithaca, NY: Cornell University Press.

Turner, V. W. (1969). *The ritual process: structure and anti-structure*. Chicago: Aldine.

Uecker, J. E., Regnerus, M. D. & Vaaler, M. L. (2007). Losing my religion: the social sources of religious decline in early adulthood. *Social Forces* 85: 1667–1692.

Walker, D. (1990). The Black Muslims in American society: from millenarian protest to transcontinental relationships. In: G. W. Trompf (ed.) *Cargo cults and millenarian movements: transoceanic comparisons of new religious movements*, pp. 343–390. New York: Mouton de Gruyter.

Waller, B. M. & Dunbar, R. I. M. (2005). Differential behavioural effects of silent bared teeth display and relaxed open mouth display in chimpanzees (*Pan trogolodytes*). *Ethology* 111, 129–142.

Wellman, H. M., Cross, D. & Watson, J. (2001). Meta-analysis of theory-of-mind development: the truth about false belief. *Child Development* 72(3): 655–684.

Whitehouse, H. (1996). Rites of terror: emotion, metaphor, and memory in Melanesian initiation cults. *Journal of the Royal Anthropological Institute* (N.S.) 2(4): 703–715.

Whitehouse, H. (2008). Cognitive evolution and religion: cognition and religious evolution. In: J. Bulbulia, R. Sosis, E. Harris, R. Genet, C. Genet & K. Wyman (eds) *The evolution of religion: studies, theories, and critiques*, pp. 31–41. Santa Margarita, CA: Collins Foundation Press.

Whiten, A. & Byrne, R. (1997). *Machiavellian intelligence II*. Cambridge: Cambridge University Press.

Youngblade, L. M. & Dunn, J. (1995). Individual differences in young children's pretend play with mother and sibling: links to relationships and understanding of other people's feelings and beliefs. *Child Development* 66: 1472–1492.

15

Some Functions of Collective Forgetting

PAUL CONNERTON

COERCED FORGETTING was one of the malign features of the 20th century. Forgetting as repressive erasure appeared in its most brutal form in the history of totalitarian regimes where, in the words of Milan Kundera, the struggle of man against power is the struggle of memory against forgetting. The testimonies of Primo Levi and Elie Wiesel, of Alexander Solzhenitsyn and Nadezhda Mandelstam, were written in defiance of that threat of forgetting. Their testimonies were at once political and therapeutic acts. Political acts, because to write was to denounce the injustice which they had survived or escaped. And therapeutic acts, because for them to write was a way of making sense of a destructive, violent past, one in which they had been victims, and of triumphing over that experience, of turning it into a motivation for living and working. Germany after Hitler, France after Pétain, Spain after Franco, Chile after Pinochet, Greece after the colonels, Argentina after the generals, South Africa after apartheid, the post-socialist states of central and eastern Europe—all these societies had a difficult past and needed to take up some explicit position with regard to that past.

We may, therefore, say that there was an ethics of memory at the end of the 20th century, in the sense that there had not been an ethics of memory at the end of the 19th, 18th or 17th centuries. This structure of feeling has cast a shadow over the context of intellectual debate on memory, in the shape of the widely held if not universal view that remembering is usually a virtue and that forgetting is necessarily a failing. Yet forgetting is not always a failure, and it is not always something about which we should feel culpable. Indeed, forgetting can sometimes be a success; and I want to distinguish three types of forgetting which are successful, in the sense that they establish and enhance social bonds.

Proceedings of the British Academy **158**, 309–316. © The British Academy 2010.

PRESCRIPTIVE FORGETTING

The first type is what I would call *prescriptive* forgetting. This is precipitated by an act of state and is believed to be in the interests of all the parties to the previous dispute; it can therefore be acknowledged publicly. Its aim is to prevent a chain of retribution for earlier acts from running on endlessly.

The Ancient Greeks provide us with a prototype of this type of forgetting. They were acutely aware of the dangers entailed in remembering past wrongs because they well knew about the endless chains of vendetta revenge to which this so often led. And since the memory of past deeds threatened to sow division in the whole community and could lead to civil war, they saw that not only those who were directly threatened by motives of revenge but all those who wanted to live peacefully together in the polis had a stake in not remembering. This thought was famously expressed in 403 BC. In that year the Athenian democrats, after having suffered defeat at the hands of the dictatorship, re-entered the city of Athens and proclaimed a general reconciliation. Their decree contained an explicit interdiction: it was forbidden to remember all the crimes and wrongdoing perpetrated during the immediately preceding period of civil strife. This interdict was to apply to all Athenians, to democrats, to oligarchs, and to all those who had remained in the city as non-combatants during the period of the dictatorship. Perhaps more remarkable still was the fact that the Athenians erected on the acropolis, in their most important temple, an altar dedicated to Lethe—that is, to forgetting. The installation of this altar meant that the injunction to forget, and the eradication of civil conflict which this was thought to promote, was seen as the very foundation of the life of the polis (Meier 1996).

Ernest Renan shared the same sentiment. In his essay of 1882, 'What is a nation?', he argued that a shared amnesia is at least as essential for the development of what we now consider a nation as is the ability to invoke common memories. He cited as his example the fact that every French citizen must have forgotten the anniversary of Saint Bartholomew. He saw no necessity to explain to his readers what 'Saint Bartholomew' meant; only the French could be assumed to know that it referred to the anti-Huguenot pogrom launched on 24 August 1572 by Charles X and his Florentine mother. To remember that event vividly would be to recall that the French body politic was once riven by murderous hatred. Better instead to remain in a paradoxical position; Renan's readers were being told to 'have already forgotten' what Renan's words assumed they naturally remembered.

Nor was Renan alone in this conviction. Whether at the resolution of civil conflict or after international conflict, the formulation of peace terms has frequently contained an explicit expression of the wish that past actions should be not just forgiven but forgotten. The Treaty of Westphalia, which brought the Thirty Years' War to an end in 1648, contained the injunction that both sides should forget forever all the violence, injuries and damage that each had inflicted on the other. After Charles II ascended the English throne in 1660 he declared 'An act of full and general pardon, indemnity and forgetting'. And when Louis XVIII returned to occupy the French throne in 1814 he declared in his constitutional charter that he sought to extinguish from his memory all the evils under which France had suffered during his exile, that all research into utterances of opinion expressed before his restoration was to be forbidden, and that this rule of forgetting was enjoined upon both the law courts and the citizens of France (Frisch 1979).

Or to cite a 20th-century example: Paloma Aguilar (1999) contrasts what she calls the 'pathological amnesia of the Spanish' regarding the civil war in the political sphere with the many representations of the same topic in the fields of film and literature. The prolonged period of political repression under Franco had brought about a generational break. Veteran *mujeres libres*, who had been militants in the organization founded by anarchist women in 1936, and young ones who took up the name of the organization when they began to mobilize themselves after the death of Franco, found that they were unable to work together or even to speak to each other without their exchanges degenerating into mutual recriminations and misunderstandings. The protracted repression of the Franco regime was responsible for this generational rupture. But for this loss there was a compensating gain. In the period of transition after Franco's death in 1975 there was a widespread feeling in Spain that it was essential in political life to forget the rancour of the past if democracy was to be consolidated. The silence about the Franco period, while it was the site of a generational break, made it possible to avoid the use of the past as a weapon in contemporary struggles.

This demonstrates that sometimes at the point of transition from conflict to conflict resolution there may be no explicit requirement to forget, but that the implicit requirement to do so is nonetheless unmistakable. Societies where democracies are regained after a recent undemocratic past, or where democracy is newly born, must establish institutions and make decisions that foster forgetting as much as remembering. Not long after the defeat of Nazism, it became evident that West Germany could not be returned to self-government and civil administration if the purge of Nazis continued to be pursued in a sustained way. So the identification and punishment of active Nazis had become a forgotten issue in Germany by the early 1950s, just as the number of convicted persons was kept to a minimum in Austria and France. For what was necessary after 1945, above all, was to restore a minimum level of cohesion to civil society and to re-establish the legitimacy of the state in societies where authority, and the very bases of civil behaviour, had been obliterated by totalitarian government; the overwhelming desire was to forget the recent past (Judt 1992).

FORGETTING AS CONSTITUTIVE IN THE
FORMATION OF A NEW IDENTITY

A second type of forgetting is that which is *constitutive in the formation of a new identity*. One ingredient in a sense of identity is the feeling of being committed to certain patterns of action. Specific narratives sometimes play a role in shaping people's dispositions to act in certain ways, whether directly or by giving rise to stereotypes of right action; and socially shared dispositions which function in this way are likely to be connected with narratives preserved by collective memory. The narratives preserved by collective memory may play a causal role in influencing people's dispositions; or they may play a normative role, by providing criteria by which models of action can be shaped.

When a new identity is in process of formation some of these older narratives may fall into abeyance. We might think of this as a loss but it is not necessarily so. The forgetting which is entailed in the formation of a new identity is not so much the loss involved in being unable to retain certain things as rather the gain that accrues to those who know how to discard memories that serve no practicable purpose in the management of one's current identity and ongoing purposes. Forgetting then becomes part of the process by which newly shared memories are constructed, because a new set of memories is frequently accompanied by a set of tacitly shared silences. Many small acts of forgetting, which these silences help to enable over time, are not random but patterned. There is, for instance, the forgetting of details about grandparents' lives, which in some cases are not transmitted to grandchildren, whose knowledge about grandparents might not be conducive to, but rather detract from, the effective implementation of their present intentions; or there is the forgetting of details about previous marriages or sexual partnerships, which, if attended to too closely, could impair a present marriage or partnership; or again there are the details of a life formerly lived within a particular religious or political affiliation which has been superseded by embracing an alternative affiliation. Not to forget might in all these cases provoke too much cognitive dissonance. So pieces of knowledge which are not passed on come to have a negative significance by allowing other narratives of identity to come to the fore. They are, so to speak, like pieces of an old jigsaw puzzle which if retained would prevent a new jigsaw puzzle from fitting together. Or to put the matter in another way, unlike prescriptive forgetting this second type of forgetting is unmarked.

The cognatic societies of South East Asia exemplify the way in which this type of forgetting provides living space for present projects. Ethnnographic studies of these societies, in Borneo, Bali, the Philippines and rural Java frequently remark upon the absence of knowledge about ancestors. Knowledge about kinship stretches outwards into degrees of siblingship rather than backwards to predecessors; it is, as it were, horizontal rather than vertical. It is not so much a retention of relatedness as rather a creation of relatedness between those who were previously unrelated. The crucial precipitant of this type of kinship, and the characteristic form of remembering and forgetting attendant upon it, is the high degree of mobility between islands in the South East Asian area. With great demographic mobility it is no longer vital to remember ancestors in the islands left behind, whose identity has become irrelevant in the new island setting, but it becomes crucial instead to create kinship through the formation of new ties. Newcomers to islands are transformed into kin through hospitality, through marriage and through having children. The details of their past diversity, in the islands they have now left, cease to be part of their mental furniture. Forgetting them may be unacknowledged, it is probably only gradual and implicit, and no particular attention is drawn to it. But it is necessary nevertheless. Forgetting is here part of an active process of creating a new and shared identity in a new setting (Carsten 1996).

In much the same sense, no narrative of modernity as a historical project can afford to ignore its subtext of forgetting (Koselleck 1985). That narrative has two interrelated components, one economic, the other psychological. There is, first, the objective transformation of the social fabric unleashed by the advent of the capitalist world market, which tears down feudal and ancestral limitations on a global scale. And there is, second, the subjective transformation of individual life chances, the emancipation of individuals increasingly released from fixed social status and role hierarchies. These are two gigantic processes of discarding. To the extent that these two interlocked processes are embraced, to that extent certain things must be forgotten because they have to be discarded. This long-term forgetting, this casting into forgetting in the interests of forming a new identity, is signalled by two types of semantic evidence, of which one is the emergence of a new type of vocabulary, while the other is the disappearance of a now obsolete vocabulary. On the one hand, certain substantives, which refer at once to historical movements in the present and to projects for the future, enter the currency: History, Revolution, Liberalism, Socialism, Modernity itself. On the other hand, certain words previously employed by writers in English cease to be used and are no longer easily recognizable: memorous (memorable), memorious (having a good memory), memorist (one who prompts the return of memories), mnemonize (to memorize), mnemonicon (a device to aid the memory) (Casey 1987). Could there be a more explicit indication than that signalled in these two semantic shifts of what is thought desirable and what can be cast into oblivion?

FORGETTING AS ANNULMENT

A third type of forgetting might be called *annulment*. This is a possible response to a surfeit of information. Paradoxically we live in a throwaway society and in one where memory is archival. No epoch has deliberately produced so many archives as ours, with our museums, libraries, depositories and centres of documentation.

This development has been brought about in two phases. The first was the great archivalization which was an essential ingredient in the formation of the modern state. We routinely assume now that no state power can possibly exist without its administrative machinery of documents, files and memoranda—even if it sometimes happens that a few of these go missing. Habsburg Spain was a spectacular pioneer of the modern state in this sense. The overwhelming mass of documentation generated by the Spanish administration in the 16th and 17th centuries, installed in the great state archive in Simancas, was the first and possibly the most voluminous of such storehouses in Europe. At a later date the administrative core of the British Empire was built around knowledge-producing institutions like the British Museum, the Royal Geographical Survey, the

India Survey, the Royal Society, and the Royal Asiatic Society, all of which institutions together formed what was thought of as an imperial archive, collected in the service of the state and empire (Richards 1993).

The idea of an imperial archive foreshadowed a later historical development, namely, the spread at immense speed throughout the globe of new information technologies in the two decades between the mid 1970s and the mid 1990s. Of course, large segments of the world's population, in the American inner cities, in French banlieues, in African shanty towns, in deprived rural areas of India, remain cut off from these innovations. But the dominant groups and territories across the globe had become interlinked by the end of the millennium in a new technological system that had begun to take shape only in the 1970s. Taken together, the great archivalization and the new information technologies have brought about such an informational surfeit that the concept of discarding may come to occupy as central a role in the 21st century as the concept of production did in the 19th.

To say that something has been stored, in an archive or computer, is in effect to say that, though it is in principle always retrievable, we can afford to forget it. We now live in a society that has access to too much information and in the foreseeable future the problem can only get worse. Genuine skill in knowing how to manage one's life may come to reside less in knowing how to gather information and more in knowing how to discard it.

This need to discard is felt most acutely, of course, in the natural sciences. As long ago as 1963 it was calculated that 75 per cent of all citations in the field of physics were taken from publications that were less than ten years old. Every scientist needs to learn how to forget in this way if his research activity is not to be crippled by chronic over-information at the outset. Indeed, Kuhn's (1962) concept of the scientific paradigm is an idea about forgetting. Kuhn sees the development of science as one in which every shift in scientific evolution unburdens scientific memory, where every demise of a paradigm is always an act of forgetting of great importance for the economy of scientific effort. The paradigm that has been surpassed is the one that can be forgotten. This is why Kuhn observed that almost always the men who achieve fundamental scientific discoveries leading to a new paradigm have either been very young or very new to the field whose paradigm they change: in other words, their scientific imagination has been unburdened by too much scientific memory.

Even if the historical disciplines are not susceptible to such a drastic process of in-built obsolescence, they too have been marked by a paradigm shift and a corresponding collective forgetting. Fifty years ago historians would often attempt large-scale narratives mapping the course of historical change over long periods, and history was taken to mean politics, the constitution, diplomacy and warfare. Now the flowering of microhistory involves the intensive study of small communities and single events on the model of Emmanuel le Roy Ladurie's *Montaillou* and Carlo Ginzburg's *The cheese and the worms*, and historians seize upon every aspect of human behaviour and experience, from childhood to old age, from dress to table manners, from smells to laughter, from shopping to barbed wire. The old narratives and the old core stories slowly become effaced. No doubt there are a number of reasons for this change, but one at least is the wish to circumvent the problems of informational overload which flows from a sheer excess of knowledge.

   None of these three types of forgetting—prescribed forgetting, forgetting in the interests of shaping a new identity, and forgetting as annulment—represents a failure. All of them are successful, in the sense that they conduce to the establishment and enhancement of social bonds.

REFERENCES

Aguilar, P. (1999). Agents of memory: Spanish Civil War veterans and disabled soldiers. In: J. Winter & E. Sivan (eds) *War and remembrance in the twentieth century*. Cambridge: Cambridge University Press.

Carsten, J. (1996). The politics of forgetting: migration, kinship and memory on the periphery of the Southeast Asian state. *Journal of the Royal Anthropological Institute* (ns) 1: 317–335.

Casey, E. S. (1987). *Remembering: a phenomenological study*. Bloomington: Indiana University Press.

Frisch, J. (1979). *Krieg und Frieden im Friedensvertrag: Eine universalgeschichtliche Studie über Grundlagen und Formelemente des Friedensschlusses*. Stuttgart: Klett-Cotta.

Ginzburg, C. (1980). *The cheese and the worms*, trans. J. Tedeschi and A. Tedeschi. London: Routledge.

Judt, T. (1992). The past is another country: myth and memory in postwar Europe. *Daedalus* 121: 83–118.

Koselleck, R. (1985). *Futures past: on the semantics of historical time*. Cambridge, MA: Harvard University Press.

Kuhn, T. (1962). *The structure of scientific revolutions*. Chicago: University of Chicago Press.

Ladurie, E. L. (1978). *Montaillou*, trans. B. Bray. Harmondsworth: Penguin.

Meier, C. (1996). Erinnern—Verdrängen—Vergessen. *Merkur* 50: 937–952

Richards, T. (1993). *The imperial archive: knowledge and the fantasy of empire*. London: Verso.

16

What is Cognition? Extended Cognition and the Criterion of the Cognitive

THE MIND EXTENDED AND EMBEDDED

ACCORDING TO THE VIEW known variously as the *extended mind* (Clark & Chalmers 1998), *vehicle externalism* (Hurley 1998; Rowlands 2006), *active externalism* (Clark & Chalmers 1998), *locational externalism* (Wilson 2004) and *environmentalism* (Rowlands 1999), at least some token cognitive processes extend into the cognizing organism's environment in that they are composed, partly (and, in most versions, contingently), of manipulative, exploitative and transformative operations performed by that subject on suitable environmental structures. More precisely, what I shall refer to as the thesis of the *extended mind* (*ExM*) is constituted by the following claims:

- The world is an external store of information relevant to processes such as perceiving, remembering, reasoning, etc.
- Cognitive processes are hybrid—they straddle both internal and external operations.
- The external operations take the form of *action*: manipulation, exploitation and transformation of environmental structures— ones that carry information relevant to the accomplishing of a given task.
- At least some of the internal processes are ones concerned with supplying the subject with the ability to use relevant structures in its environment appropriately.

Proceedings of the British Academy **158**, 317–337. © The British Academy 2010.

As I shall understand it, therefore, the thesis of the extended mind is (1) an *ontic* thesis, of (2) *partial* (3) *composition* of (4) *some* mental processes.[1]

Let us deal with condition (4) first, since it is fairly obvious. *ExM* does not make a blanket claim about all mental processes. The thesis can view with equanimity the strong likelihood that the composition of some, even many, mental processes is exclusively neural. *ExM* claims only that exclusive neural composition is not true of all mental processes. Indeed, the focus, until recently, has largely been on a sub-category of mental processes: cognitive processes.[2]

Considering the remaining conclusions, *ExM* is an *ontic* thesis (1) in the sense that it is a thesis about what (some) mental processes *are*, as opposed to an *epistemic* thesis about the best way of *understanding* mental processes. This ontic claim, of course, has an epistemic consequence: it is not possible to understand the nature of at least some mental processes without understanding the extent to which that organism is capable of manipulating, exploiting and transforming relevant structures in its environment (Rowlands 1999). However, this epistemic consequence is not part of *ExM* itself. Indeed, the epistemic claim is compatible with the denial of *ExM*.[3]

ExM claims that (some) token mental processes are, *in part*, made up of the manipulation, exploitation or transformation of environmental structures (2). There is always an irreducible internal—neural, and sometimes also wider bodily—contribution to the constitution of any mental process. No version of *ExM* will claim that a mental process can be composed entirely of manipulative, exploitative or transformative operations performed on the environment.

ExM is a claim about the *composition* or *constitution* of (some) mental processes (3). Composition is a quite different relation than *dependence*. Thus, *ExM* is a stronger and more distinctive claim than one of environmental embedding; and the thesis of the extended mind must be clearly distinguished from that of the *embedded* mind (*EmM*). According to *EmM*, some mental processes function—and indeed have been designed to function—only in tandem with certain environmental

---

[1] There are other possible ways of understanding *ExM*, but this was the status of the thesis I developed and defended in Rowlands (1999).

[2] For extension of this idea to conscious experiences, see Hurley (1998), Rowlands (2002) and Noë (2004).

[3] This is because this epistemic claim is also a corollary of a weaker claim to be discussed shortly: the thesis of the *embedded mind*.

structures, so that in the absence of the latter the former cannot do what they are supposed to do or work in the way they are supposed to work. Thus for *EmM* some mental processes are dependent, perhaps essentially dependent, for their operation on the wider environment. *ExM*, on the other hand, does not simply claim that mental processes are *situated* in this way in a wider system of scaffolding, a system that facilitates—perhaps in crucial ways—the operation of these processes. That would be a claim of dependence. Rather, *ExM* claims that things we do to this wider system of scaffolding in part compose or constitute (some of) our mental processes.

OBJECTIONS TO THE EXTENDED MIND

ExM has attracted a number of objections:

(1) *The differences argument.* This type of objection points to the significant differences between internal cognitive processes and the external processes that *ExM* alleges are also cognitive. This casts doubts on the claim that both processes should be regarded as belonging to a single psychological kind (Rupert 2004).

(2) *The coupling-constitution fallacy.* This objection claims that *ExM* confuses cognition with its extraneous causal accompaniments. More precisely, it confuses those structures and processes constitutive of cognition with those in which cognition is (merely) causally embedded. This type of objection has been developed by Adams and Aizawa (2001, in press) and Rupert (2004).

(3) *The mark of the cognitive objection.* According to this objection, *ExM* should be rejected on the grounds that it is incompatible with any plausible mark of the cognitive; that is, any criterion that specifies the conditions under which a process qualifies as cognitive. This objection is developed by Adams and Aizawa (2001, in press).

As we shall see, these three objections all reduce to a certain kind of worry: that the arguments for *ExM* in fact only establish *EmM*. That is, the arguments that purport to show that cognition is extended only really show that cognition is embedded. This chapter has two primary goals. The first is to show that this worry can be assuaged by the provision of an adequate and properly motivated criterion of the cognitive. The second is to provide such a criterion.

THE DIFFERENCES ARGUMENT:
PARITY AND INTEGRATION IN *ExM*

ExM is often thought to be grounded in the concept of *parity*: roughly speaking, the *similarity* between the external processes involved in cognition and internal processes that are widely accepted as cognitive. *ExM*'s reliance on this notion of parity is often thought to be embodied in, and demonstrated by, Clark and Chalmers' deployment of what they call the *parity principle*:

> If, as we confront some task, a part of the world functions as a process which, *were it done in the head*, we would have no hesitation in recognizing as part of the cognitive process, then that part of the world is (so we claim) part of the cognitive process. (Clark & Chalmers 1998, 9, emphasis theirs)

Critics of *ExM* have, without exception, understood the parity principle as introducing a *similarity-based criterion* of when an external process or structure is to be understood as cognitive—that is, as a genuinely cognitive part of a cognitive process: if an external process is sufficiently similar to an internal cognitive process, then it too is a cognitive process. It is this interpretation of the role of the parity principle that underwrites the *differences argument*. Thus Rupert, in connection with my argument for extended memory (Rowlands 1999), outlines his strategy as follows:

> I argue that the external portions of extended 'memory' states (processes) differ so greatly from internal memories (the process of remembering) that they should be treated as distinct kinds; this quells any temptation to argue for HEC [hypothesis of extended cognition] from brute analogy (viz. extended cognitive states are like wholly internal ones; therefore, they are of the same explanatory cognitive kind; therefore there are extended cognitive states). (Rupert, 2004, 407)

The operative assumption is that the function of the parity principle is to introduce a similarity-based criterion of when a cognitive process such as remembering can be extended into the world. Rupert then argues that since external processes involved in memory are, in fact, *not* sufficiently similar to internal cognitive processes, then they are *not* cognitive processes.

This *differences argument*, however, rests on a failure to properly understand the arguments for *ExM*. *ExM* does not rely on a similarity-based criterion of when a cognitive process may legitimately be regarded as extended. The notion of parity is indeed, I shall argue, an important one for *ExM*. However, equally important is the notion of *integration*: the meshing of disparate types of process that, *precisely because* of their disparate character can enable a cognizing organism to accomplish tasks that it would not be able to achieve by way of either type of process alone (Menary 2006, 2007; Sutton in press). From this *integrationist* perspective, the *differences* between internal and external processes are as important as, or even more important than, the similarities. The reason cognition extends into the environment is precisely because, with respect to the accomplishing of certain cognitive tasks, external processes can do things that internal processes cannot do. External structures and processes possess quite different properties from internal ones, and it is precisely this difference that affords the cognitive agent the opportunity to accomplish certain tasks that it could not, or might not, be able to accomplish purely by way of internal cognitive processes. Without these differences, the external processes would be *otiose*.

Thus, for example, extended models tend to emphasize the relative *stability* of relevant external structures, and the enhanced possibilities for manipulation and exploitation that this stability engenders (Donald 1991; Noë 2004; O'Regan & Noë 2001; Rowlands 1999, 2003). These possibilities, it is argued, have little or no echo in the case of internal processes, and they underwrite the abilities of organisms to accomplish certain cognitive tasks that they could not accomplish by way of internal processes alone. *ExM* tends also to emphasize the distinctive *structure* of external items (e.g. linguistic or combinatorial), structure that, again, has (arguably) no echo in internal items (Donald, 1991; Hurley, 1998; Rowlands, 1999). In each case, it is precisely the *different* properties of external structures that allow the cognitive agent to accomplish things that it either could not, or does not, accomplish by way of internal processes alone.

Given the central role played by the notion of integration in *ExM*, one cannot predicate, as does the *differences argument*, an objection to *ExM* simply by citing differences between internal and external processes. *ExM*, properly understood, both *predicts* and *requires* such differences. Understood on its own terms, therefore, the differences argument fails.

However, the integrationist's emphasis on the *differences* between the internal and external processes involved in cognition does leave *ExM* vulnerable to another objection. If *ExM* requires significant differences between internal processes and the external processes that it regards as cognitive, what reason is there for supposing that the latter really are part of cognition rather than merely an external accompaniment to real, internal, cognitive processing? This is the worry outlined at the beginning of the chapter. That is, the emphasis on integration leaves *ExM* vulnerable to the charge that the arguments canvassed in its favour only actually support embedded rather than extended cognition. This worry can be avoided if we are able to provide an adequate and properly motivated *criterion of the cognitive*: a criterion that would allow *ExM* to justify the claim that the external processes involved in cognition are indeed cognitive processes. This will be the task of the second half of this chapter.

THE COUPLING-CONSTITUTION FALLACY

The *coupling-constitution fallacy* objection can take slightly different forms. According to Adams and Aizawa:

> This is the most common mistake that extended mind theorists make. The fallacious pattern is to draw attention to cases, real or imagined, in which some object or process is coupled in some fashion to some cognitive agent. From this, they slide to the conclusion that the object or process constitutes part of the agent's cognitive apparatus or cognitive processing. (Adams & Aizawa 2001, 408)

Rupert expresses a similar objection, albeit in more cautious terms. Referring, again, to my version of *ExM*, he writes:

> Rowlands, however, does not make clear why the use of an internally represented code applied to the contents of an external store implies HEC, rather than what it would seem to imply: HEMC. (Rupert 2004, 408)

HEC is the *hypothesis of extended cognition*, which Rupert, correctly, distinguishes from HEMC, the *hypothesis of embedded cognition*. What reason do we have, Rupert asks, for regarding the external processes as part of cognition rather than simply a form of extraneous scaffolding in which *real*—internal—cognitive processes can be causally embedded? This is, once again, the worry advertised at the outset of this chapter.

It is, however, implausible to suppose that *ExM* is guilty of simply *confusing* constitution and causal coupling. Far from *confusing* constitution and causal coupling, the most natural way of understanding the arguments for *ExM* are precisely as *arguments* for reinterpreting what had traditionally been regarded as extraneous causal accompaniments to cognition as, in fact, part of cognition itself. And, in general, to *argue* for the identification of X and Y, when X and Y had hitherto been regarded as distinct types, is not to *confuse* X and Y.

Consider, for example, my argument for extended memory cited by Rupert. I argued that, in certain cases, the external processes involved in cognition—bodily manipulation and exploitation of information-bearing structures in the cognizer's environment—possess certain abstract, general, features of processes commonly regarded as cognitive, while also differing in the sorts of concrete ways required by the integrationist underpinning of *ExM*. Thus, these external processes are employed in order to accomplish cognitive tasks. They involve information processing—the manipulation and transformation of information-bearing structures. This processing results in the making available to organisms of information that was previously unavailable, and so on. That is, I *argued* for the cognitive status of external processes of these sorts by trying to show that they satisfy a certain criterion of the cognitive. One can, I think, legitimately question whether I rendered this criterion sufficiently explicit, and even if it were explicit whether it was adequate. But one can hardly accuse me of *confusing* causation and constitution. And if I were in possession of an adequate and properly motivated criterion of the cognitive, and if the sorts of external processes I identify were to satisfy this criterion, then I would have, in fact, made it clear why my view implies HEC rather than HEMC.

Thus, like the differences argument, the coupling-constitution fallacy objection is derivative on the mark of the cognitive objection. If *ExM* can provide an adequate criterion of the cognitive, and demonstrate that the external processes it regards as cognitive satisfy this criterion, then there is no substance to the charge that it confuses constitution and mere coupling.

THE MARK OF THE COGNITIVE

According to the mark of the cognitive objection, *ExM* should be rejected on the grounds that it is incompatible with any plausible mark or criterion of the cognitive. The goal of the second half of this chapter is to supply such a criterion, and argue that, far from contradicting the claims of *ExM*, it actually supports those claims. Therefore, if the other objections to *ExM* are indeed derivative on the mark of the cognitive objection, then provision of this criterion will serve to defuse these objections also.

Some are sceptical about the need for a mark of the cognitive. Do we need, they ask, a mark of the biological in order to do biology—or, for that matter, a mark of the physical in order to do physics? (The question is intended as rhetorical.)

Underlying this attitude is the idea that science simply does what it does—identifies its laws and constructs its theories—and, as long as it can do this, has no need for any deeper understanding of what it is doing. Thus, it might be argued, we have an adequate intuitive grasp of what counts as cognitive, and this grasp is sufficient for us to adjudicate the claims of *ExM*.[4] There is another way of thinking about science—as a form of self-interpreting activity—according to which a gradual deepening of the understanding of what a science is doing is built into the scientific project itself (see, for example, Heidegger 1962 [1927]). The sort of philosophy of psychology that attempts to understand what it is for a process to be cognitive is built on this alternative vision of the scientific enterprise. I do not propose to adjudicate between these two conceptions of science. However, it is worth pointing out that in the case of *ExM* at least, it is not only the mark of the cognitive objection that is at stake. If the arguments of the first half of the chapter are correct, then *all* of the objections to *ExM* can be solved through the provision of an adequate mark of the cognitive. This might be enough to at least convince defenders of *ExM* that a criterion of the cognitive is something worth investigating.

In the prevailing dialectical situation it is clear *why ExM* needs a criterion of the cognitive; but it is not yet clear precisely *what* sort of thing this criterion should be. The criterion I shall defend does not try to give a reductive definition of 'the cognitive' in terms that are exclusively non-cognitive. Rather, the goal of the criterion is to provide a means of demarcating, with a reasonable but not necessarily indefeasible level of precision, those processes that count as cognitive from those that do not.

The criterion I shall defend provides a *sufficient* condition for a process to count as cognitive, not (I wish to emphasize) a *necessary* condition. That is, if a process satisfies the criterion it thereby qualifies as cognitive. However, if a process does not satisfy the criterion, it does not automatically follow that it is not cognitive. Moreover, it is a sufficient condition that, I shall argue, any *critic* of *ExM* would have to accept. This is crucial: my strategy is to give the critic of *ExM* everything in a criterion of cognition that he or she could reasonably want, and show that *ExM still* follows. The idea underpinning the criterion is that if we wish to understand what cognitive processes are, then we should pay close attention to the sorts of things cognitive scientists regard as cognitive. That is not to say that we must restrict ourselves to the pronouncements or

---

[4] I am grateful for conversations with Andy Clark for this point.

determinations of cognitive scientists, or that we should regard these as decisive, but merely that we should be prepared to use these as our starting point. A significant part of the criterion I shall defend can be extracted from a careful examination of cognitive-scientific *practice*— *internalist* cognitive-scientific practice. When we examine such practice, I shall argue, what we find is an implicit mark of the cognitive that looks like this. A process *P* is a *cognitive* process if:

(1) *P* involves information processing—the manipulation and transformation of information-bearing structures.

(2) This information processing has the *proper function* of *making available* either to the *subject* or to *subsequent processing operations* information that was (or would have been) unavailable prior to (or without) this processing.

(3) This information is made available by way of the production, in the subject of *P*, of a *representational* state.

(4) *P* is a process that *belongs* to the *subject* of that *representational state*.

Before motivating and defending this criterion, it is necessary to remark on these four conditions in turn.

Condition (1)

The idea that cognition involves information processing is now commonplace. In its classical form, cognitive science was understood to involve the postulation of internal configurations of an organism or system, configurations that carry information about extrinsic states of affairs. The concept of information employed is, in essence, that elaborated by Claude Shannon, or a close variant thereof. According to Shannon, information is to be understood in terms of relations of conditional probability. On the version championed by Shannon, a receptor *r* carries information about a source *s* only if the probability of *s* given *r* is 1 (see Dretske 1981). Other, less sanguine, versions associate the carrying of information with an increase in conditional probability, although not necessarily to the value of 1. That is, *r* carries information about *s* only if the probability of *s* given *r* is greater than the probability of *s* given not-*r* (see Lloyd 1989).

Whichever explication of the concept of information is employed, the underlying vision of cognition is unaffected. Cognitive processes are understood as a series of transformations performed on information-bearing structures. These transformations will be effected according to certain rules or principles—principles that effectively define the character of the type of cognitive process in question.

Condition (2)

The second condition relies heavily on the concept of *proper function*. I shall understand this in the etiological sense championed by Millikan (1984, 1993), among others. In both cases, the appeal to proper function reminds us that the concept of cognition is, in part, a normative one. Cognitive processes can function well or badly, properly or improperly: they are defined in terms of what they are *supposed* to do, not what they *actually* do. A cognitive process might have a function that it fails to fulfil in particular cases. Indeed, it might never fulfil this function, due to faults in the mechanisms that realize it or in surrounding mechanisms. Moreover, in addition to doing what it is supposed to do, it might also do various things that are not its proper function. A process might have a proper function only in relation to a given environmental contingency, and this contingency might fail to obtain, etc.

The distinction between making information available to a *subject* and making it available to *subsequent processing operations* is also important. Roughly, and with appropriate clarifications to follow shortly, it corresponds to the distinction between *personal* and *sub-personal* cognitive processes. Processes that make information available to a subject are personal-level processes, and this is true whether they also make information available to subsequent processing operations. However, processes that make information available *only* to subsequent processing operations are sub-personal cognitive processes.

Condition (3)

The notion of a representational state is not co-extensive, still less synonymous, with the notion of a *semantically evaluable* state. It would be implausible to suppose that all representational states are semantically evaluable: such states must possess *adequacy conditions*, but they need not possess *truth-conditions*. Mental models, or cognitive maps, possess adequacy conditions but not truth-conditions. The concept of truth is constitutively connected—for familiar Davidsonian reasons—with the logical connectives, and mental models do not relate to these connectives in the same way as sentences, external or internal. Thus, for example, the negation of a sentence is another *specific* sentence, but to the extent that it makes sense to speak of the negation of a map or model, this can mean nothing more than a distinct, but non-specific, map or model. Once we understand the connection between truth and the logical connectives, I take it that this point is incontrovertible, though often oddly neglected. However, nothing much will turn on it in the arguments to follow.

I shall assume that the type of representational state invoked in (3) is one that possesses *non-derived* content. Derived content is content, possessed by a given state, that derives from the content of other representational states of a cognizing subject or from the social conventions that constitute that agent's linguistic milieu.[5] Non-derived content is content that is not derived from *other* content—it is not content that is irreducible or *sui generis*:[6] it is *what* content is derived from that is crucial. It can, for example, derived from, and be explained in terms of, the history or informational-carrying profile of the state that has it. The existence of non-derived content is controversial (see, for example, Dennett 1987). However, there is one very good reason why we should restrict the sort of content possessed by the representational state designated in (3) to non-derived content. The claim that non-derived content is central to cognition has been used to attack *ExM*. For example, Adams and Aizawa (2001) attack Clark and Chalmers' (1998) claim that the sentences in Otto's notebook constitute a subset of his beliefs precisely on the grounds that these sentences possess only derived content. Therefore, without the restriction to non-derived content, the proposed criterion would be regarded as question-begging by the critics of *ExM*. If one is chary about this sort of deployment of the concept of non-derived content, then one should recall that the proposed criterion is intended only as providing a *sufficient* condition for cognition. The strategy pursued in this chapter, one should remember, is to give the critic of *ExM* enough rope to hang himself: to grant everything he could reasonably require—and then show that *ExM* still follows.

---

[5] Adherence to such conventions might be taken to involve some kind of intentional action on the part of the agent, and therefore also invoke the content of other representational states, merely at one step removed.

[6] In their invocation of non-derived content, Adams and Aizawa (2001) sometimes refer to it as 'intrinsic content'. This is a deeply unfortunate locution, even more misleading than 'non-derived content'. No content is intrinsic. As Dretske once quipped, one might as well talk of an *intrinsic grandmother*.

Condition (4)

I shall argue that anything that is to count as a cognitive process must belong to some or other representational subject (broadly construed). There are no un-*owned* cognitive processes. Understanding the sense in which cognitive processes have an owner is, I think, one of the hardest tasks in understanding the nature of cognition. It would not be possible to undertake that task in this chapter. Here my goals are more modest. I shall argue that understanding the sense in which a cognitive process is owned by a subject is just as problematic for internalists with regard to cognition as it is for defenders of *ExM*. A problem for both is not a problem specifically for one. While this 'solution' is not ideal, it is the only strategy permitted within the constraints imposed by a chapter of this length.

For reasons that will become clear, I shall motivate and defend conditions (1)–(3) separately from condition (4).

DEFENDING THE CRITERION:
COGNITIVE-SCIENTIFIC PRACTICE

I shall defend conditions (1)–(3) of the criterion by showing that they can be extracted, in a relatively straightforward manner, from examination of cognitive-scientific practice. The guiding principle is that if we want to identify a mark of the cognitive, then we should pay close attention to the sorts of processes that cognitive scientists regard as cognitive, and then try to identify the general features of processes of these kinds. However, to avoid the charge that the criterion is motivated by *ExM*-aforethought, the cognitive-scientific practice in question must be *internalist* cognitive science—and the more paradigmatic or archetypal the form of internalism the better. Therefore, I will focus here on David Marr's (1979) theory of vision. While many of the details of this theory are now starting to look a little quaint, the general approach adopted by Marr has dominated internalist-inspired theorizing in cognitive science.

For Marr, visual perception begins with the formation of an informationally impoverished retinal image. The function of properly perceptual processing is to transform this retinal image into, successively, the raw primal sketch, the full primal sketch, and the 2½D sketch, the culmination of properly perceptual processing. At each stage in the operation, one information-bearing structure is transformed into another. The retinal image, reputedly, contains very little information, but it does contain some. The retinal image is made up of a distribution of light intensity values across the retina. Since the distribution of intensity values is nomically dependent on the way in which light is reflected by the physical structures that the organism is viewing, the image carries some information about these structures. Then this information-bearing structure is transformed into the raw primal sketch. In the raw primal sketch, information about the edges and textures of objects has been added. Application of various grouping principles (e.g. proximity, similarity, common fate, good continuation, closure and so on) to the raw primal sketch results in the identification of larger structures, boundaries and regions. This more refined representation is the full primal sketch. And so on.

Abstracting from the details, a very definite picture of visual perception emerges. First of all, perception involves information processing: the transformation of information-bearing structures (condition (1)). The retinal image is transformed into the raw primal sketch. Further processing operations then transform this into the full primal sketch and so on. The result of these transformations is the making available to subsequent processing operations of information that was previously unavailable (condition (2)). Thus, in the transformation of the retinal image into the raw primal sketch new information becomes available for subsequent processing—information that was not present in the retinal image. And in the transformation of the raw primal sketch into the full primal sketch, further information becomes available, information that was not available in the raw sketch. The culmination of the perceptual process is the 2½D sketch. This sketch carries information that is available for further processing operations—the post-perceptual operations that result in the formation of *3D object representations* (which are, in turn, available to play a further role in belief formation, etc.). The general picture is clear: at each stage in the operation, it is possible to identify a new structure, one which carries novel information that is available to subsequent processing operations. Marr's theory thus provides a graphic illustration of condition (2).

Each identified stage in the operation culminates in a new representational state (condition (3)). The retinal image, while impoverished, does carry some information about the environment. The goal of visual processing is to successively transform this into an item sufficiently rich in informational content to provide the basis of visual perception and post-perceptual judgements. Each stage of the process, therefore, culminates in a state that carries more information about the environment than its predecessor. Once we leave retinal image behind, each successive state is *normative* in at least the following, minimal, sense: given that the state is instantiated with the properties it has, the world is *supposed* to be a certain way. With the retinal image, there is no distinction between the way the world is and the way it is supposed to be: the retinal image is caused by whatever causes it. However, the raw primal sketch contains new information—information contributed by the first stage of perceptual processing. This, in effect, is the brain's 'guess' about the way the world would have to be in order to have produced the retinal image being processed. As such, given the 'guess', the world is supposed to be a certain way; and if it is not the 'guess' was mistaken. At each successive stage of processing, therefore, we find a state that carries information and makes normative claims on the world. That is, we find basic representational states. Moreover, the content they carry as representational states does not derive from the content of representational states that lie outside the particular processing stream. That is, while the content of the 2½D sketch derives from that of the full primal sketch which, in turn, derives from that of the raw primal sketch, the content involved in the successive transformations that constitute this processing stream does not derive from the content of representational states that lie outside this stream. The content embodied in this particular processing stream is, therefore, *non-derived* content.

EXTENDING COGNITION

With this general model in mind, consider, once again, the extended account of memory I developed in *The body in mind* (Rowlands 1999). The account was based around certain central illustrative examples pertaining to our reliance on external information storage structures in the constitution of memory. The Peruvian *kvinu* officer who employs a system of knots to store information employs his biological memory in a very different way from that of the envoy of a culture in which external forms of information storage have not been invented (Rowlands 1999, 134–136). The latter must rely on biological memory to retain information, and must do so afresh for each item of information he needs to retain. But the *kvinu* officer need deploy his biological memory only in the remembering of the 'code' that allows him to tap into the information contained in each knot. Once he does this, a potentially unlimited amount of information becomes available to him through his abilities to manipulate and exploit such external structures.

The knot is an information-bearing structure that exists outside the skin of the subject that deploys it: it is, in this sense, external to the subject. Deployment of knots can take various forms: one can tie them, one can modify them, one can read them, and one can use the information they contain as an aid in the construction of further knots. These are all ways in which the knots can be manipulated or exploited. When one ties a knot, for example, or modifies a knot that has already been tied (in order, for example, to register some change in pertinent information), then one is manipulating or transforming an information-bearing structure. Thus, the deployment of knots by the *kvinu* officer satisfies condition (1) of the criterion of the cognitive.

The result of this manipulation or transformation of knots is the making available to the cognitive subject of information that was previously unavailable. Indeed, not only does the knot do this: it is its proper function to do this. We are, of course, dealing with a case of remembering, rather than the transferral of novel information to a distinct individual. So, the relevant scenario would look something like this: the person who ties the knot would otherwise have forgotten the information that the knot contains, due to, let us suppose, other demands on her biological memory resources. But when she picks the knot up again—the next day, for example—the information it contains is once again available to her. In this case, the knot has the proper function of making available to the subject information that would have been, without the tying of the knot, unavailable. It thus satisfies condition (2) of the proposed criterion of the cognitive.

The way in which this process of manipulating or exploiting knots makes information available to the subject is in the form of the production in that subject of a representational state: a perception of the knot, and subsequent belief-based representations of the informational content contained therein. It is, as I emphasized earlier, no part of *ExM* to claim that processes entirely external to (i.e. outside the skin of) a cognizing subject can count as cognitive. For *ExM*, cognitive processes are entirely internal or are coupled wholes composed of operations occurring both inside and outside the subject's skin. That is, according to *ExM*, cognitive processes always contain a non-eliminable internal element. It is here that we find representational states that possess non-derived content. Manipulation of the knot, an external information-bearing structure, thus makes information available to the subject by way of its production in that subject of representational states that possess non-derived content. Therefore, this manipulation of an external information-bearing structure satisfies condition (3) of the proposed criterion of the cognitive.

Therefore the kinds of manipulation, exploitation and transformation of external information-bearing structures employed in a process of remembering satisfy conditions (1)–(3) of the criterion of the cognitive in precisely the same way as the manipulation of internal information-bearing structures described by Marr for the process of perceiving. Therefore, if (1)–(3) do indeed partly delineate what it is for a process to qualify as cognitive, then with respect to these conditions at least, external operations of the sort invoked by *ExM* seem to qualify as cognitive in the same way that classical internal operations qualify as cognitive.

It is obviously not possible, in a chapter of this sort, to exhaustively examine all possible internalist and extended models of various cognitive processes to establish that they satisfy conditions (1)–(3). Indeed, it may well be that not all versions of *ExM* can satisfy these conditions. However, I hope to have shown that *ExM* can at least make a *prima facie* case for the idea that the sorts of processes it claims are cognitive are cognitive precisely because they satisfy a plausible criterion of the cognitive. This is a criterion of the cognitive implicated in paradigmatic examples of internalist cognitive theorizing. And all of the principal objections to *ExM* are based on its purported failure to satisfy such a criterion.

However, to complete this case, there is one further condition that needs to be discussed: the *ownership* condition.

OWNERSHIP AND THE PROBLEM OF BLOAT

Suppose I am using a telescope.[7] The telescope is, let us suppose, a *reflector*, and therefore works by transforming one mirror image into another. Mirror images are information-bearing structures—their properties are systematically determined by a mapping function determined by the specific properties of the mirror and the properties of the visual environment. Therefore, the operation of the telescope is based on the transformation of information-bearing structures, and so it satisfies condition (1). The processes occurring inside the telescope are, in combination with other processes, of the sort normally capable of yielding a

[7] My thanks to Richard Samuels for this example.

representational state. This is true even when the content of this state is non-derived. Thus, in combination with other processes—ones occurring inside *me*—the processes can yield a representational state; for example, my visual perception of Saturn's rings. This is a representational state with non-derived content. Therefore, the processes occurring inside the telescope satisfy condition (3). And the proper function of the processes occurring inside the telescope is making information available, both to me and to subsequent processing operations within me (for example, processes of inference), of information that was previously unavailable (for example, the current orientation relative to earth of Saturn's rings), and thus satisfy condition (2). Therefore, the processes occurring inside the telescope satisfy conditions (1)–(3) of our criterion of cognition. If these conditions were sufficient for cognition, then the intra-telescopic processes would have to be classified as cognitive.

Relevantly similar examples can be easily generated. How can we rule out, for example, processes occurring inside my calculator, or my computer, from counting as cognitive ones? They seem to involve the transformation of information-bearing structures (1). They are also the sort of processes that, when combined with other processes, can produce representational states (3). Thus, when combined with operations occurring inside my brain, the processes occurring inside the calculator can produce a representational state in me—for example, when I read off the result of their operations from the screen. And the proper function of these processes is, it seems, to make information available to me, information that I might subsequently employ in further processing operations, where this information was not available prior to the operations of the calculator or computer (2). Therefore, the processes occurring inside the calculator and computer seem to satisfy conditions (1)–(3), and, without further constraints, would therefore count as cognitive.

This, in essence, is a problem of *cognitive bloat*—the unbridled expansion of the realm of the cognitive beyond the bounds of plausibility. We sidestep this problem if we refuse to allow the existence of *subjectless* cognitive processes. Cognitive processes always have an owner, and this owner is an *individual* of some form.[8] This is the import of condition (4) of the criterion.

Explaining the sense in which a subject owns his, her, or perhaps its, cognitive processes is, I think, far more difficult than it seems. It is not the

---

[8] To say that they their owner is an individual is, of course, *not* to say, necessarily, that this is a person.

sort of project that can be addressed in a chapter of this length. Accordingly, in the rest of the chapter I want to pursue only a more modest aim. I shall argue that explaining ownership of cognitive processes is just as much of a problem for internalist accounts of cognition as it is for extended accounts. There is, therefore, no *special* problem faced by extended accounts in accounting for the ownership of cognitive processes. Therefore, the presence of condition (4) in the criterion of cognition would count against extended accounts no more than it does against internalist models.

Traditionally, cognitive processes are thought of as spatially contained within the boundaries of a cognizing subject. Extended cognitive processes are not thus contained. Therefore, one might suppose that the traditional conception is at a distinct advantage over the extended alternative with respect to explaining ownership of such processes: we explain their ownership by a subject in terms of their spatial containment within that subject. A cognitive process *P* belongs to subject *S* just in case *P* occurs inside *S*. However, this, I shall argue, will not work. Indeed, I doubt that spatial containment is plausible criterion of ownership for *any* of the primary bodily processes we undergo; *a fortiori* this is true of cognitive processes

To see this, consider, as an example of a non-cognitive biological process, *digestion*. It may seem obvious that what makes a digestive process mine, and not anyone else's, is the fact that it occurs inside of me and not anyone else. This claim, however, should be resisted: spatial containment is only a fallible guide to the ownership of digestive processes. Imagine a case whereby one's digestive processes become *externalized*. Suppose, for example, one cannot produce enough of the relevant enzymes in one's digestive tract. The solution, drastic and implausible, but nonetheless a solution, is to reroute one's tract into an external device where the relevant enzymes are added, before routing the tract back into one's body where it finishes its work in the usual way. The most natural way of understanding this scenario is, I think, as a case where *my* digestive processes pass outside my body and receive the required external aid. The processes do not stop being mine just because they are, for a time, located outside my body.

Underlying this intuition is (1) the idea that digestive processes are defined by way of their proper function, and (2) that what makes a digestive process mine is that it fulfils this proper function with respect to *me*. Thus, the proper function of digestive processes is to break down food and release it into the body in the form of energy. And a digestive process is *mine* if it breaks down food *I* have ingested and releases energy into *my* body.

If this is correct, then the specific character of the external device is largely irrelevant—as long as it permits this proper function to be realized. Suppose, for example, that the external device were the body of someone else. That is, suppose my digestive tract were temporarily rerouted through the tract of someone else. We will suppose that the food contents of each tract are kept separate, but that the coupling allows the other person's digestive enzymes to pass over into my tract, thus aiding in the digestion of food that I ingested. Afterwards, my tract passes back into my body where it culminates in the usual manner. This would appear to be a case where *my* digestive processes are spatially located inside someone else's body, and indeed make use of someone else's digestive enzymes. And, once again, what underwrites this intuition is the idea that a digestive process is mine if the proper function of digestion is being fulfilled with respect to *me*: it is *my* food that is being broken down, and energy is being released into *my* body. The connection between ownership and location of a digestive process is merely contingent.

Ownership of digestive processes seems to be determined not by spatial containment but by a kind of *integration*. For a digestive process to be mine, it is necessary and sufficient for it to be integrated into my other biological processes in the right way. For example, it is integrated into my *ingestive* processes to the extent that it consists in the breaking down of food that I have taken in. And it is integrated into my other *respiratory* processes to the extent that it releases energy that enables those processes to continue. The criterion of appropriate integration is determined by proper function: a digestive process is appropriately integrated into my other biological processes when it is fulfilling its proper function with respect to those processes.

This, I think, provides the right model for understanding ownership of cognitive processes. Ownership is to be understood in terms of the appropriate sort of integration into the life—and in particular, the psychological life—of a subject. However, in the case of cognitive processes, specification of the appropriate sort of integration will be complicated by the possibility of a distinction that has no real echo in the case of biological processes such as digestion: the distinction between *personal* and *subpersonal* cognitive processes. Very roughly, this is the distinction between processes occurring between processes that are conscious, or under the conscious control of the subject, and those that are not. This distinction is reflected in condition (2) of the criterion of cognition. My suspicion—

although this is not something I can defend here, nor is it something upon which the arguments developed here depend—is that ownership of sub-personal cognitive processes will prove to be derivative upon ownership of personal-level cognitive processes: for cognitive processes, integration is ultimately integration into the conscious life of a subject.

However, whether or not this turns out to be the case, the important point is that there is no reason for thinking that explaining the relevant notion of integration will be any more problematic for *ExM* than it will be for traditional internalist accounts. That is, there is no reason for supposing that a subject's use of external resources—its manipulation, transformation and exploitation of external information-bearing struc-tures— will be any more difficult to integrate into that subject's overall psychological economy than will be cognitive processes in the traditional internal sense. The only reason for supposing that there will be an addi-tional problem for *ExM* is a residual commitment to the containment criterion of ownership, and that criterion is, I think, untenable.

CONCLUSION

I have argued that all of the principal objections to *ExM* reduce, in one way or another, to the mark of the cognitive objection. Underlying this objection is the worry that the arguments for extended cognition only establish the claim of embedded cognition. However, far from falling foul of any plausible criterion of the cognitive, I have argued that *ExM* is com-patible with a criterion of the cognitive that emerges in a fairly straightfor-ward way from analysis of standard internalist cognitive-scientific practice. Indeed, not only is *ExM* compatible with such a criterion, this cri-terion actually seems to be implicit in at least one well-known development of *ExM*. There is every reason to suppose that *ExM* satisfies conditions (1)–(3) of the criterion of the cognitive proposed here. And there is no rea-son for supposing that it will have any more difficulty satisfying condition (4) than will internalist accounts of cognitive processes.

REFERENCES

Adams, F. & Aizawa, K. (2001). The bounds of cognition. *Philosophical Psychology*
    14: 43–64.

Adams, F. & Aizawa, K. (in press). Why the mind is still in the head. In R. Menary (ed.) *The extended mind*. Cambridge, MA: MIT Press.

Clark, A. & Chalmers, D. (1998). The extended mind. *Analysis* 58: 7–19.

Dennett, D. C. (1987). *The intentional stance*. Cambridge, MA: MIT Press.

Donald, M. (1991). *Origins of the modern mind*. Cambridge, MA: Harvard University Press.

Dretske, F. (1981). *Knowledge and the flow of information*. Cambridge, MA: MIT Press.

Heidegger, M. (1962 [1927]). *Being and time*, trans. J. Macquarie and E. Robinson. Oxford: Blackwell.

Hurley, S. (1998). *Consciousness in action*. Cambridge, MA: Harvard University Press.

Lloyd, D. (1989). *Simple minds*. Cambridge, MA: MIT Press.

Marr, D. (1979). *Vision*. New York: W. H. Freeman.

Menary, R. (2006). Attacking the bounds of cognition. *Philosophical Psychology* 19(3): 329–344.

Menary, R. (2007). *Cognitive integration: attacking the bounds of cognition*. Basingstoke: Palgrave.

Menary, R. (in press). *The extended mind*. Cambridge, MA: MIT Press.

Millikan, R. (1984). *Language, thought and other biological categories*. Cambridge, MA: MIT Press.

Millikan, R. (1993). *White queen psychology, and other essays for Alice*. Cambridge, MA: MIT Press.

Noë, A. (2004). *Action in perception*. Cambridge, MA: MIT Press.

O'Regan, K. & Noë, A. (2001). A sensorimotor account of vision and visual consciousness. *Behavioral and Brain Sciences* 23: 939–973.

Rowlands, M. (1999). *The body in mind: understanding cognitive processes*. Cambridge: Cambridge University Press.

Rowlands, M. (2002). Two dogmas of consciousness. In: A. Noë (ed.) *Is the visual world a grand illusion?* Special edition of *Journal of Consciousness Studies* 9(5–6): 158–180.

Rowlands, M. (2003). *Externalism*. Stocksfield: Acumen.

Rowlands, M. (2006). *Body language: representation in action*. Cambridge, MA: MIT Press.

Rupert, R. (2004). Challenges to the hypothesis of extended cognition. *Journal of Philosophy* 101: 389–428.

Sutton, J. (in press). Exograms and interdisciplinarity: history, the extended mind, and the civilizing process. In: R. Menary (ed.) *The extended mind*. Cambridge, MA: MIT Press.

Wilson, R. (2004). *Boundaries of the mind*. Cambridge: Cambridge University Press.

PART V

**TESTING THE PAST:
ARCHAEOLOGY AND THE
SOCIAL BRAIN IN PAST ACTION**

17

Firing Up the Social Brain

JOHN GOWLETT

THE MASTERY OF FIRE is one of the great human achievements. In modern life, technology and consciousness of health and safety build naked fire out of our lives, but even then, 'living flames' and candles hint at its symbolic significance. In this chapter I address the wider importance of fire, arguing that it is part of a fundamental nexus of human evolution, deeply tied into our biology as well as our economy and technology, and indeed a main motor of the social brain.

We know of several great developments which run side by side through the last 2 million years (Figure 17.1): the evolution of the large

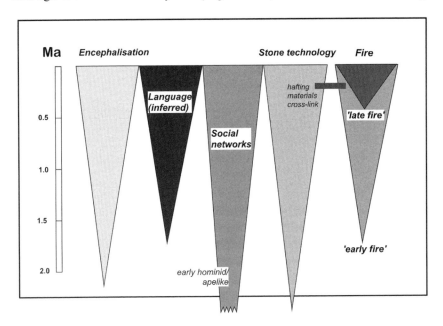

Figure 17.1. Major domains of evidence in the Pleistocene record, showing 'traditional' uncertainties in the fire record. The chapter argues that the weight of evidence points to accepting the early dates for fire as working hypothesis.

Proceedings of the British Academy **158**, 341–366. © The British Academy 2010.

human brain; the evolution of language; the evolution of complex social networks; the evolution of technology. Fire use is generally taken to be an 'add-on' to technology. Its presence is harder to document than that of stone tools, so the general assumption is that it appears later. Fire control is often thought to represent some cognitive advance. Debate then focuses on the point of arrival. Here I argue for a quite different approach: that fire is a natural resource which has played a large part in shaping humanity across several of the domains already mentioned. It is part of the nexus of human evolution: biological, cultural, economic, technical and symbolic.

FIRE AMONG THE MAJOR DOMAINS
OF HUMAN EVOLUTION

When we consider the several domains of Figure 17.1, a central question is 'How far do these pillars of evolution co-evolve?' The likelihood is that these great factors do affect one another, with looping feedback effects—but these are often difficult to trace in detail. However difficult it is for us to find cross-links between these domains, the issues matter: we need to know whether fire control appears at, say, 1.5 million years or 0.5 million years ago, because fire affects other interpretations.

This question must be addressed if we are to achieve a framework for investigating hominin use of fire. Events in some of the major domains are well-documented—especially changes in brain size (Aiello & Dunbar 1993; Dunbar 1998; Lee & Wolpoff 2003) and the development of stone technology (Gowlett 1992; Hallos 2005; Klein 1999; Semaw 2000), but we have very few cross-ties between them. Wood and stone technologies are linked by microwear studies, phytoliths and hafting (Dominguez-Rodrigo et al. 2001; Keeley & Toth 1981; Thieme 1999). Anatomy gives hints of language in brain structure, control of breathing and the tuning frequencies of ear canals (Holloway 1972; Martinez et al. 2004; Tobias 2005).

At the moment we have a good outline picture of the emergence and development of *Homo*, but doubt—perhaps in the range of half a million years or more—surrounds the first appearance of many key characters through the course of the Quaternary (the last 2.6 million years). That very fact demonstrates that we do not understand all the interrelationships of explanatory loops. Fire itself is one of the clearest examples. If we did not know whether fire use first appeared 1.5 million years ago, a million years ago or half a million years ago, we would not understand how much of a part fire played in changing diet, nor even its relationship with wood technology.

Many models of Pleistocene incremental change rely on positing cycles of positive feedback, whether social or social-technical (Alexander 1979; Gowlett 1984; Huxley 1955). These must always be set in motion by an earlier instability or 'kick', and a gradual development from that state must be favoured by selection at every stage. Such evolution happens in complex systems, but to examine it we may have to take single evidence categories as exemplars. To evaluate what might happen with wood, or fire, we can use the much better-known record of stone technology for assessing something of the nature of trends and feedback.

After hominins had made the initial discovery that sharp stone cuts, we might envisage a constant long-term selective pressure for improvement, but not necessarily a strong one. There are signs of a trend towards improvements promoting efficiency and lowering cost. As André Leroi-Gourhan (1993) demonstrated, these serve to achieve a greater length of sharp edge from a given amount of stone. Along the general trend, hafting of stone tools would be a major leap, a step change (Barham ch. 18 this volume). No doubt hafting would have been useful a million years earlier (its first signs appear about 400,000 years ago) but it required not just the idea, but also an efficient technical solution—and some of that came via a fire technology, as employed in preparing gypsum or pitch mastic (Friedman et al. 1995; Koller et al. 2001). These were complex tasks operable only in a shared social context.

Fire itself would be a key point in such transmission of ideas, as it has been in more recent pyrotechnology: a crossroads for new solutions, illustrating the potential for chance conjunctions of ideas occasionally to race ahead of immediate pressures. There are two points to extract here: the first, central, one is that where we can see past evidence for any new developments in detail through the Pleistocene, there is generally a first visible competence, followed by a slow intensification and eventual acceleration. We might postulate that model for fire-control. Second, in the social milieu of human evolution, feedback loops that bring about these intensifications need not operate in a single domain. They cross boundaries, so that we need to look for cross-ties to gain fuller understanding of how biological, social and technical factors interrelate.

I argue that, from the perspective of the social brain, we do know enough to fit fire into the picture, but that to do so requires a new approach less centred on a 'yes-no' evaluation of individual hearths, and more on a broad multidisciplinary view.

THE FUNDAMENTAL IMPORTANCE OF FIRE

Fire occurs widely in nature, but most animals do not use it a great deal. This very contrast to modern humans makes our pervasive fire control particularly important in any effort to achieve a comparative perspective. Unusually, we have little chance to learn from other primates, except in two important factors where they differ from us—their use of time, and their patterns of diet and eating.

Modern humans are notable for living long days and sleeping short nights. All humans sleep around eight hours per night—to the point that sleeping for more than this becomes a marker of morbidity (Burazeri et al. 2003). They are awake for 16 hours, in inverse proportion to the activity cycle of almost all other mammals. For example, the gorilla rises at dawn, forages, naps in the middle of the day, forages again, then goes to sleep at dusk (Schaller 1963) (Figure 17.2a and b).

Adrian Kortlandt has also commented on the way that chimps go to sleep as humans begin their evening activities (pers. comm.). The differences from human activity patterns are so systematic and predictable that undoubtedly they have a biological basis. Strong evidence for this comes from the human circadian rhythm. In the human circadian cycle, lowest activity occurs around 4.00 a.m., and peak alertness is in early evening when other animals are going to sleep. We thus achieve four hours or more of crucial evening activity which is denied to other primates. We achieve that with no more than minor phase shifts almost regardless of actual day-length, which varies so much with latitude and season (Lavie 2001; Yoneyama et al. 1999).

The consistency of this pattern strongly suggests that this is a biological shift with a genetic underpinning. Such genetic changes are more than probable: in thirty years of extensive research into the circadian rhythm itself, mutations in single genes have provided the major tool of investigation, often leading to changes of four hours or more in the cycle (Takahashi 2004). Many genes are involved in maintaining the circadian rhythm, but a mutation in one can have a major effect. In human evolution the effects *within* rather than *of* the circadian rhythm have clearly been crucial. How has the far longer day been obtained?

The most notable observation is that two key parameters—core body temperature (CBT) and cerebral blood flow (CBFV) run out of phase in humans, having moved apart by six hours—a 90 degree rotation (see

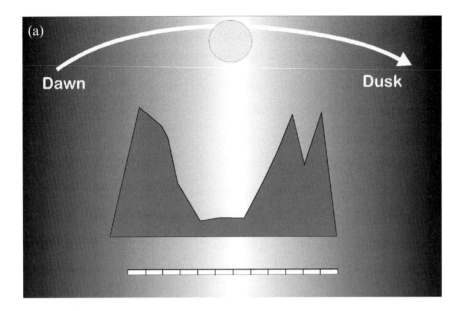

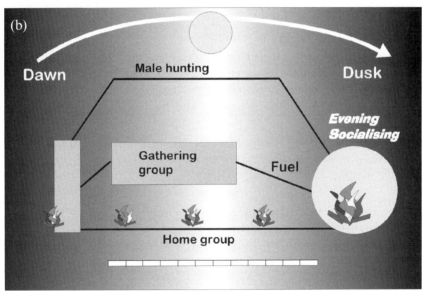

Figure 17.2(a). The gorilla day, following Schaller (1963). The day is limited by daylight, and consists largely of foraging periods separated by a midday nap. **(b).** The extended human day showing the typical complexity of foraging patterns and fire use among hunter-gatherers. (Barscales indicate approximate tropical daylight hours, 0600–1800.)

Conroy et al. 2005). If the two are rotated into synchrony, they show a very similar pattern, differing mainly in a 'kick' of CBFV which starts the day. This rapid rise may result from the abrupt change of physical activity in getting up, and correlates with a peak in the occurrence of strokes in modern populations (Stergiou et al. 2002).

The striking change in sleep patterns has many ramifications, both metabolic and social. It provides major benefits, but they are hard-earned. Longer waking hours may provide more effective defence for a group, as well as more scope for social interaction, but the brain must be fuelled at a waking rate for more hours of the day (leading to observable performance deficits which may be a detriment, although chiefly in a modern society). Infants cannot maintain this cycle and children need to sleep 10–12 hours a night until their teens, their sleep time moving towards that of adults in a predictable curve (Iglowstein et al. 2003). In other words, *the extended day that allows a longer, fuller social life also necessitates a more complex social life*, with a need to accommodate the different patterns of different age groups. The changes may thus be part of a single complex of developments, including greater generational length, extended lifespan and roles for grandparents, particularly as these might also have the effect of increasing local group size (cf. O'Connell et al. 1999).

There is little doubt that fire has played a central role in effecting these crucial changes. Fire is often seen as a means of extending the day, and the timing of peak activity would suggest more than this: that fire actually makes possible a crucial part of the day—around four hours of evening—and that for humans there has been a restructuring of the day, with different activities taking place at different times. Feedback loops come into play again as fire also helps to provide the higher-grade nutrition which allows the larger social brain (Aiello & Dunbar 1993; Dunbar 1998).

The focus of social brain studies was initially centred on group size (e.g. Dunbar 1998), but is increasingly being seen as about complexity (Dunbar ch. 8 this volume)—a theme argued before for culture (Gowlett 1979). Here then is a new opportunity for social brain studies—to investigate patterns of timing that are distinctive to humans, especially in the daily cycle, and to explore their evolutionary significance. Fire provides a good lead, because it is a fundamental part of the equation, interacting with other cultural threads and very clearly tied to changes which may leave archaeological evidence.

FIRE THE NATURAL RESOURCE

Fire is a widely available and sometimes frightening natural resource—
the term 'wildfire' conveys menace, contrasting with the comfort of
'hearthfire'. Like other resources it had variable affordance—in this, fire
is not really different from stone raw material sources. Our intuitive
Western impression is that fire was only sporadically available to early
hominins, and very hard to keep and apply: hence, fire control is often
seen as requiring a cognitive leap. However, if fire were relatively easily
available and offered simple immediate returns, the position would be different—and in some environments, in fact, fire would be available in just
this way.

By far the most common agent of natural fire regimes is lightning. As
lightning strikes seem sporadic, it has traditionally been thought that
early hominids would have great difficulty in harnessing their effects. But
lightning storms occur in predictable patterns, at least to 50 degrees
north, and in most areas there are several strikes per square kilometre per
year (Huffines & Orville 1999; Johnson 1992). These ground strikes create fires with predictable regularity in some circumstances, especially
when a first storm follows a long period of warm dry weather (Gisbourne
1926, 1931; Huffines & Orville 1999), although the match between lightning frequency and fires is by no means complete (Figure 17.3). Lightning
is most frequent in the tropics, but rarely causes fires in the rainforest
habitats of apes, while savannah zones have high frequencies of both
lightning and fires, especially in those first storms following a dry season
(Beringer et al. 2007; Sankaran et al. 2005; Scott 2000). Arid zones to the
north and south have fewer ground strikes, and less susceptible vegetation, while temperate forests tend to have spring-summer or spring and
fall fire regimes, depending on latitude (Lafon et al. 2005; McCarthy
1923). Most thunderstorms occur in high summer, but vegetation sometimes catches fire more easily in the earlier and later storms. Again, fire
weather is predictable and especially well-studied in parts of North
America (Gisbourne 1926, 1931; Huffines & Orville 1999; Johnson 1992).
Further north, probability drops rapidly because of the rarity or absence
of thunderstorms and of easily ignited vegetation. In glacial periods,
lightning strikes were probably even less common in the north, so that fire
was hardest to attain from nature in the areas where it was most needed.

A brief mention should be made of other sources of fire: vulcanism,
spontaneous combustion in matted vegetation and friction fires (Bond &
Keeley 2005). In general these are far less common than lightning strikes.

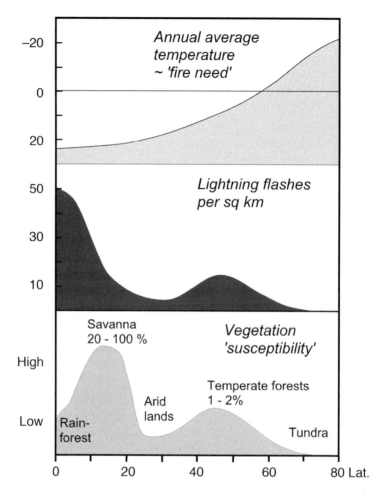

Figure 17.3. An approximate profile by latitude of major factors affecting fire generation and use. From 60 degrees north there is a great need for fire, but little chance of it being generated by natural means (compiled from a variety of sources).

Volcanoes such as Etna, however, would undoubtedly furnish fire continually for early humans living near them, potentially stimulating cultural knowledge and behaviour that could be transmitted further afield in other circumstances.

Natural fire does not just occur predictably: it also leads to predictable patterns of burning, and thus to predictable patterns of 'resource enhancement'. Fire signals its presence by smoke. It exposes roots, tubers, small animals and their burrows, birds' nests and eggs, sometimes ready-cooked, and leads afterwards to regeneration of young vegetation, which may be edible or attract game. There is a vast bibliography of hunter-gatherer fire use, perhaps highlighted best in Rhys Jones' classic paper on Australian 'firestick farming' (Jones 1969), but many examples are also given by Pyne (2001), Goudsblom (1992) and Perlès (1977).

HUMAN USES—THE MODERN COMPARATIVE VIEW

Fire is a universal in the modern human world, with several major benefits as outlined in Table 17.1. Hunters and gatherers offer a bridge between the archaeological evidence and past lives, because of the localized scale of their activity and their closeness to the natural world. As in every other aspect of their behaviour, there is great variety in fire use (as for example Barnard [1992] discusses among southern African hunters and gatherers and pastoralists).

An idealized outline of a hunter-gatherer day might be that individuals of a hunter-gatherer band wake in the morning; they revive fires; they begin to prepare for the day (Figure 17.2b). Then there tends to come a division, which is often tripartite, as some males depart to forage; a group of women and children also may leave to forage and collect firewood; and some other group members stay in camp, often maintaining a fire through the day. Members of the different groups tend to fuse again in late afternoon. If not already burning, fires will be lit before dusk, and social activities will continue around them perhaps into the night.

This simple scenario does not fully encompass the variety which we see. The Hadza may set a fire at a kill site far from their camp to render parts of the carcass on the spot, making immediate use of marrow and offal especially (O'Connell et al. 1988). Lewis Binford's classic studies of Nunamiut fires are partly based on those lit by small task groups while waiting for game (Binford 1983). Thus the setting and duration of individual fires may depend on many factors.

Table 17.1. The major benefits of fire

Protection	against large predators
Warmth	especially in high latitudes
Food preparation	especially cooking of meat and starch
Tool preparation	especially of stone and wood (but also mastic, and all later pyrotechnologies)
Social focus	group interactions, ritual, language

As noted, comparisons of other simple technologies now benefit from being able to include chimpanzee activity (Lycett et al. 2007; McGrew 1992, 1998; Whiten et al. 1999). In the case of fire it is harder to establish such an out-group, since chimpanzees do not use it. There is anecdotal evidence suggesting that chimpanzees in the wild may be habituated to fire occurrences (MacKinnon 1978), and it is well known that captive chimpanzees may become fascinated by fire although having difficulty in lighting it (Brink 1957).

Although there is no extensive comparative picture, fire is regularly exploited by certain animals, demonstrating that such use would be well within the cognitive capacities of early hominids. Animals use fire opportunistically, as when birds hover near a fire front ready to pounce on fleeing creatures: both in South America and Africa these 'fire followers' comprise several species, including hawks, swifts, storks, bee-eaters and corvids (Berthold et al. 2001). The main lesson these examples offer is that a variety of species makes a ready association between the occurrence of fire and resource-gaining opportunities.

MODELLING THE PAST

If fire is so important, why do we have so little preserved? As Catherine Perlès (1975) has remarked, fire differs from other artefacts in that the evidence tends to destroy itself immediately. But we can evaluate the record of fire in parallel with other essential materials—stone and wood. This comparison illustrates large differences in sampling density, as well as in conventional approaches to interpretation. The stone tool record is quite dense, distributed across three continents and 2.6 millions of years, and its presence or absence is not usually at issue, except in rare circumstances. In contrast, the record of wood, which was probably used by humans at least as often as stone, is exceptionally sparse as it decays so easily. Even so, wood is found preserved at key Middle Pleistocene sites such as Kalambo Falls in Zambia, Gesher Benot Ya'aqov in Israel and Schöningen in Germany (Alperson-Afil 2008; Clark 2001; Goren-Inbar et al. 2004; Thieme 1996, 1999). From these few sites we feel free to postulate very widespread past use of wood.

In contrast again, evidence for fire occurs somewhat more frequently, but its interpretation has been much more contentious. In the past, archaeologists have been cautious in assuming that such occurrences are more likely to represent wildfire than controlled fire. Nevertheless, there is

Box 17.1. The context of fire

```
Before 2.6 million years—no indication
First visible (stone) technology at 2.6 Ma
Brain size growth from around 2.5–2.0 Ma
Wide hominid distribution at 1.7 Ma
Visible evidence of fire on sites at 1.5 Ma
Fire broadly accepted, hearthfire at 0.7 Ma
Hearths widespread at 0.4 Ma
Fire used on wooden tools at 0.4 Ma
Hearths related to structures visible within ca. 0.2 Ma
```

a remarkable coincidence of occurrence: the sites where fire is found are, by and large, those where wood is also found, demonstrating the great force of sampling/preservational factors and highlighting biases in conceptual approach. That is, it appears more permissible to extrapolate from wood than fire, even though there is a very strong link in terms of their preservational contexts.

Although fire histories make many useful points (Goudsblom 1992; Perlès 1977; Pyne 2001), it is easier to sketch in the likely past role of fire than to arrive at a general model. Almost the only model specifically directed towards early hominids is that of Wrangham (e.g Wrangham 2007; Wrangham & Peterson 1996; Wrangham et al. 1999), which stresses the dietary needs imposed on early hominids by savannah environments as a force for rapid change. In place of the predictable fruit and herb sources of the rainforests, hominins would be compelled to rely far more on meat-eating and tubers (USO—underground storage organs), especially during dry seasons. There is no doubt that many starchy foods are almost inedible without cooking (Peters & O'Brien 1981). Ideally, the early dietary model and archaeological evidence would be evaluated separately to see whether they converge.

This is not the place to discuss archaeological methodologies, which are treated by several authors (e.g. Bellomo 1993, 1994; Gowlett in prep.; James 1989; Perlès 1977; Rolland 2004). The very best evidence consists of part-burnt artefacts, which demonstrate human presence and argue against a general conflagration. Yet such specific evidence will be so rare that it can restrict a general view. To provide some kind of initial framework it seems logical to offer and develop a three-stage model (Figure 17.4; cf. Gowlett in prep; and NB Barnard ch. 12 this volume for a tripartite approach to kinship).

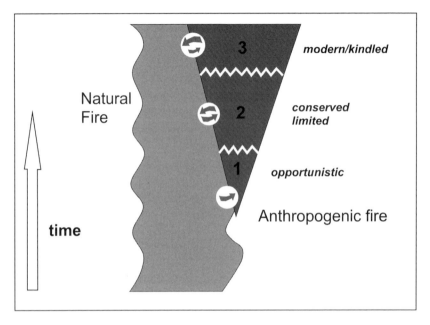

Figure 17.4. A general outline for the development of fire use, showing its emergence from and interchanges with natural (wild) fire.

(1) Opportunistic use—searching for fire events, coupled with exploita-
    tion of their immediate opportunities. Available to hominins living
    in savannahs and temperate forests.
(2) Concentrated use, in controlled fires. Necessitates social coopera-
    tion and considerable investment in fuel (division of labour).
(3) Full control with kindling of fire at will, and use in processes
    beyond immediate subsistence, such as complex tool-making, as
    well as conceptual use of fire as a social focus.

These stages are useful for analysis, but are also likely to be part of a
mosaic of continuous gradations.

TESTING THE EVIDENCE

Whatever its limitations, archaeology provides the key evidence from the
past, alongside which the evidence of anatomy and ecological modelling
must be evaluated.

Lower Pleistocene

We take in one sweep the period from earliest tool-making (2.6 million years ago) to about 1 million years ago. We now know that there was widespread occupation to 40 degrees north as much as 1.7 million years ago by hominins that were still relatively small-brained (600–700 cc), and small-bodied. We see them best at Dmanisi in Georgia (Gabunia et al. 2000, 2001) but there are early dates in the Nihewan basin of China (Zhu et al. 2004) and in the west at Atapuerca in Spain (Carbonell et al. 2008). Fire evidence is also widespread, considering how few sites are preserved. It occurs at Chesowanja in East Africa, Swartkrans in South Africa and Bogatyri north of the Black Sea (Bosinski 2006; Brain 2005; Brain & Sillen 1988; Gowlett 1999; Gowlett et al. 1981). The common feature is association with bone (charred at Swartkrans and Bogatyri). At Swartkrans many pieces of bone also demonstrate cutmarks made by stone tools, otherwise unknown from the early South African sites. There are no proven hearth concentrations, but at the east African sites there are limited baked patches at Koobi Fora, and a localized distribution of burnt clay at Chesowanja (Gowlett 1999; Gowlett et al. 1981; Harris & Isaac 1997).

This earliest evidence for fire can be seen in the context of two other major points. First, the highly selective transport and management of raw materials for stone tools shows a detailed knowledge of their properties, and a detailed knowledge of resource geography as early as 2.6 million years ago at Hadar (Semaw 2000). The transport across distances of 10–20 km indicates a high degree of knowledge, social collaboration and investment of effort for a return. In addition, this early record shows a repeated focus on large animal carcasses, often elephants, in both Africa and Asia (Surovell et al. 2005), an association which implies a preoccupation with meat, and successful competition with large carnivores.

The abilities demonstrated in these two task activities are very much those that are also necessary for simple fire use. As the early record is similar in these features wherever found, it appears that earliest culture was robust in its form, serving partly to 'equalize' in the face of a varying world. Fire, more strictly necessary in some areas than others, may have had a similarly equalizing force.

If we accept the evidence for fire in this early period, it can be seen as a facilitator in a triangle of *diet change—detailed environmental knowledge—social collaboration*, and becomes a prime candidate for fuelling the growth in brain size from about 500 to 1,000 cc between 2 and 1 million years ago.

Middle Pleistocene

The Middle Pleistocene, from about 800,000 years ago, provides much more definite evidence of hearths. Good examples are provided by Beeches Pit and Schöningen in northern Europe, both dating to ca. 400,000 years ago (Gowlett 2006; Gowlett et al. 2005; Preece et al. 2006; Thieme 1996, 1999, 2005). Each of these sites shows several hearth features, associated with corroborative artefact evidence. Beeches Pit in East Anglia provides the earliest evidence yet of an individual working by a fireside, perhaps as one of a group, but certainly in a social context. That person was making a tool, an Acheulean hand-axe. In the manufacture of this tool, two stone flakes fell forward into the fire and were burnt red. They provide a striking demonstration of highly localized fire. The hand-axe was discarded before completion because of a flaw in the flint. Nearby are several other bifaces, of varied form and size, belonging to the same phase of occupation and suggesting the practice of varied tasks, probably by more than one individual. The Beeches Pit hearths were large, burnt at high temperatures, and were set repeatedly over several days at least, perhaps several weeks. Their size, around a metre across by 10 to 20 cm deep, indicates fires which needed 50 kg of wood or more, and which must have been fed by a collaborative effort. Animal bones identified include horse, deer and rhinoceros (Gowlett et al. 2005; Preece et al. 2006).

At Schöningen, as at Beeches Pit, hearths seem to be on a strandline somewhat removed from the main occupation. The presence of a wooden stave charred at one end can be taken as artefactual proof of controlled human fire use (Thieme 1999).

The earlier site of Gesher Benot Ya'aqov in Israel is highly useful for extending this detailed picture further back in time, to around 700,000 years ago (Goren-Inbar et al. 2004). Again, the record seems to show several hearths—in this case smaller ones—and repeated occurrences of fire (Alperson-Afil 2008). The hearth evidence is not as securely linked with large burnt artefacts as at Beeches Pit and Schöningen, but the repeated episodes of burning at separate levels and the highly selective burning of organic materials such as wood and seeds (less than 5% of the entire organic remains are burnt), show clearly that these are not general conflagrations.

Gesher dates from approximately the time of the common ancestors of Neanderthals and modern humans—estimated to be in the approximate range 1.0 million to 700,000 years ago (Green et al. 2006; Krause et al. 2007; Krings et al. 1997). Adding together this early evidence with that of the northern sites such as Beeches Pit and the southern sites such as Kalambo Falls, where there are also charred seeds and charred wood (Clark 2001), it would not be surprising to find that the humans of the north and the humans of the south had similar fire records subsequently. This appears to be the case: as later hearths are common both in Neanderthal and modern human contexts, and as there is a 'deep root' to both, it seems most economical to postulate that the common ancestor did indeed have fire use.

There is a good deal of other Middle Pleistocene evidence, sometimes controversial, so that some authors emphasize fire as a new appearance (in Europe: de Lumley 2006; Rolland 2004), and sometimes its lack of specific hearth features as at Zhoukoudian in China (Binford & Ho 1985; Goldberg et al. 2001; Weiner et al. 1998). The larger frame of argument has now moved beyond the local detail. In total, the Middle Pleistocene record offers proof of certain points: that humans made use of fire in repeated events in one place; that they made large recurrent investments in fuel collection; and that for them fire now had both social and technical functions.

Upper Pleistocene

A hearth of the last interglacial at Florisbad in South Africa ushers in the Upper Pleistocene record (from about 125,000 years ago) (Henderson 2001). Hearths are now widespread geographically, occur in varied con-texts—including caves and open sites—and are found as repeated events through long sequences, for example at Kebara Cave in Israel (Bar-Yosef et al. 1992). In general pattern, they resemble earlier hearths, with the occasional addition of hearthstones, as in the Caucasus (Golovanova & Doronichev 2003). Thus we could say that by about 100,000 years ago, the main story is over. Everyone is using fire, with considerable skill and application—and we have the modern phenomenon of Phase 3 fire use. But there are still points to extract.

First, there remains a similarity in the evidence wherever found. Florisbad is similar to Wallertheim in Germany, both set at the centre of spreads of stone tools and associated with animal remains (Adler & Conard 2005; Henderson 2001).

Second, there is early evidence of an intensive industrial focus to fire—but it comes from the Neanderthal domain, at Königsaue in east-ern Germany (Koller et al. 2001). Here pitch has survived, enough to show that Neanderthals were able to prepare the material in quantity from birch bark at high temperature, although we have no direct knowledge of them using containers (cf. Gamble ch. 2 this volume). For modern humans and the Upper Palaeolithic we do not find anything comparably illuminating until the loess sites of Moravia, about 30,000 years ago, where baked ceramic figurines demonstrate both a technical capability and a symbolic sense (Otte 1981; Svoboda 1994).

Third, different kinds of hearth appear side by side or close to one another. Those of Abríc Romaní in north-east Spain resemble the hearths of Beeches Pit in size, but at nearby Roca del Bous there are far smaller examples (Martinez-Moreno et al. 2004; Vallverdú et al. 2005; Vaquero & Pastó 2001).

Although this record shows a great ease of use of fire, there is no direct evidence for kindling. Perhaps relevant is the new dating of pierced beads back to the last interglacial 125,000 years ago (Vanhaeren et al. 2006). They show the existence of threads and cordage, whether of plant materials or sinew, technology that would make possible the bow and the firedrill. Tanged stone points of the Aterian in North Africa—mainly in the time-range ca. 130,000–60,000 BP—indicate a new refinement in projectile points and the possibility that the bow was in use. Kindling can, however, be achieved with other friction apparatus.

The later Upper Palaeolithic documents the full range of modern fire behaviour, sometimes in brilliant detail as at Verberie and Pincevent in northern France, where the social context of reindeer processing by hearths is vividly apparent (Audouze & Enloe 1997; Julien et al. 1987; Leroi-Gourhan & Brézillon 1972).

BUILDING A SOCIAL BRAIN

If we have an agreed basic picture—that fire use developed somewhere during the Pleistocene—does it matter when? It does, because of the deep interrelationships between biological, social and cultural factors already noted. A late development of fire technologies would mean that colonization, encephalization, diet change, use of combustible materials, had all run for more than a million years before fire was routinely used. That interpretation now seems implausible if to achieve it we have to write off fire evidence from a number of early sites, even though hominids were demonstrating the necessary cultural capacities in other respects, and even though these various chains of activity are very much interlinked at later dates.

This chapter explicates the case that fire has a vital role in allowing and fuelling the longer day, also generating genetic changes which allow humans to exploit this 'time colonization' through modified circadian rhythms. In this way fire both constructs and structures social space to a remarkable degree. It also features in altering equations about group sizes by providing a longer day with more scope for interactions, and stretching adult wakefulness to the point that young children, in particular, must operate on a different (protected) time regime.

At the moment our theoretical framework and factual data are insufficient to provide truly hard answers about 'first fire'. It is also the case that 'conventional' archaeological approaches are limited to testing very sporadic evidence on very specific terms, struggling to build up a broader picture. It is exciting then that we can now begin to put together a composite picture based on several lines of evidence.

First, there is a strong 'clade-based' argument that the common ancestor of Neanderthals and modern humans had fire control, as both descendant species did so and the Gesher finds sit close to the time of their common ancestry. These findings alone prise fire use well away from any connection with revolutions of *Homo sapiens*. Second, there is a remarkable complex of changes which occur at about 2.3–1.7 million years ago, the time of the emergence of the genus *Homo*. There is a 50 per cent increase in encephalization, changes in brain organization, marked reduction in tooth size, the adoption of stone technology, of larger ranges, dispersal across Eurasia and a marked preoccupation with meateating (Aiello & Wheeler 1995; Dominguez-Rodrigo & Pickering 2003; Stiner 2002), seen at its peak in the Neanderthals (Bocherens et al. 1999).

In this light, assuming that changes in biological day length must be fire-driven, it becomes a useful hypothesis that they are so fundamental that they may go back to the first major leap in encephalization 2.3–1.7 million years ago, especially as this period is now linked with dispersal to northern latitudes. In turn, increased day length and altered sleeping patterns link to all the extensive social changes that have already been discussed. Then, in a comparative sense, the steady development of other technologies—wood, bone and stone—coupled with the existing evidence of early fire, would suggest a long slow development, starting more than 1.5 million years ago. In short, the indirect aspects would tally with the more direct information which we have about encephalization, human dispersal and the circadian rhythms of modern humans, as well as with the evidence of diet and nutrition (Aiello & Wheeler 1995; Wrangham 2007).

It might be enough here to show that fire simply *fuelled* the great enlargement and reorganization of the brain, but clearly it had other functions. Our key question is, what roles did fire play in *stimulating* a social brain and its higher faculties? It is clear that these roles are multiple. Repeated fires mark 'home'. They offer centres for tasks. Above all, they give structure to human interactions. Controlled fire liberates energy, but in return for considerable work. Fire, there in front of you, has a measurable value. Almost immediately it demands a division of labour, and agreed social arrangements.

At a technical level (the technology being socially mediated) fire performs two notable functions. First, it transforms materials, so that even early hominins might see its generalizing effect: meat becomes cooked, tubers become roasted, resin can change to pitch, wood to charcoal. Humans would be given insights by these processes. Fire is, after all, at the core of most new technologies which have arisen through the last few thousand years (Wertime & Wertime 1982), and the same seems likely at earlier dates. As mentioned, at Beeches Pit several discarded hand-axes lie around the hearth where the stone knapper was making a new specimen. As they were not made at the site, very probably they were used there for other functions, of butchery or wood working. Here then is the social and imaginative force of the fire. It brings together processes: different operational chains cross at this point. The effective hafting of wood to stone by pitch or gypsum was made possible only through use of a fire-rendered material, and its properties had to be discovered before there could be a solution. Just as with ores in later times, first accidental burnings probably paved the way—then fire weaves the nexus of ideas that can come together.

This materials argument can be transferred to the more purely ideational, in myth and religion. I have hinted at the links of fire with imagination and symbolism. On the latter aspect, the messages are mixed. There were the fire festivals of Europe (Frazer 1922), or Lévi Strauss's emphasis on the raw and the cooked (Leach 1970), but some well-known anthropology books also fail to mention fire in this light at all (Kroeber 1948 gives one practical example; there is no mention in the index of Lee & Daly 1999). Yet fire can be linked with language (Ronen 1998): conversation takes place around the fire, paralleling the material processes, perhaps carrying on through the evening as the concentration for tool-making tasks fades. Then it can pass to other topics with a more social focus.

A last key development may be the elaboration of sharing and division, which we see in the plethora of small hearths often found in more recent settlements, and traceable at Pincevent around 12,000 years ago (Leroi-Gourhan & Brézillon 1972). The single large fire made to roast a larger animal is too big to allow conversation across and around it; it requires much fuel, and breaks routine. It cannot be fuelled every day without great effort, as available wood around camp becomes rapidly used up. Smaller hearths reflect smaller family groups within a band, and probably shared spoils and real conversation groups. Much more work is necessary to see whether there is a general shift from large earlier hearths to later smaller fires through the Middle Pleistocene, but that is a possibility.

CONCLUSIONS

This chapter argues centrally that fire use was not an 'add on', but a vital force or motor in human evolution. There are three problems which have hindered a fuller picture from emerging, including the complexity of fire, both natural and artificial; the disappearing act of fire and the difficulty of its identification in the archaeological record; and the straitjacket of a somewhat simplistic presence/absence debate.

Fire may have been used in many ways on different scales (Figure 17.5), so restricting the question of control to preserved *hearths* provides only a limited grasp of the issues. Any occurrence of fire on an archaeological site proves its availability as a resource, but the positive side of that observation has been little noted. In summary:

(1) Fire was a widely present resource.
(2) Simple use did not require a cognitive leap over other technology.
(3) Use and preservation of other technologies give clues about the likely nature of fire use, especially as fire becomes tied to them later on.
(4) There is a huge dietary benefit to fire use.
(5) There is a huge technical benefit to fire, proven by later technologies, with an emphasis on heat control and process.

Above all, there is a vital social and ideational side to fire: not only did it do much to fuel the social brain, it served as a focus for bringing together insights and ideas, eventually in a strong context of language. Through the Pleistocene, probably from beginning to end, it has played a major part in linking the social and technical, firing the brain and also its imagination.

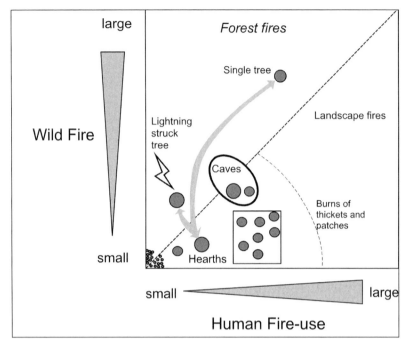

Figure 17.5. The scale complexities of fire evidence, natural and humanly controlled. These create ambiguities, but direct association of part-burnt artefacts with fires gives a very clear indication of human involvement with controlled fire. The variety of possible fire uses militates against judgements that take a simple 'yes/no?' view of fire control.

Note. I am grateful for support from the British Academy for the excavations at Beeches Pit, and also within the 'Lucy to Language' project; also to the Arts and Humanities Research Council and Forest Enterprise for additional support in the Beeches Pit project, and to my colleagues at these sites: Richard Preece, David Bridgland, Simon Lewis and Simon Parfitt, and at Chesowanja, especially J. W. K. Harris.

REFERENCES

Adler, D. S. & Conard, N. J. (2005). Tracking hominins during the last interglacial complex in the Rhineland. In: C. S. Gamble & M. Porr (eds) *The hominid individual in context: archaeological investigations of Lower and Middle Palaeolithic landscapes, locales and artefacts*, pp. 133–153. London: Routledge.

Aiello, L. C. & Dunbar, R. I. M. (1993). Neocortex size, group size, and the evolution of language. *Current Anthropology* 34(2): 184–193.

Aiello, L. C. & Wheeler, P. (1995). The expensive tissue hypothesis: the brain and the digestive system in human and primate evolution. *Current Anthropology* 36: 199–221.

Alexander, R. D. (1979). *Darwinism and human affairs*. London: Pitman.

Alperson-Afil, N. (2008). Continual fire-making by Hominins at Gesher Benot Ya'aqov, Israel. *Quaternary Science Reviews* 27: 1733–1739

Audouze, F. & Enloe, J. G. (1997). High resolution archaeology at Verberie: limits and interpretations. *World Archaeology* 29(2): 195–207.

Barnard, A. (1992). *Hunters and herders of southern Africa: a comparative ethnography of the Khoisan peoples*. Cambridge: Cambridge University Press.

Bar-Yosef, O., Vandermeersch, B., Arensberg, B., Belfer-Cohen, A., Goldberg, P., Laville, H. et al. (1992). The excavations in Kebara Cave, Mount Carmel. *Current Anthropology* 33: 497–550.

Bellomo, R. V. (1993). A methodological approach for identifying archaeological evidence of fire resulting from human activities. *Journal of Archaeological Science* 20: 525–555.

Bellomo, R. V. (1994). Methods of determining early hominid behavioural activities associated with the controlled use of fire at FxJj20 Main, Koobi Fora, Kenya. *Journal of Human Evolution* 27: 173–195.

Beringer, J., Hutley, L. B., Tapper, N. J. & Cernusak, L. A. (2007). Savanna fires and their impact on net ecosystem productivity in North Australia. *Global Change Biology* 13: 990–1004.

Berthold, P., Bauer, H. G. & Westhead, V. (2001). *Bird migration: a general survey*. Oxford: Oxford University Press.

Binford, L. R. (1983). *In pursuit of the past*. London: Academic Press.

Binford, L. R. & Ho, C. K. (1985). Taphonomy at a distance: Zhoukoudian, the cave home of Beijing man? *Current Anthropology* 26: 413–442.

Bocherens, H., Billiou, D., Mariotti, A., Patou-Mathis, M., Otte, M., Bonjean, D. et al. (1999). Palaeoenvironmental and palaeodietary implications of isotopic biogeochemistry of last interglacial Neanderthal and mammal bones in Scladina Cave (Belgium). *Journal of Archaeological Science* 26: 599–607.

Bond, W. J. & Keeley, J. E. (2005). Fire as global 'herbivore': the ecology and evolution of flammable ecosystems. *Trends in Ecology and Evolution* 20: 387–394.

Bosinski, G. (2006). Les premiers peuplements de l'Europe centrale et de l'Est. In: H. de Lumley (ed.) *Climats, cultures et sociétés aux temps préhistoriques, de l'apparition des Hominidés jusqu'au Néolithique*. *Comtes Rendus Palevol* 5(1–2): 311–317.

Brain, C. K. (2005). Essential attributes of any technologically competent animal. In: F. d'Errico & L. Backwell (eds) *From tools to symbols: from early hominids to modern humans*, pp. 38–51. Johannesburg: Witwatersrand University Press.

Brain, C. K. & Sillen, A. (1988). Evidence from the Swartkrans cave for the earliest use of fire. *Nature* 336: 464–466.

Brink, A. S. (1957) The spontaneous fire-controlling reactions of two chimpanzee smoking addicts. *South African Journal of Science* 53: 241–247.

Burazeri, G., Gofin, J. & Kark, J. D. (2003). Over 8 hours of sleep—marker of increased mortality in Mediterranean population: follow-up population study. *Croatian Medical Journal* 44: 193–198.

Carbonell, E., Bermúdez de Castro, J. M., Parés, J. M., Pérez-González, A., Cuence-Bescos, G., Ollé, A. et al. (2008). The first hominin of Europe. *Nature* 452: 465–470.

Clark, J. D. (ed.) (2001). *Kalambo Falls*, vol. 3. Cambridge: Cambridge University Press.

Conroy, D. A., Spielman, A. J. & Scott, R. Q. (2005). Daily rhythm of cerebral blood flow velocity. *Journal of Circadian Rhythms* 3(1): 3.

Domínguez-Rodrigo, M. & Pickering, T. R. (2003). Early hominid hunting and scavenging: a zooarcheological review. *Evolutionary Anthropology* 12: 275–282.

Domínguez-Rodrigo, M., Serrallonga, J., Alcalá, L. & Luque, L. (2001). Woodworking activities by early humans: a plant residue analysis on Acheulian stone tools from Peninj (Tanzania). *Journal of Human Evolution* 40: 289–299.

Dunbar R. I. M. (1998). The social brain hypothesis. *Evolutionary Anthropology* 6: 178–190.

Frazer, J. G. (1922). *The golden bough*. London: Macmillan.

Friedman, E., Goren-Inbar, N., Rosenfeld, A., Marder, O. & Burian, F. (1995). Hafting during Mousterian times: further indication. *Journal of the Israel Prehistoric Society* 26: 8–31.

Gabunia, L., Vekua, A. & Lordkipanidze, D. (2000). The environmental context of early human occupation in Georgia (Transcaucasia). *Journal of Human Evolution* 34: 785–802.

Gabunia, L., Antón, S. C., Lordkipanidze, D., Vekua, A. Justus, D. et al. (2001). Dmanisi and dispersal. *Evolutionary Anthropology* 10: 158–170.

Gisbourne, H. T. (1926). Lightning and forest fires in the northern Rocky Mountain region. *Monthly Weather Review* 54(7): 281–286.

Gisbourne, H. T. (1931). A five-year record of lightning storms and forest fires. *Monthly Weather Review* 59(4): 139–149.

Goldberg, P., Weiner, S., Bar-Yosef, O., Xu, Q. & Liu, J. (2001). Site formation processes at Zhoukoudian, China. *Journal of Human Evolution* 41: 483–530.

Golovanova, L. V. & Doronichev, V. B. (2003). The Middle Palaeolithic of the Caucasus. *Journal of World Prehistory* 17: 71–140

Goren-Inbar, N., Alperson, N., Kislev, M. E., Simchoni, O., Melamed,Y., Ben-Nun, A. et al. (2004). Evidence of hominin control of fire at Gesher Benot Ya'aqov, Israel. *Science* 304: 725–727.

Goudsblom, J. (1992). *Fire and civilization*. London: Penguin.

Gowlett, J. A. J. (1979). Complexities of cultural evidence in the Lower and Middle Pleistocene: news and views. *Nature* 278: 14–17.

Gowlett, J. A. J. (1984). Mental abilities of early man: a look at some hard evidence. In: R. A. Foley (ed.) *Hominid evolution and community ecology*, pp. 167–192. London: Academic Press.

Gowlett, J. A. J. (1992). Tools—the Palaeolithic record. In: R. Martin, D. Pilbeam & S. Jones (eds) *The Cambridge encyclopaedia of the human evolution*, pp. 350–360. Cambridge: Cambridge University Press.

Gowlett, J. A. J. (1999). Lower and Middle Pleistocene archaeology of the Baringo Basin. In: P. Andrews & P. Banham (eds) *Late Cenozoic environments and hominid evolution: a tribute to Bill Bishop*, pp. 123–141. London: Geological Society.

Gowlett, J. A. J. (2006). The early settlement of northern Europe: fire history in the context of climate change and the social brain. In: H. de Lumley (ed.) *Climats, cultures et sociétés aux temps préhistoriques, de l'apparition des Hominidés jusqu'au Néolithique. Comtes Rendus Palevol* 5(1–2): 299–310.

Gowlett, J. A. J. (in prep). Focus of the hearth.

Gowlett, J. A. J., Harris, J. W. K., Walton, D. & Wood, B. A. (1981). Early archaeo-logical sites, hominid remains and traces of fire from Chesowanja, Kenya. *Nature* 294: 125–129.

Gowlett, J. A. J., Hallos, J., Hounsell, S., Brant, V. & Debenham, N. C. (2005). Beeches Pit—archaeology, assemblage dynamics and early fire history of a Middle Pleistocene site in East Anglia, UK. *Eurasian Prehistory* 3: 3–38.

Green, R. E., Krause, J., Ptak, S. E., Briggs, A. W., Ronan, M. T., Simons, J. F. et al. (2006). Analysis of one million base pairs of Neanderthal DNA. *Nature* 444: 330–336.

Hallos, J. (2005). '15 minutes of fame': exploring the temporal dimension of Middle Pleistocene lithic technology. *Journal of Human Evolution* 49(2): 155–179.

Harris, J. W. K. & Isaac, G. L. (1997). Sites in the Upper KBS, Okote, and Chari mem-bers: reports. In: G. L. Isaac & B. Isaac (eds) *Koobi Fora research project*, vol. 5: *Plio-Pleistocene archaeology*, pp. 115–223. Oxford: Clarendon Press.

Henderson, Z. (2001). The integrity of the Middle Stone Age horizon at Florisbad, South Africa. *Navorsinge van die nasionale Museum Bloemfontein* 17(2): 26–52.

Holloway, R. L. (1972). Australopithecine endocasts, brain evolution in the Hominoidea, and a model of human evolution. In: R. Tuttle (ed.) *The functional and evolutionary biology of primates*, pp. 185–203. Chicago: Aldine.

Huffines, G. R. & Orville, R. (1999). Lightning ground flash density and thunder-storm duration in the continental U.S. *Journal of Applied Meteorology* 38: 1013–1019.

Huxley, J. (1955). Evolution, cultural and biological. In: *Yearbook of Anthropology* 2–25.

Iglowstein, I., Jenni, O. G., Molinari, L. & Largo, R. H. (2003). Sleep duration from infancy to adolescence: reference values and generational trends. *Pediatrics* 111: 302–307.

James, S. R. (1989). Hominid use of fire in the Lower and Middle Pleistocene: a review of the evidence. *Current Anthropology* 30(1): 1–26.

Johnson, E. A. (1992). *Fire and vegetation dynamics: studies from the North American boreal forest*. Cambridge: Cambridge University Press.

Jones, R. (1969). Firestick farming. *Australian Natural History* 16: 224–228.

Julien, M., Karlin, C. & Bodu, P. (1987). Pincevent: ou en est le modèle théorique aujourd'hui? *Bulletin de la Société Préhistorique Française* 84: 335–342.

Keeley, L. H. & Toth, N. (1981). Microwear polishes on early stone tools from Koobi Fora, Kenya. *Nature* 293: 464–465.

Klein, R. G. (1999). *The human career: human biological and cultural origins*, 2nd edn. Chicago: University of Chicago Press.

Koller, J., Baumer, U. & Mania, D. (2001). High-tech in the Middle Palaeolithic: Neandertal-manufactured pitch identified. *European Journal of Archaeology* 4: 385–397.

Krause, J., Lalueza-Fox, C., Orlando, L., Enard, W., Green, R. E., Burbano, H. A. et al. (2007). The derived FOXP2 variant of modern humans was shared with Neandertals. *Current Biology* 17: 1–5.

Krings, M., Stone, A., Schmitz, R. W., Krainitzki, H., Stoneking, M. & Pääbo, S. (1997). Neandertal DNA sequences and the origin of modern humans. *Cell* 90: 19–30.

Kroeber, A. L. (1948). *Anthropology*. London: Harrap.

Lafon, C. W., Hoss, J. A. & Grissino-Mayer, H. D. (2005). The contemporary fire regime of the central Appalachian mountains and its relation to climate. *Physical Geography* 26: 126–146.

Lavie, P. (2001). Sleep-wake as a biological rhythm. *Annual Review of Psychology* 52: 277–303.

Leach, E. (1970). *Lévi-Strauss*. London: Fontana/Collins.

Lee, R. B. & Daly, R. (1999). *The Cambridge encyclopaedia of hunters and gatherers.* Cambridge: Cambridge University Press.

Lee, S.-H. & Wolpoff, M. H. (2003). The pattern of evolution in Pleistocene human brain size. *Paleobiology* 29: 186–196.

Leroi-Gourhan, A. (1993). *Gesture and speech*, trans. A. B. Berger. Cambridge, MA: MIT Press.

Leroi-Gourhan, A. & Brézillon, M. (1972). *Fouilles de Pincevent: essai d'analyse ethnographique d'un habitat Magdalénien (la section 36)*. VII Supplement to *Gallia Préhistoire*. Paris: Editions CNRS.

de Lumley, H. (2006). Il y a 400,000 ans: la domestication du feu, un formidable moteur d'hominisation. In: H. de Lumley (ed.) *Climats, cultures et sociétés aux temps préhistoriques, de l'apparition des Hominidés jusqu'au Néolithique. Comptes Rendus Palevol* 5(1–2): 149–154.

Lycett, S. J., Collard, M. & McGrew, W. C. (2007). Phylogenetic analyses of behaviour support existence of culture among wild chimpanzees. *Proceedings of the National Academy of Science USA* 104: 17588–17592.

McCarthy, E. F. (1923). Forest fire weather in the southern Appalachians. *Monthly Weather Review* 51(4): 182–185.

McGrew, W. C. (1992). *Chimpanzee material culture: implications for human evolution.* Cambridge: Cambridge University Press.

McGrew W. C. (1998). Culture in nonhuman primates? *Annual Review of Anthropology* 27: 301–328.

MacKinnon, J. (1978). *The ape within us*. London: Collins.

Martínez, M., Rosa, M., Arsuaga, J.-L., Jarabo, T., Quam, R., Lorenzo, C. et al. (2004). Auditory capacities in Middle Pleistocene humans from the Sierra de Atapuerca in Spain, *Proceedings of the National Academy of Science USA* 101: 9976–9981.

Martínez-Moreno, J., Mora, R. & Torre, I. de la (2004). Methodological approach for understanding Middle Palaeolithic settlement dynamics at La Roca dels Bous (Noguera, Catalunya, north-east Spain). In: N. J. Conard (ed.) *Settlement dynamics of the Middle Paleolithic and Middle Stone Age*, vol. 2, pp. 393–413. Tübingen: Kerns Verlag.

O'Connell, J. F., Hawkes, K. & Blurton-Jones, N. B. (1988). Hadza hunting, butchering and bone transport and their archaeological implications. *Journal of Anthropological Research* 44: 113–161.

O'Connell, J. F., Hawkes, K. & Blurton-Jones, N. B. (1999). Grandmothering and the evolution of *Homo erectus. Journal of Human Evolution* 36: 481–485.

Otte, M. (1981). *Le Gravettien en Europe Centrale*. Brugge: Dissertationes Archaeologicae Gandenses, vol. 20.

Perlès, C. (1975). L'homme préhistorique et le feu. *La Recherche* 6: 829–839.

Perlès, C. (1977). *La préhistoire du feu.* Paris: Masson.

Peters, C. R. & O'Brien, E. M. (1981). The early hominid plant-food niche: insights from an analysis of plant exploitation by *Homo, Pan* and *Papio* in eastern and southern Africa. *Current Anthropology* 22: 127–140.

Preece, R. C., Gowlett, J. A. J., Parfitt, S. A., Bridgland, D. R. & Lewis, S. G. (2006) Humans in the Hoxnian: habitat, context and fire use at Beeches Pit, West Stow, Suffolk, UK. *Journal of Quaternary Science* 21: 485–496.

Pyne, S. J. (2001). *Fire: a brief history.* London: British Museum Press.

Rolland, N. (2004). Was the emergence of home bases and domestic fire a punctuated event? A review of the Middle Pleistocene record in Eurasia. *Asian Perspectives* 43(2): 248–280.

Ronen, A. (1998). Domestic fire as evidence for language. In: T. Akazawa (ed.) *Neanderthals and Moderns in Asia,* pp. 439–445. New York: Plenum Press.

Sankaran, M., Hanan, N. P., Scholes, R. J., Ratnam, J., Augustine, D. J., Cade, B. S. et al. (2005). Determinants of woody cover in African savanna. *Nature* 438: 846–849.

Schaller, G. B. (1963). *The mountain gorilla: ecology and behavior.* Chicago: University of Chicago Press.

Scott, A. C. (2000). The pre-Quaternary history of fire. *Palaeogeography, Palaeoclimatology, Palaeoecology* 164: 297–334.

Semaw, S. (2000). The world's oldest stone artifacts from Gona, Ethiopia: their implications for understanding stone technology and patterns of human evolution between 2.6–2.5 million years ago. *Journal of Archaeological Science* 27: 1197–1214.

Stergiou, G. S., Vernmos, K. N., Pliarchopoulou, K. M., Synetos, A. G., Roussias, L. G. & Mountokalakis, T. D. (2002). Parallel morning and evening surge in stroke onset, blood pressure, and physical activity. *Stroke* 33: 1480–1486.

Stiner, M. (2002). Carnivory, coevolution, and the geographic spread of the genus *Homo. Journal of Archaeological Research* 10: 1–63.

Surovell, T., Waguespack, N. & Brantingham, P. J. (2005). Global archaeological evidence for proboscidean overkill. *Proceedings of the National Academy of Sciences* 102: 6231–6236.

Svoboda, J. (1994). *Paleolit Moravy a Slezska [The Paleolithic of Moravia and Silesia].* Brno: The Dolní Věstonice studies, vol. 1.

Takahashi, J. S. (2004). Finding new clock components: past and future. *Journal of Biological Rhythms* 19: 339–347.

Thieme, H. (1996). Altpaläolithische Wurfspeere aus Schöningen, Niedersachsen— ein Vorbericht. *Archäologisches Korrespondenzblatt* 26(4): 377–393.

Thieme, H. (1999). Altpaläolithische Holzgeräte aus Schöningen, Lkr. Helmstadt. *Germania* 77: 451–487.

Thieme, H. (2005). The Lower Palaeolithic art of hunting: the case of Schöningen 13 II-4, Lower Saxony, Germany. In: C. S. Gamble & M. Porr (eds) *The hominid individual in context: archaeological investigations of Lower and Middle Palaeolithic landscapes, locales and artefacts,* pp. 115–132. London: Routledge.

Tobias, P. V. (2005). Tools and brains: which came first? In: F. d'Errico & L. Backwell (eds) *From tools to symbols: from early hominids to modern humans,* pp. 82–102. Johannesburg: Witwatersrand University Press.

Vanhaeren, M., d'Errico, F., Stringer, C., James, S. L., Todd, J. A. & Mienis, H. K. (2006). Middle Paleolithic shell beads in Israel and Algeria. *Science* 312: 1785–1788.

Vallverdú, J., Allué, E., Bischoff, J. L., Cáceresa, I., Carbonell, E., Cebrià, A. et al. (2005). Short human occupations in the Middle Palaeolithic level i of the Abric Romaní rock-shelter (Capellades, Barcelona, Spain). *Journal of Human Evolution* 48: 157–174

Vaquero, M. & Pastó, I. (2001). The definition of spatial units in Middle Palaeolithic sites: the hearth related assemblages. *Journal of Archaeological Science* 28: 1209–1220.

Weiner, S., Xu, Q., Goldberg, P., Lui, J. & Bar-Yosef O. (1998). Evidence for the use of fire at Zhoukoudian, China. *Science* 281: 251–253.

Wertime, T. A. & Wertime, S. F. (eds) (1982). *Early pyrotechnology: the evolution of the first fire-using industries*. Washington, DC: Smithsonian Institution Press.

Whiten, A., Goodall, J., McGrew, W. C., Nishida, T., Reynolds, V., Sugiyama, Y. et al. (1999). Cultures in chimpanzees. *Nature* 399: 682–685.

Wrangham, R. W. (2007). The cooking enigma. In: P. S. Ungar (ed.) *Evolution of the human diet: the known, the unknown and the unknowable*, pp. 308–323. Oxford: Oxford University Press.

Wrangham, R. & Peterson, D. (1996). *Demonic males: apes and the origins of human violence.* London: Bloomsbury.

Wrangham, R. W., Jones, J. H., Laden, G., Pilbeam, D. & Conklin-Brittain, N. (1999). The raw and the stolen: cooking and the ecology of human origins. *Current Anthropology* 40: 567–594.

Yoneyama, S., Hashimoto, S. & Honma, K. (1999). Seasonal changes of human circadian rhythms in Antarctica. *American Journal of Physiology* 277: 1091–1097.

Zhu, R. X., Potts, R., Xie, F., Hoffman, K. A., Deng, C. L., Shi, C. D. et al. (2004). New evidence of the earliest human presence at high northern latitudes in northeast Asia. *Nature* 431: 559–562.

18

A Technological Fix for 'Dunbar's Dilemma'?

LAWRENCE BARHAM

Only through imitation do we develop toward originality.

(John Steinbeck)

DEFINING DUNBAR'S DILEMMA

THE 'SOCIAL BRAIN HYPOTHESIS' (Dunbar 1998, 2003) offers a persuasive functional argument for the evolution of large primate brains, and in particular the relatively recent expansion of neocortex size in humans. According to this hypothesis, the formation and maintenance of complex social relationships has been the driving selective force in primate cognitive evolution. The neocortex has expanded according to its involvement in higher cognitive functions associated with enhanced memory and information processing. More recently, Dunbar (2007) has argued that modern human behaviour is defined by the ability to form imaginative worlds, as exhibited in communal religion and storytelling, and that these behaviours are ultimately rooted in the social domain. According to Dunbar (2007, 97), the computational demands of such abstractions as belief in supernatural forces or in fictional characters require a well-developed level of intentionality which evolved recently with the earliest anatomically modern humans (~135 ka). If we accept the premise that the manipulation of imaginary states is an essentially human capacity, then its appearance should be recognizable in the archaeological record in the form of accepted indicators of symbolically structured societies (Henshilwood & Marean 2003). The archaeological evidence of external symbolic storage (art, artefact style and structured use of social space), however, post-dates the proposed evolution of imaginary realms, and the even earlier evolution of language ca. 500 ka (Aiello & Dunbar 1993).

Proceedings of the British Academy **158**, 367–389. © The British Academy 2010.

The discrepancies between the predictions of the social brain hypothesis and the archaeological evidence of first appearances pose a methodological and conceptual dilemma of which Dunbar is well aware: if we are 'to insist on the primacy of the artefact record . . . we might seriously underestimate the true historical depth of the modern human mind . . .' (2007, 92). He sidesteps the apparent limitations of much of the more mundane Palaeolithic record of stone tools by arguing that technology is a by-product of the social brain rather than central to its development: 'Not only are tool-making and tool-use less cognitively demanding than navigating one's way through the minefields of the social world, but a case can be made that tools play only a modest part in the everyday lives of modern humans . . .' (2007, 93). As Dunbar recognizes, most current interpretations of the archaeological record do not support a pre-*sapiens* emergence of language and personal beliefs, or a later development of communal religion ca. 200 ka. Archaeologists can be forgiven for considering the predictions of the social brain hypothesis as precocious or simply flawed in the face of the material evidence. The two research communities are, as a result, able to dismiss each other's interpretations as marginal or misguided and merrily carry on with their own agendas— the 'Lucy to Language' project and this conference volume are the rare exceptions to the norm. Alternatively, we can respond to the challenge of the social brain predictions and consider the social and neural processes involved in tool-making and use. Relevant ethnographic and experimental data, though limited, does exist (Bamforth & Finlay 2008), and the field of neuroscience is just beginning to offer insights into the neural foundations of the co-evolution of the brain and technology (Grove & Coward 2008; Stout & Chaminade 2006). However, very few Palaeolithic archaeologists have made an effort to integrate their analyses of stone tools with the conceptual framework of the social brain hypothesis (though see e.g. Hallos 2005; McNabb 2007).

Dunbar's dilemma remains unresolved, but there is a way forward through a reconsideration of the archaeological evidence of the cognitively demanding behaviours embedded in certain forms of technology. This chapter takes one category of tool-making—composite technology—that developed about 300,000 years ago (possibly earlier in Europe and Africa), and uses it as an example of the skeins of social interaction intertwined in its creation, use and transmission across generations. The conceptual foundations of this technology potentially involve imaginary schemata that differ from those needed to visualize and execute hand-held tools, and which could be extended to other spheres of social life.

The transformational quality inherent in composite technology is analogous to the anticipatory element of higher levels of social intentionality, and may indirectly have contributed to the development of social differentiation based on craft skills. The following brief overview of the social brain hypothesis makes clear the predictions for the archaeological record and the limited role attributed to technology in managing social relations. This section is followed by a summary of what is currently the most widely accepted archaeological evidence for symbolically structured cultures. The making of composite tools is described as a transformative process, and as such an indicator of a cognitively demanding behaviour that involves elements of the distributed mind framework. As well as offering practical benefits, this technology also has the potential to carry and transmit subtle messages about the human ability to transform physical and social environments. The conclusion is that technology is embedded in social life, and that it participated in and perhaps even initiated changes in social relations

THE SOCIAL BRAIN HYPOTHESIS

Brain tissue is recognized as highly demanding to maintain in terms of energy costs (Aiello & Wheeler 1995). The evolution of large brains relative to body size among primates, in particular among humans, requires an adaptive or functional explanation to account for the maintenance of such a costly organ. Proponents of the social brain hypothesis argue that the selective stimulus for increased brain size lies in the cognitive demands associated with social living, especially those resulting from the management of bonds between individuals under the pressures of increasing group size (Barton 1996; Dunbar 1998, 2003; Shultz & Dunbar 2007). Ecological challenges are met communally or through social learning rather than individually (Shultz & Dunbar 2007, 207), and technology represents a by-product rather than an essential element of sociality (Dunbar 2007, 91). The highly enlarged human neocortex enables individuals to anticipate the desires, wishes, beliefs and intentions of others, both for personal advantage and for creating and maintaining social bonds. Among non-human primates, social bonds are maintained through grooming, but such intensive physical communication places a constraint on potential group size as it competes for time with other essential activities such as feeding and reproducing. Increasing group size also places demands on the information processing capacity of the brain (neocortex), and a comparison of mean group size with neocortex ratios (neocortex volume/remaining brain volume) across monkeys, apes and humans shows a strong linear relationship (Dunbar 2007, Figure 8.1). Humans have transcended the physical and cognitive limitations of grooming through language, with modern humans able to manage social networks of up to 125–150 individuals, beyond which we struggle to maintain personal knowledge (Dunbar 2003).

Neocortex ratios calculated from fossil hominin cranial volumes have provided an evolutionary scale of estimated cognitive changes from Pliocene australopithecines to contemporary *H. sapiens* (Dunbar 1996, 2003, 2007). An exponential increase in both brain and group size took place in the mid-Pleistocene (~500 ka), with the evolution of a nearly fully modern cranial capacity among 'archaic *sapiens*' as represented by *Homo heidelbergensis* (Aiello & Dunbar 1993). The evolution of language is implicated, given the limitations of physical grooming on group size. The social brain hypothesis also predicts that the mid-Pleistocene witnessed the evolution of fission-fusion social systems, male–female pair-bonding, and personal and social religion (Aurelli et al. 2008; Dunbar 2007). The latter is of particular interest because of the implications of religion for symbol-based behaviours. Dunbar (2007) argues that the rapid increase in group size predicted after 500 ka increased the social stresses of main-taining group bonds against the problem of free-riders—those willing to benefit from group living in terms of added protection, but not pay the costs in terms of sacrificing individual interests. Communal religion arose about 200 ka, with the evolution of *Homo sapiens*, as a means of cement-ing social bonds through a shared identity, but also as a shared belief in the threat of unseen and long-term punishment for those who shirked their social responsibilities.

Before assessing these predictions against the archaeological evidence, mention needs to be made of an important framework of the social brain, and that is the principle of theory of mind based on intentionality. Intentionality refers to conscious awareness of one's own state of mind and the beliefs, desires and intentions held. The ability to attribute these states to the minds of other individuals marks a theory of mind. Degrees of insight and attribution can be ordered into increasingly complex states of causal awareness, or levels of intentionality, that depend on the size of the neocortex for holding and processing information (Dunbar 2000). Second-order intentionality, the basis of theory of mind, is essential for forming and managing social relationships and for planning (Barrett et al. 2003), and possibly exists among chimpanzees (Dunbar 2004). It is also essential for language and is the foundation for imagining alternative states of existence, including the past and future. In turn, abstractions such as art and religion, as well as personal identity and a sense of belonging to a group that includes unrelated individuals, depend on believing that you understand the minds of others, and they yours. Without language, we are limited to second-order intentionality as, regardless of whether one can imagine multiple layers of intentionality, they cannot be communicated and agreement reached (Gärdenfors 2003). Based on estimated neocortex size alone, *Homo heidelbergensis*—a likely immediate ancestor of *Homo sapiens*—would have been capable of fourth-order intentionality, which is well within the modern human range and is the foundation for complex beliefs in the supernatural and the creation of symbols (Dunbar 2007, Figure 8.3).

THE 'STANDARD' ARCHAEOLOGICAL RECORD

An emerging consensus among archaeologists, at least those working in Africa, is that only with evidence for the material expression of symbolic thought (in the combined forms of art, artefact style and socially constructed use of space) can we say with certainty that we have recognizably modern behaviours. Collectively these are forms of external symbolic storage, providing indirect indicators that societies existed in which social relations were actively structured using symbols (Henshilwood 2007; Henshilwood & Marean 2003). This view, labelled here as the 'standard' model—though it has its vocal detractors (McBrearty 2007)—highlights the earliest expressions of symbol-based behaviours associated with *Homo sapiens*. The capacity to use symbols, which may have existed earlier, was only enacted fully in the late Pleistocene by anatomically modern humans (~135 ka). The evidence comes from south-western Asia (Skhūl Cave 135–90 ka; Vanhaeren et al. 2006), northern Africa (Taforalt Cave 88 ka, Bouzouggar et al. 2007) and southern Africa (Blombos Cave ~77 ka, Henshilwood 2007), with marine shell beads a common link across this broad geographical range (d'Errico & Vanhaeren 2007). In terms of the social brain hypothesis, beads as forms of personal ornamentation signal individual and potentially group identity, and as such represent at least a second-order level of intentionality and the probable existence of language in the negotiation of identities. This, then is the earliest widely accepted evidence for symbol-based behaviours indicative of the modern mind as defined by the social brain hypothesis, with a clear disparity evident between predictions of cognitive evolution based on neocortex ratios versus the earliest unequivocal archaeological signatures. The disparity lessens somewhat if a less restrictive set of criteria is applied that accepts the appearance of individual elements of external symbolic storage rather than the full complement. Ethnographic and archaeological records, taken together, show the importance of environmental, demographic and other historical processes on when and to what extent symbolic behaviours are expressed in material form (Barham 2007). That contingency is reflected by tantalizing glimpses of potentially symbol-based social conventions in the African record, including the post-mortem modification of the Herto crania at 160 ka (White et al. 2003), the geographically diverse distribution of ochre use between 300 and 200 ka (Barham 2002) and the emergence of the first distinctive regional artefact styles (265 ka) (Barham 2000). The latter two precede the evolution of anatomically modern humans, but uncertainty remains about how reliable of each of these claimed extensions of the standard model might be, either because of alternative functional explanations or the limitations of the chronological controls. For the time being, the search continues for ever older archaeological markers of external symbolic storage, but the prospects of reaching the predicted social brain targets of 500 ka for language and 200 ka for communal religion still seem distant.

A TECHNOLOGICAL FIX?

A considerable theoretical literature has developed in recent years around the theme of material culture as an active participant in structuring social life (e.g. Gamble 1999; Gell 1998; Gosden & Marshall 1999; Hodder 1991; Ingold 2007). Whether artefacts possess agency independent of their makers (e.g. Gosden 2005) is not a relevant issue here, but their embedded role in mediating social relations between individuals is well attested by anthropologists and ethnoarchaeologists working in non-Western and pre-industrial societies (Killick 2004). Tool-making and use plays more than the 'modest' role suggested by Dunbar (2007, 93) in hunter-gatherer societies, with macro-scale latitudinal clines of technological elaboration linked to climate and micro-scale variations reflecting social processes of decision-making (Hayden & Gargett 1988; Torrence 2001). At either scale, technology is essential to the lives of people who extract energy directly from the environment and as such is inevitably incorporated into the cognitively demanding arena of socio-politics. Also demanding in terms of social responsibilities and time is the training of new generations of artisans to make the objects on which social life depends. In the case of stone tools, years of practice are required to combine specific motor skills and knowledge of materials with the strategic reasoning involved in problem-solving (Bamforth & Finlay 2008). How that learning takes places is the focus of cultural transmission theory (Boyd & Richerson 1985; Hewlett & Cavalli-Sforza 1986; Richerson & Boyd 2005), with various options available for learning, including through observation or teaching, in family contexts or in the more formal settings of apprenticeships (Stout 2002). Variations on these general contexts occur with gender, age and group size, the latter in particular affecting opportunities for learning from a broader spectrum of individuals beyond the immediate family (Shennan 2001; Shennan & Steele 1999).

From an evolutionary perspective, studies of social learning among communities of tool-using chimpanzees highlight the importance of a developed theory of mind as an underpinning for teaching and imitation, which are relatively rare behaviours among these primates (Tomasello 1999). The non-human primate data also points to the importance of stable social environments for the retention of learned skills, and highly sociable communities as contexts in which innovation is more likely to arise through interaction and take hold (van Schaik & Pradham 2003). The ecological and social contexts that stimulate innovation and support social learning are important in understanding the regionally diverse repertoires of tool-making found among chimpanzees (McGrew 2004; Whiten et al. 1999). These ethological studies also highlight the fundamental sociality of technology in its learning and use. The making and use of stone tools among humans, as with other learned crafts, provides arenas of interaction between individuals that encourage the development of cognitive empathy and perception of others as self-equivalent beings, as well as the recognition that individual differences exist in levels of skill and knowledge (Grove & Coward 2008, 383). (Apprenticeships as structured and long-term systems of learning would not be possible without considerable cognitive empathy as a foundation for the high levels of intentionality involved.)

Increased relative neocortex size, which equates with enhanced capacities for information processing and memory, correlates with rates of innovation and social learning (Reader & Laland 2002). Based on the relatively rapid brain expansion that took place ~600 ka associated with *Homo heidelbergensis* (Rightmire 2004) and increased estimated group sizes (social brain hypothesis prediction), we could expect to see archaeological evidence of increased rates of innovation from this time onwards, and also indirect evidence of language among communities of presumably highly sociable pre-*sapiens*. With regard to the African archaeological data, the period between ~600 and 300 ka is indeed one of change that includes evidence for innovations such as prepared core technology, an extended range of small retouched tools (Kleindeinst 1961) and increased use of soft-hammer flaking to refine bifaces (Clark 2001b; Texier 1996). Long-distance movement of raw materials up to 150 km (Clark 2001b) is rare but indicative of increased levels of planning and, by extension, intentionality. It is impossible to say with certainty that language was essential for any of these developments, but undoubtedly the learning and use of these technologies, as well as the formation of extended resource (= social?) networks would be greatly enhanced by language. This interval of technological and presumed social change coincides with the onset of enhanced climatic variability in the Middle Pleistocene, linked to shifts in the duration and amplitude of global glacial cycles after 430 ka (EPICA 2004). Technology as a socially derived behaviour offered an important buffer to ecological shifts in resource distribution, with a potential selective advantage offered to those groups able to foster innovations and their transmission. The absence of unequivocal signals of external symbolic storage at this time may be a reflection of small, dispersed populations not needing to invest in costly signalling, rather than any inherent lack of cognitive capacity (Barham 2007; Shennan 2001).

About 300 ka, a technological transition began in eastern and southern Africa (and in Europe; see Bridgland et al. 2006) that marked a shift in emphasis in tool-making away from hand-held tools (Mode 2) towards a greater reliance on hafted tools (Mode 3) made of multiple components (Mode 2/3 transition; Barham & Mitchell 2008). Clark (1989) drew attention to the practical advantages of composite technology in terms of risk-reducing behaviours, greater efficiency of raw material use and improved hunting abilities (Table 18.1). These benefits can translate into increased inclusive fitness through greater security of high-quality foods for offspring and reduced personal exposure to physical risks for adults in their reproductive prime. Composite technology represents more than a set of functional benefits; it marks a conceptual shift and one possibly sup-

---

[1] Composite technology as defined here is conceptually distinct from observations of chimpanzees using two or more tools in sequence to achieve a goal, or pushing two sticks together to form an extended tool (Parker & McKinney 1999, 55). The emphasis here is on the integration of materials with differing properties to create a single tool, a series of actions not yet observed among non-human primates.

Table 18.1. The practical and social consequences of hafting (based on Clark 1989 and Barham & Mitchell 2008)

Greater leverage, processing efficiency
Increased wounding/killing efficiency
Reduced contact with biological hazards
Reduced muscle mass, skeletal robustness and metabolic needs
Increased flexibility of tool design (technological buffer)
Greater raw material efficiency
Haft as vehicle of communication—personal, group identity
Craft specialization, more effective division of labour

ported by developments in the neocortex that have not yet been appreciated fully by evolutionary psychologists or archaeologists—myself included.

Before considering the conceptual implications of composite technology, a summary is needed of the cognitive operations involved in making multi-component tools. As a technology, it is far more intellectually demanding than generally credited (e.g. Bickerton 2007, 99). The craft involves integrating materials, typically with differing physical properties, to make a working whole.[1] The haft, as the supporting element, needs to be designed to withstand the stresses that will be placed on the working bits in relation to the dominant motion of the activity. Scraping, adzing, sawing, slicing, piercing, drilling and puncturing as separate actions place different stresses on the haft as well as on the inserts. Among the four types of haft used prehistorically and observed ethnographically (juxtaposed, inclusion, cleft and composite hafts; Figure 18.1), each has its own tolerances in relation to the angle and force of use plus hardness of contact materials (Rots et al. 2006). The deceptively simple inclusion haft, which involves inserting a working bit into a pre-shaped hole, will invariably lead to the snapping of the bit if the fit is too tight (N. Taylor pers. comm.). Through experience, observation or teaching, the craftsperson learns to allow some play in this form of haft. The craftsperson also needs to consider the properties of the raw material used to make the haft in relation to the intended function. Woods, for example, vary in their responses to force, in their durability, weight and ease of shaping, as do other organic hafting materials such as bone (green/fresh or dry), antler, shell and horn. For armature, such as spear shafts, the haft's weight and aerodynamic properties also need to be considered. Further decisions have to be made about the means of attaching the bit to a haft. The hafting process may simply involve the insertion of the bit into a carefully pre-shaped hole, or include a binding on its own or one integrated with an

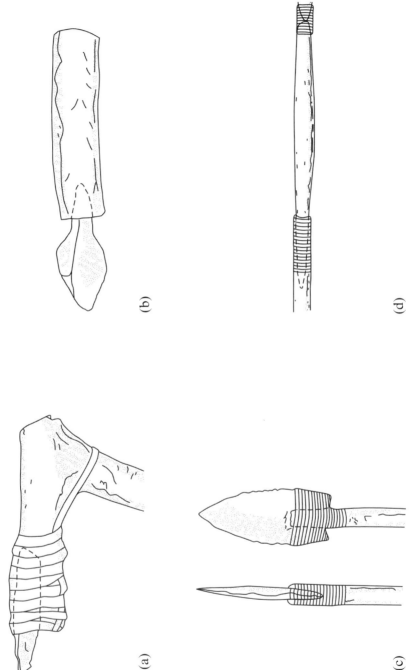

Figure 18.1. Four forms of hafting generally recognized by archaeologists: (a) juxtaposed; (b) inclusion or male; (c) cleft; (d) composite haft

adhesive. Binding materials, whether plant- or animal-based, have differing properties (flexibility, durability) and preparation steps (e.g. soaking, stripping, pounding). As with the haft, the binder needs to be matched to the intended purpose of the complete tool. Adhesives represent yet another set of cognitive operations based on an understanding of the properties of the material matched to the design needs of the tool. Like binders, adhesive can be plant- or animal-based (bitumen as a natural hydrocarbon is the rare exception), with varying properties of elasticity, durability and responses to heat, cold and damp. Pitch and other resin-based adhesives are typically heated to make a pliable but sticky filler for application to the haft and insert. Binding is necessary with pitch to ensure a secure hold. A drying agent can be added to minimize cracking as the resin hardens. These agents, usually coarse-textured, can include ground charcoal, ochre, ash, beeswax, powdered stone and dry dung (Callahan 1999). Taken together, the knowledge invested in hafts, binders and adhesives—not to mention the design of the inserts and use of the tool itself—represents a considerable social investment in learning through trial and error.

Perhaps the most significant development represented by this technology was the creation of conceptually new forms of tools made from a *combination* of materials that did not exist previously. Earlier tools, such as hand-axes, though undoubtedly complex in design and execution (Lycett & Gowlett 2008), were essentially created by linear reductive processes rather than hierarchical additive ones. The same description of linearity can be applied to any tools made of a single material, such as wooden spears or bone awls. They may vary in the length of the *chaînes opératoires* involved, but not in their conceptual framework. By contrast, composite tools, as hierarchical creations, mark something new technologically and cognitively. Envisaging a composite tool involves integrating constellations of material knowledge into a functional whole. The process is transformative and ultimately imaginative.

The creative act of imagining new forms and applications of composite technology also involves the kind of analogical reasoning that underpins complex language (Szathmáry & Számadó 2008). A proto-language as defined by Bickerton (2007, 101–102) would be unable to support the trains of thought necessary to create the conceptual innovation represented by composite tool forms. Syntactic language, as a hierarchical structure based on potentially infinite and recursive combinations of embedded phrases and clauses (Gibson 2007, 68), would support the thought structure inherent in composite technology. New tool forms would also presumably have required new names or categorization to share their identification for purposes of manufacture, use, development as well as teaching. A socially distributed expertise in the retention and transmission of these spheres of knowledge would not only spread the cognitive load, but also contribute to further innovation, and perhaps incipient craft specialization. Once the analogical, recursive reasoning involved in complex language (and composite technology) had evolved, it could be applied to other socially demanding contexts, such as the creation and extension of kinship classifications (Barnard 2008; Gamble 2008). With language came the potential for a ratchet effect on human social evolution as ideas could be shared readily between individuals, and transmitted between generations (Tomasello 1999). Composite tools embody this ratchet effect, not just in the social learning involved in their making and use, but also as communal rather than individual responses to solving ecological problems. The integration and transformation of organic and inorganic materials into new forms offers a forum for the exchange of knowledge between individuals. Such a focal point also has the potential to foster cognitive empathy through close physical proximity and shared experiences in the processes of making and using tools (Grove & Coward 2008; Iriki 2006). As an aside, the general observation can be made that because so few Westerners are engaged in the processes of tool-making in their daily lives, we underestimate the role of technology in small-scale societies as an arena for social bonding and learning (e.g. Stout 2002).

We can speculate that the evolution of working memory as an emergent property of the neocortex and its subcortical connections would have been central to the development of composite technology. Working memory involves the capacity to hold information in mind, making it available for application to problem-solving by facilitating the anticipation of future states, making conceptual connections and executing complex action sequences that engage long-term memory (Wynn & Coolidge 2003). These capacities of working memory would be involved in the production and use of composite tools, just as they are in the production of complex language, symbol use and the negotiation of social interactions. Neural imaging studies are beginning to reveal the networks involved in the conception of simple tools and their use, along with their linkages to language areas and other cortical fields (Stout & Chaminade 2006). The neural involvement with composite technology is likely to be even more extensive, though just a few genetic changes may be involved in enabling an extended working memory to operate as a scaffold for recursive thinking (Read 2008).

THE EVIDENCE

Having made the argument for hierarchical thought as integral to composite technology as well as language and imagination, plus the broader point that technology is deeply embedded in human social life, the archaeological record then provides the means of reassessing the predictions of the social brain hypothesis. In brief, composite technology was not an invention so much as an innovation derived from existing knowledge of organic and inorganic materials, but brought together for the first time as integrated tools. Bone-working has considerable time-depth, with early regional traditions in southern and eastern Africa ca. 1.8–1.5 Ma, associated with one or more early hominins including *Homo erectus* (Backwell & d'Errico 2005). Bone bifaces are also known from the later European Acheulean of ~500–400 ka (Gaudzinski et al. 2004; Villa 1991), associated with *Homo heidelbergensis*, as is the use of antler as a soft hammer to finely shape flint hand-axes (Roberts & Parfitt 1999). Wood-working appears to occur as early as bone-working in Africa, based on the evidence of plant residues (*Acacia* phytoliths) adhering to stone bifaces from Peninj, Tanzania (~1.6 Ma; Domínguez-Rodrigo et al. 2001). Wood was also probably used by the makers of later Acheulean bifaces (~780 ka and later) as a soft hammer for thinning and final shaping (Clark 2001b; Sharon & Goren-Inbar 1999). Direct evidence for wood-working comes from waterlogged deposits at Gesher Benot Ya'aqov (Israel) dated to 780 ka (Goren-Inbar et al. 2002) and possibly from the waterlogged levels at the later site of Kalambo Falls in Zambia at ~400 ka (Clark 2001a).

The earliest claim for direct evidence of hafting comes from Schöningen (Germany, 400 ka), where exceptional preservation provides evidence for the working of spruce, pine and fir into a variety of pointed tools (spears, throwing sticks and a fire hook) and perhaps cleft hafts for holding small flint flakes (Thieme 2003). Three branches of fir have diagonal grooves cut into one end and a fourth bears notches at both ends (Thieme 2003, 10). As cleft hafts, these tools would require some kind of binding, or combined mastic with binding, to support stone inserts; alternatively, these could be struts or supports unrelated to hafting. Microscopic and trace element analyses of the clefts and exterior surfaces may provide more conclusive evidence of the forms of use, but in the interim these and the other wooden tools at Schöningen demonstrate a developed understanding of the properties of wood as a raw material. The hominin involved would most likely have been *Homo heidelbergensis*.

The earliest evidence for the use of mastic or adhesives comes from patches of birch tar preserved on stone flakes from fluvial deposits in central Italy (Mazza et al. 2006). Pitch mastic on its own, as mentioned above, would not be strong enough to form a secure bond, with some form of binding required. The age of these deposits, as estimated from associated fauna, is probably at least ~220 ka, which suggests that *Homo neanderthalensis* was the likely maker.

Given the rarity of organic preservation in the Palaeolithic, most inferences for the use of hafts derive from indirect indicators, including wear traces and artefact morphology and size. The thinning of the bases of late Acheulean hand-axes and cleavers may indicate some kind of hafting in the African record, but in the absence of experimental replication work this hypothesis remains untested and these tools are still assumed to be hand-held (Phillipson 1997). Small bifacially retouched points typical of the African Middle Stone Age (Mode 3) are generally assumed to have been inserts as spear points (Shea 2006), or knife blades. As spear points, these tools would probably have been inserted into inclusion or cleft hafts, as demonstrated experimentally on later southern African assemblages (Lombard 2005; Villa et al. 2008). The transition from hand-held to hafted tools in Africa was under way by ~285 ka and seems to have occurred relatively rapidly from eastern to southern Africa, but the dated evidence comes from a very small number of sites (Barham & Mitchell 2008). Wear traces indicative of hafting (using juxtaposed hafts; Figure 18.2) are associated with core-axes of the Lupemban industry of central Africa (Van Peer et al. 2004). Small blunted, snapped or backed pieces also occur in the Lupemban, and, given their size and deliberate preparation, are assumed to have been inserts in hafted tools (Barham 2002), probably cleft hafts. The earliest of these Lupemban assemblages is dated to ~265 ka from the site of Twin Rivers, Zambia, and includes one bifacial point with a notched base (Figure 18.3) (Barham 2001). The notch, if intentional, would have facilitated binding in a cleft haft. Further replication experiments are needed to test these speculations about the variety of haft forms used, but in the interim the existing indirect evidence leads to the conclusion that in Africa juxtaposed hafts—with bindings—were being used before the evolution of *Homo sapiens* (~195 ka), and possibly as early as 285 ka. Other forms of hafts also were probably in use with backed pieces and points, but the supporting experimental evidence is lacking for the earliest phases. In Europe, the traces of pitch from Italy are roughly comparable in age to the African evidence for hafting, and imply a comparable knowledge of binding materials. The Schöningen

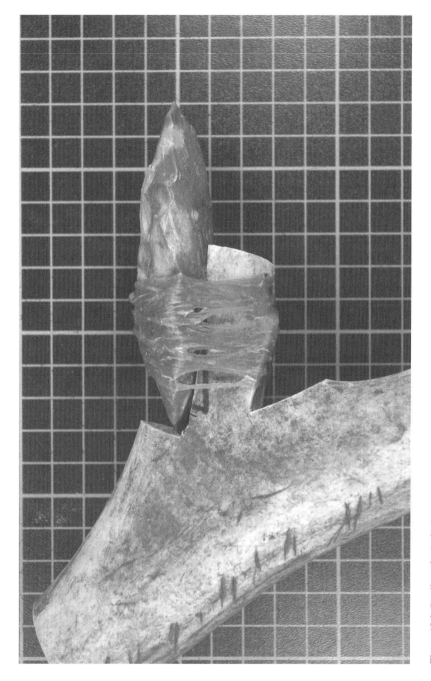

Figure 18.2. Replica of a hafted Lupemban core-axe from Kalambo Falls (juxtaposed haft) (Courtesy of Nick Taylor)

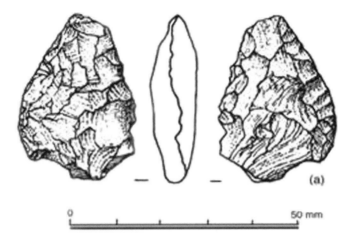

Figure 18.3. Mode 3 (Middle Stone Age) point from the Lupemban levels of Twin Rivers cave, Zambia, showing a notched base presumably intended for strengthening a cleft or inclusion haft (reproduced with permission of the Western Academic & Specialist Press)

cleft pieces suggest an even earlier development of a technology based on integrated organic and inorganic elements, though the evidence requires verification through closer analysis combined with replication studies.

The combined evidence for early composite technology, though limited, indicates a Middle Pleistocene origin and implicates *Homo heidelbergensis* as the likely innovator. This species—as the last common ancestor of Neanderthals in Eurasia and modern humans in Africa (Rightmire 2004)—seems to have had the cognitive capacity to engage in complex technology and, by implication, language and intricate social relations. The apparently coeval occurrence of composite technology on both continents suggests either parallel but separate technological developments, or their spread from a source area.[2] A model of separate, unrelated origins could be based on the premise of a common cognitive capacity for hierarchical thinking and language that enabled convergent responses to similar adaptive pressures. The social brain hypothesis predicts just such a capacity for language roughly 500,000 years ago, based on the evolution of large-brained pre-*sapiens*, and there is a growing body of anatomical evidence that by this time *Homo heidelbergensis* already

---

[2] An alternative explanation for the co-occurrence of Mode 3 or hafted technology in Africa and Europe relies on identifying an earlier area of innovation in Africa and the subsequent spread of this technology into Europe with the dispersal of a shared ancestral hominin (*Homo helmei*) from Africa (Lahr & Foley 2001; but see also White & Ashton 2003).

possessed the bony structures involved in speech production (hyoid) and perception (outer and middle ear) (Martínez et al. 2004, 2008). In terms of relative brain size, *Homo heidelbergensis* had only a marginally smaller brain than modern humans, from which inferences can be drawn about the evolution of new specialized cortical fields that underpinned the expansion of the neocortex and the potential for new behaviours (Neill 2007). Genetic support is also emerging for *Homo heidelbergensis* as the ancestral source of mutations in the gene *FOXP2*, which is involved in the production of speech and development of other neural circuitry. These mutations are found in the ancient DNA of Neanderthals as well as in modern humans, suggesting a shared inheritance through a last common ancestor (Krause et al. 2007).

BEYOND BEADS, PIGMENTS AND BURIALS

By taking a fresh perspective on the archaeological record and integrating fossil, neural and genetic data, we can resolve at least part of Dunbar's dilemma. A Middle Pleistocene origin for language ~500 ka no longer seems unsupportable. The hierarchical neural processing involved in syntax would have been available for application to other demanding behavioural areas, such as the creation of extended social networks through kinship. Technology as an extension of social relations would also benefit from the development of hierarchical thought. The innovation of composite technology offers one echo of an increasingly complex social world ultimately founded on language. A network of interacting effects co-evolved with language, supported by selection for those networks of genes that underpin complex behaviours (Szathmáry & Számadó 2008). That other part of Dunbar's dilemma, the evolution of higher levels of intentionality necessary for creating imaginary worlds, also now seems less problematical. By at least 200 ka, *Homo sapiens* and Neanderthals were capable of imagining new tool forms constructed of combinations of materials that do not exist in nature. If, as has been argued, complex behaviours develop in tandem as part of neural and behavioural networks rather than as isolated traits, then we have a conceptual framework with which to explore the archaeological record for those hints of the real cognitive capacities of both species. The conceptual gap closes between hierarchical technology, based on imagination, and the capacity to create imaginary worlds. As argued elsewhere (Barham 2007), we should look to combinations of technological and social behaviours for evidence of the fuller expression of the cognitive potential of pre- and non-*sapiens*. A narrowly focused search for the beginnings of symbol use overlooks the historical processes that may influence the timing and forms of this and other complex behaviours (Gamble 2007). Dunbar's worry that we might 'seriously underestimate the true historical depth of the modern human mind' (2007, 92) risks fulfilment under the current *status quo*.

The integrated approach advocated here arguably leads to resolution of the chronological and evidential dilemmas arising from the predictions of the social brain hypothesis. In doing so, it allows other equally intriguing issues to return to centre stage. Foremost among these are the separate developmental histories of modern humans within and outside Africa, and of Neanderthals in Eurasia. If both species inherited comparable cognitive capacities, then how do we explain their respective behavioural differences? The question is certainly not new (see Lahr & Foley 2001 for summary), but if we can accept a common starting point grounded in complex language, and learn to recognize the behavioural potentials of Neanderthals (e.g. d'Errico 2003) as well as those of pre-*sapiens* in Africa, then we are certain to develop more regionally tuned models of behavioural diversity. More broadly, the challenges posed by Dunbar's dilemma have brought about a closer integration of archaeology with evolutionary psychology and neurobiology, and for that incremental step we should be grateful for a problem well-raised.

Note. I thank the organizers of the British Academy Centenary Research Project, 'Lucy to Language: The Archaeology of the Social Brain', for their invitation to contribute to this volume and the conference on which it was based. Thanks also to Nick Taylor for conversations on the intricacies of bindings and hafts.

REFERENCES

Aiello, L. C. & Dunbar, R. I. M. (1993). Neocortex size, group size and the evolution of language. *Current Anthropology* 34: 184–193.

Aiello, L. C. & Wheeler, P. (1995). The expensive tissue hypothesis: the brain and digestive system in human and primate evolution. *Current Anthropology* 36: 199–221.

Aurelli, F., Schaffner, C. M., Boesch, C., Bearder, S. K., Call, J., Chapman, C. A. et al. (2008). Fission-fusion dynamics. *Current Anthropology* 49: 627–654.

Backwell, L. & d'Errico, F. (2005). The origin of bone tool technology and the identification of early hominid cultural traditions. In: F. d'Errico & L. Backwell (eds)

From tools to symbols: from early hominids to modern humans, pp. 239–275. Johannesburg: University of Witwatersrand Press.

Bamforth, D. B. & Finlay, N. (2008). Introduction: archaeological approaches to lithic production skill and craft learning. *Journal of Archaeological Method and Theory* 15: 1–27.

Barham, L. (2000). *The Middle Stone Age of Zambia, south-central Africa*. Bristol: Western Academic & Specialist Press.

Barham, L. (2001). Central Africa and the emergence of regional identity in the Middle Pleistocene. In: L. Barham & K. Robson-Brown (eds) *Human roots: Africa and Asia in the Middle Pleistocene*, pp. 65–80. Bristol: Western Academic & Specialist Press.

Barham, L. (2002). Systematic pigment use in the Middle Pleistocene of south central Africa. *Current Anthropology* 43:181–190.

Barham, L. (2007). Modern is as modern does? Technological trends and thresholds in the south-central African record. In: P. Mellars, K. Boyle, O. Bar-Yosef & C. Stringer (eds) *Rethinking the human revolution*, pp. 165–176. Cambridge: McDonald Institute Monographs.

Barham, L. & Mitchell, P. (2008). *The first Africans: African archaeology from the earliest toolmakers to most recent foragers*. Cambridge: Cambridge University Press.

Barnard, A. (2008). The co-evolution of kinship and language. In: N. Allen, H. Callan, R. Dunbar & W. James (eds) *Early human kinship: from sex to social reproduction*, pp. 232–244. London: John Wiley & Sons.

Barrett, L., Henzi, P. & Dunbar, R. I. M. (2003). Primate cognition: from 'what now?' to 'what if?' *Trends in Cognitive Sciences* 7: 494–497.

Barton, R. A. (1996). Neocortex and behavioural ecology in primates. *Proceedings of the Royal Society of London B* 263: 173–177.

Bickerton, D. (2007). Did syntax trigger the human revolution? In: P. Mellars, K. Boyle, O. Bar-Yosef & C. Stringer (eds) *Rethinking the human revolution*, pp. 99–106. Cambridge: McDonald Institute Monographs.

Bouzouggar, A., Barton, N., Vanhaeren, M., d'Errico, F., Collcutt, S. & Higham, T. (2007). 82,000-year-old shell beads from North Africa and implications for the origins of modern human behaviour. *Proceedings of the National Academy of Sciences* 104: 9964–9969.

Boyd, R. & Richerson, P. (1985). *Culture and the evolutionary process*. Chicago: University of Chicago Press.

Bridgland, D. R., Antoine, P., Limondin-Lozouet, N., Santisteban, J. I., Westaway, R. & White, M. (2006). The Palaeolithic occupation of Europe as revealed by evidence from rivers: data from IGCP 449. *Journal of Quaternary Science* 21: 437–455.

Callahan, E. (1999). A word on pitch. In: D. Westcott (ed.) *Primitive technology: a book of earth skills*, p. 190. Salt Lake City, UT: Gibbs-Smith Publishers.

Clark, J. D. (1989). The origins and spread of modern humans: a broad perspective on the African evidence. In: P. Mellars & C. Stringer (eds) *The human revolution*, pp. 565–588. Edinburgh: Edinburgh University Press.

Clark, J. D. (2001a). *Kalambo Falls prehistoric site*, vol. III. Cambridge: Cambridge University Press.

Clark, J. D. (2001b). Variability in primary and secondary technologies of the Later Acheulian in Africa. In: S. Milliken & J. Cook (eds) *A very remote period indeed: papers on the Palaeolithic presented to Derek Roe*, pp. 1–18. Oxford: Oxbow Books.

d'Errico, F. (2003). The invisible frontier: a multiple species model for the origin of behavioural modernity. *Evolutionary Anthropology* 12: 188–202.

d'Errico, F. & Vanhaeren, M. (2007). Evolution or revolution? New evidence for the origin of symbolic behaviour. In: P. Mellars, K. Boyle, O. Bar-Yosef & C. Stringer (eds) *Rethinking the human revolution*, pp. 275–286. Cambridge: McDonald Institute Monographs.

Domínguez-Rodrigo, M., Serralonga, J., Juan-Treserras, J., Alcala, L. & Luque, L. (2001). Wood working activities by early humans: a plant residue analysis on Acheulian stone tools from Peninj, Tanzania. *Journal of Human Evolution* 40: 289–299.

Dunbar, R. I. M. (1996). *Grooming, gossip, and the evolution of language*. Cambridge, MA: Harvard University Press.

Dunbar, R. I. M. (1998). The social brain hypothesis. *Evolutionary Anthropology* 6: 178–190.

Dunbar, R. I. M. (2000). Causal reasoning, mental rehearsal and the evolution of primate cognition. In: C. Heyes & L. Huber (eds) *Evolution of cognition*, pp. 205–231. Cambridge, MA: MIT Press.

Dunbar, R. I. M. (2003). The social brain: mind, language and society in evolutionary perspective. *Annual Review of Anthropology* 32: 163–181.

Dunbar, R. I. M. (2004). *The human story*. London: Faber & Faber.

Dunbar, R. I. M. (2007). The social brain and the cultural explosion of the human revolution. In: P. Mellars, K. Boyle, O. Bar-Yosef & C. Stringer (eds) *Rethinking the human revolution*, pp. 91–98. Cambridge: McDonald Institute Monographs.

EPICA community members. (2004). Eight glacial cycles from an Antarctic ice core. *Nature* 429: 623–628.

Gärdenfors, P. (2003). *How Homo became sapiens: the evolution of thinking*. Oxford: Oxford University Press.

Gamble, C. (1999). *The Palaeolithic societies of Europe*. Cambridge: Cambridge University Press.

Gamble, C. (2007). *Origins and revolutions: human identity in earliest prehistory*. New York: Cambridge University Press.

Gamble, C. (2008). Kinship and material culture: archaeological implications of the human global diaspora. In N. Allen, H. Callan, R. Dunbar & W. James (eds) *Early human kinship: from sex to social reproduction*, pp. 27–40. London: John Wiley & Sons.

Gaudzinski, S., Turner, E., Anzidei, A. P., Álvarez-Fernández, E., Arroyo-Cabrales, J., Cinq-Mars, J. et al. (2004). The use of Proboscidean remains in every-day Palaeolithic life. *Quaternary International* 126: 179–194.

Gell, A. (1998). *Art and agency: towards an anthropological theory*. Oxford: Clarendon Press.

Gibson, K.R. (2007). Putting it all together: a constructionist approach to the evolution of human mental capacities. In: P. Mellars, K. Boyle, O. Bar-Yosef &

C. Stringer (eds) *Rethinking the human revolution*, pp. 67–78. Cambridge: McDonald Institute Monographs.

Goren-Inbar, N., Werker, E. & Feibel, C. S. (2002). *The Acheulian site of Gesher Benot Ya'aqov, Israel, I: The wood assemblage.* Oxford: Oxbow Books.

Gosden, C. (2005). What do artefacts want? *Journal of Archaeological Method and Theory* 12: 193–211.

Gosden, C. & Marshall, Y. (1999). The cultural biography of objects. *World Archaeology* 31: 169–178.

Grove, M. & Coward, F. (2008). From individual neurons to social brains. *Cambridge Archaeological Journal* 18: 387–400.

Hallos, J. (2005) '15 minutes of fame': exploring the temporal dimension of Middle Pleistocene lithic technology. *Journal of Human Evolution* 49: 155–179.

Hayden, B. & Gargett, R. 1988. Specialization in the Paleolithic. *Lithic Technology* 17: 12–18.

Henshilwood, C. S. (2007). Fully symbolic *sapiens* behaviour: innovations in the Middle Stone Age at Blombos Cave, South Africa. In P. Mellars, K. Boyle, O. Bar-Yosef & C. Stringer (eds) *Rethinking the human revolution*, pp. 123–132. Cambridge: McDonald Institute Monographs.

Henshilwood, C. S. & Marean, C. (2003). The origin of modern human behavior: critique of the models and their test implications. *Current Anthropology* 44: 627–651.

Hewlett, B. S. & Cavalli-Sforza, L. (1986). Cultural transmission among Aka pygmies. *American Anthropologist* 88: 922–934.

Hodder, I. (1991). *Reading the past.* Cambridge: Cambridge University Press.

Ingold, T. (2007). Materials against materiality. *Archaeological Dialogues* 14: 1–16.

Iriki, A. (2006). The neural origins and implications of imitation, mirror neurons and tool use. *Current Opinions in Neurobiology* 16: 1–8.

Killick, D. (2004). Social constructionist approaches to the study of technology. *World Archaeology* 36: 571–578.

Kleindeinst, M.R. (1961). Variability within the late Acheulean assemblage in eastern Africa. *South African Archaeological Bulletin* 16: 35–52.

Krause, J., Lalueza-Fox, C., Orlando, L.,Enard, W., Green, R. E., Burbano, H. A. et al. (2007). The derived *FOXP2* variant of modern humans was shared with Neandertals. *Current Biology* 17: 1908–1912.

Lahr, M. M. & Foley, R. (2001). Mode 3, *Homo helmei*, and the pattern of human evolution in the Middle Pleistocene. In: L. Barham & K. Robson-Brown (eds) *Human roots: Africa and Asia in the Middle Pleistocene*, pp. 29–39. Bristol: Western Academic & Specialist Press.

Lombard, M. (2005). Evidence of hunting and hafting during the Middle Stone Age at Sibudu Cave, KwaZulu-Natal, South Africa: a multianalytical approach. *Journal of Human Evolution* 48: 279–300.

Lycett, S. J. & Gowlett, J. A. J. (2008). On questions surrounding the Acheulean 'tradition'. *World Archaeology* 40: 295–315.

McBrearty, S. (2007). Down with the revolution. In P. Mellars, K. Boyle, O. Bar-Yosef & C. Stringer (eds) *Rethinking the human revolution*, pp. 133–151. Cambridge: McDonald Institute Monographs.

McGrew, W. C. (2004). *The cultured chimpanzee: reflections on cultural primatology.* Cambridge: Cambridge University Press.

McNabb, J. (2007). *The British Lower Palaeolithic: stones in contention.* London: Routledge.

Martínez, I., Arsuaga, J. L., Jarabo, P., Quam, R., Lorenzo, C., Gracia, A. et al. (2004). Auditory capacities in Middle Pleistocene humans from the Sierra de Atapuerca in Spain. *Proceedings of the National Academy of Sciences (USA)* 101: 9976–9981.

Martínez, I., Arsuaga, J. L., Quam, R., Carretero, J. M., Gracia, A. & Rodríguez, L. (2008). Human hyoid bones from the Middle Pleistocene site of the Sima de los Huesos (Sierra de Atapuerca, Spain). *Journal of Human Evolution* 54: 118–124.

Mazza, P. P. A., Martini, F., Sala, B., Magi, M., Colombini, M. P., Landucci, F. et al. (2006). A new Palaeolithic discovery: tar-hafted stone tools in a European mid-Pleistocene bone-bearing bed. *Journal of Archaeological Science* 33: 1310–1318.

Neill, D. (2007). Cortical evolution and human behaviour. *Brain Research Bulletin* 74: 191–205.

Parker, S. T. & McKinney, M. L. (1999). *The evolution of cognitive development in monkeys, apes, and humans.* Baltimore, MD: Johns Hopkins University Press.

Phillipson, L. (1997). Edge modification as an indicator of function and handedness of Acheulian handaxes from Kariandusi, Kenya. *Lithic Technology* 22: 171–183.

Read, D. W. (2008). Working memory: a cognitive limit to non-human primate recursive thinking prior to hominid evolution. *Evolutionary Psychology* 6: 676–714.

Reader, S. M. & Laland, K. N. (2002). Social intelligence, innovation, and enhanced brain size in primates. *Proceedings of the National Academy of Sciences (USA)* 99: 4436–4441.

Richerson, P. J. & Boyd, R. (2005). *Not by genes alone: how culture transformed human evolution.* Chicago: University of Chicago Press.

Rightmire, G. P. (2004). Brain size and encephalization in early to mid-Pleistocene *Homo. American Journal of Physical Anthropology* 124: 109–123.

Roberts, M. B. & Parfitt, S. A. (1999). *Boxgrove: a Middle Pleistocene hominid site at Eartham Quarry, Boxgrove, West Sussex.* London: English Heritage.

Rots, V., Pirnay, L., Pirson, Ph. & Baudoux, O. (2006). Blind tests shed light on possibilities and limitations for identifying stone tool prehension and hafting. *Journal of Archaeological Science* 33: 935–952.

Sharon, G. N. & Goren-Inbar, N. (1999). Soft percussor use at Gesher Benot Ya'aqov Acheulian site? *Journal of the Israel Prehistoric Society* 28: 55–79.

Shea, J. (2006). The origins of lithic projectile point technology: evidence from Africa, the Levant, and Europe. *Journal of Archaeological Science* 33(6): 823–846.

Shennan, S. (2001). Demography and cultural innovation: a model and its implications for the emergence of modern human culture. *Cambridge Archaeological Journal* 11: 5–16.

Shennan, S. & Steele, J. (1999). Cultural learning in hominids: a behavioural ecological approach. In: H. Box & K. Gibson (eds) *Mammalian social learning*, pp. 367–388. Cambridge: Cambridge University Press.

Shultz, S. & Dunbar, R. I. M. (2007). Both social and ecological factors predict ungulate brain size. *Proceedings of the Royal Society (Biology)* 273: 207–215.

Steinbeck, J. (1997). *Travels with Charley.* London: Penguin Classics.

Stout, D. (2002). Skill and cognition in stone tool production: an ethnographic case study from Irian Jaya. *Current Anthropology* 5: 693–722

Stout, D. & Chaminade, T. (2006) The evolutionary neuroscience of tool making. *Neuropsychologia* 44: 1999–2006.

Szathmáry, E. & Számadó, S. (2008). Language: a social history of words. *Science* 456: 40–41.

Texier, J.-P. (1996). Evolution and diversity in flaking techniques and methods in the Palaeolithic. In: C. Andreoni, C. Giunchi, C. Petetto & I. Zavatti (eds) *Proceedings of the XIIIth Congress of the International Union of Pre- and Proto-historic Sciences*, pp. 1247–1253. Forlì: ABACO Edizioni.

Thieme, H. (2003). The Lower Palaeolithic sites at Schöningen, Lower Saxony, Germany. In: J. M. Burdukiewicz & A. Ronen (eds) *Lower Palaeolithic small tools in Europe and the Levant*, pp. 9–28. Oxford: British Archaeological Reports S1115.

Tomasello, M. (1999). *The cultural origins of human cognition*. Cambridge, MA: Harvard University Press.

Torrence, R. (2001). Hunter-gatherer technology: macro- and microscale approaches. In: C. Panter-Brick, R. H. Layton & P. Rowley-Conwy (eds) *Hunter-gatherers: an interdisciplinary perspective*, pp. 73–98. Cambridge: Cambridge University Press.

Vanhaeren, M., d'Errico, F., Stringer, C., James, S. L., Todd, J. A. & Mienis, H. K. (2006). Middle Paleolithic shell beads in Israel and Algeria. *Science* 312: 785–788.

Van Peer, P., Rots, V. & Vroomans, J.-M. (2004). A story of colourful diggers and grinders: the Sangoan and Lupemban at site 8-B-11, Sai Island, Northern Sudan. *Before Farming: the archaeology and anthropology of hunter-gatherers* 3(1): 139–166.

van Schaik, C. P. & Pradham, G. R. (2003). A model for tool-use traditions in primates: implications for the coevolution of culture and cognition. *Journal of Human Evolution* 44: 645–664.

Villa, P. (1991). Middle Pleistocene prehistory in southwestern Europe: the state of our knowledge and ignorance. *Journal of Anthropological Research* 47: 193–217.

Villa, P., Soressi, M., Henshilwood, C. S. & Mourre, V. (2008). The Still Bay points of Blombos Cave (South Africa). *Journal of Human Evolution* 36: 441–460.

White, M. & Ashton, N. (2003). Lower Palaeolithic core technology and the origins of the Levallois method in north-western Europe. *Current Anthropology* 44: 598–609.

White, T. D., Asfaw, B., DeGusta, D., Gilbert, H., Richards, G. D., Suwa, G. et al. (2003). Pleistocene *Homo sapiens* from Middle Awash, Ethiopia. *Nature* 432: 742–747.

Whiten, A., Goodall, J., McGrew, W. C., Nishidas, T., Reynolds, V., Sugiyama, Y. et al. (1999). Cultures in chimpanzees. *Nature* 399: 682–685.

Wynn, T. & Coolidge, F. L. (2003). The role of working memory in the evolution of managed foraging. *Before farming: the archaeology and anthropology of hunter-gatherers* 3(1): 68–83.

19

The Archaeology of Group Size

MATT GROVE

THE POINT OF DEPARTURE for the current chapter is Aiello and Dunbar's work (1993) on evolutionary trends in group size, which used relationships between group size and brain size in extant primates in combination with data on endocranial capacities of fossil hominins to predict prehistoric group sizes. The research reported here aims to provide an independent test of those predictions using a quite different set of data: the spatial distribution of sites and artefacts in the archaeological record. To this end, a brief review of the relevant archaeological literature is undertaken, culminating in the proposal of a new methodology for the calculation of group sizes based on archaeological site distributions. Four case studies are employed to provide a temporal trajectory of group size, and this is discussed with reference to the wider behavioural implications of the social brain hypothesis.

LAND USE IN ARCHAEOLOGY

The study of archaeological site distributions and land use patterns has a long and illustrious history in archaeology, particularly with regard to Early Stone Age sites in Africa. The central motivation of such models is to explain the association of stone tools and faunal remains in varying concentrations and at various localities in landscapes inhabited by prehistoric foragers. Thus Isaac suggested that those sites containing abundant evidence of both stone tools and animal bones might be described as 'occupation floors or campsites' (1971, 281). Such a description drew direct parallels between the site typology established by Mary Leakey at Olduvai (1971, 258) and hunter-gatherer camps known from the increasing body of ethnographic data emerging from collaborative efforts such as the 'Man the Hunter' symposium (Lee & DeVore 1968). These parallels were elaborated through the site typology developed at Koobi Fora (Isaac

Proceedings of the British Academy **158**, 391–411. © The British Academy 2010.

& Harris 1978), as well as through a series of publications in which Isaac argued that formal similarities between larger Oldowan concentrations and the increasingly well-documented campsites of the !Kung (e.g. papers in Lee & DeVore 1976) implied equivalent similarities in social behaviour.

The data available on these African 'bushmen' in particular led Isaac to observe that 'in human social groupings there exists at any time what can be called a focus in space, or "home base", such that individuals can move independently over the surrounding terrain and yet join up again' (1978, 292). Such foci are an integral feature of modern hunter-gatherer space use, yet have no parallel in chimpanzee groups; Isaac's conclusion, therefore, was that certain key elements of this derived human adaptive strategy were already present by a little after 2 million years ago. However, the social innovations Isaac initially sought to associate with home bases left little archaeological evidence, and provided an easy point of weakness for those wishing to undermine the hypothesis. Binford's early, abrasive and comprehensive critique (1981, 1984) argued that the reconstructions of hominin behaviour posited by Isaac and colleagues amounted to no more than an 'impoverished projection into the past' of modern ethnographic data (1981, 295). Binford ultimately produced a model that saw the locations of repeatedly used locales as directly deter-mined by the local ecology. According to the 'routed foraging model' (1984), cultural material would inevitably build up around lithic outcrops, waterholes, and naturally defended or sheltered places. Thus the locations of key archaeological sites were not chosen by hominin groups as places to which they would transport materials; rather, they were a response to limiting resources.

The home base and routed foraging models are two of many that seek to explain concentrations of lithic and faunal remains in the archaeolog-ical record. Both are essentially qualitative; they aim to define an over-arching strategy rather than specific aspects of forager demography or land use. The location and composition of sites is due to the confluence of generic factors such as the availability of lithics, the movements of game, and the pressures of competing with rival carnivores. Though Isaac's early (and heavily criticized) conception of the home base (e.g. Isaac 1978) carries clear social implications, these are at the level of the family rather than the general group or population. It was also precisely these implications that drew the greatest number of critics; subsequent hypotheses tended to focus less on social reconstruction and more on explicitly testable aspects of the archaeology. In particular, the develop-ment of dichotomized debates regarding hunting and scavenging or natural and cultural formation processes moved the archaeology of land use towards actualistic and experimental research, and away from synthetic treatments at the scale relevant to the current chapter.

GROUP SIZE AND RANGE AREA

While the history of land use studies in archaeology has focused on schematic models based around the qualitative reconstruction of subsistence practices, efforts to reconstruct population sizes and range areas have depended upon more quantitative approaches. Naroll (1962) suggested that population size might be calculated by reference to the total size of the dwelling floors of a settlement, and proposed that dividing this area (in square metres) by approximately 10 would provide a preliminary estimate (Figure 19.1 (A)). Later, LeBlanc (1971), using a larger dataset, cautioned against applying Naroll's scheme too readily due to the colossal confidence limits operating around his mean estimates. Wiessner (1974) was the first anthropologist to suggest the application of allometric scaling to this problem; based on Nordbeck's work on the growth of towns in urban Sweden (Nordbeck 1971) rather than upon biological data, she argued that hunter-gatherer camps are constrained to grow in a specific way around a central space. In contrast to Naroll's log-linear correlation, Wiessner's results indicated that, due to the central space, the space *per person* increases with the size of the group (Figure 19.1 (B)). This model was undoubtedly valuable in predicting population sizes of the bushman groups Wiessner was studying; however, it is hard to generalize to other populations, particularly those for whom hearth and hut structures are not known.

Other notable attempts to reconstruct generic demographic aspects of hominin populations include those of Boaz (1970), Martin (1981), and Antón and colleagues (2002). Boaz (1970) based his analysis on the density of hominin remains relative to those of other fauna in excavated assemblages; by reference to modern faunal assemblages from analogous habitats, he postulated hominin population densities of between 0.001 and 2.480 individuals per square kilometre. Martin (1981) used an existing correlation between mammalian body weight and home range in a mammalian sample to predict home ranges of *Australopithecus afarensis* at between 62 and 107,523 ha and *Paranthropus boisei* at between 130 and 287,819 ha, where the lower and upper estimates are respectively dependent upon assumptions of herbivory and carnivory (the assumption of

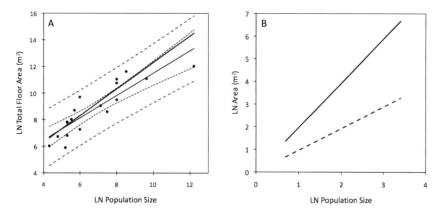

Figure 19.1. Two attempts to relate population size to the area of house floors or settlements. (A) shows the relationship found by Naroll (1962) among 18 indigenous societies from regions as diverse as North and South America, Oceania, Africa and Eurasia, from which he suggests that floor area in square metres is generally equivalent to approximately population size multiplied by 10. The thin black line represents the regression, the thick black line the relationship suggested by Naroll; dotted and dashed lines represent the confidence intervals for estimation and prediction, respectively. Note that Naroll's suggested relationship falls within the 95 per cent confidence limits for estimation throughout the range, but will under-estimate population sizes based on larger total floor areas. (B) shows the relationship found by Wiessner (1974; original data unavailable). Wiessner's allometric line, based on 16 !Kung hunter-gatherer camps, suggests a relationship of the form area $= \alpha \times$ population$^{\beta}$, with beta equal to approximately two. An important implication of this is that floor area per individual increases with the size of the settlement (dashed line), in contrast to the constant ratio implied by Naroll's analysis.

omnivory would suggest estimates between these values). Antón and colleagues (2002) again employed a correlation between range area and body weight, with a sample restricted to the primates. Their results are dubious, however, on the grounds that perfectly valid 'outliers' were excluded from the analysis, as well as the fact that six modern human groups considerably skew the slope of a regression line otherwise plotted through single-species averages. In addition to these specific weaknesses, each of these authors succeeds only in producing abstract estimates of range area or population density that are unrelated either to the group context (of what it is parsimonious to assume are social species) or to the archaeological record.

Gamble and Steele (1999) are the only previous researchers to have attempted the calculation of hominin range areas as they relate directly to archaeological sites. They employed lithic transport distances from various sources to the Lower Palaeolithic site of Caune de l'Arago and the Early Middle Palaeolithic site of Grotte Vaufrey to establish range areas via the minimum convex polygon (MCP) method, estimating ranges of 976 and 2,025 sq km, respectively (Gamble & Steele 1999, 400). While the MCP produces a flat distribution with no internal differentiation with which to interpret the structure of movements within the range, this paper represents a substantial advance relative to previous efforts, particularly in comparing sites from two different phases of the Palaeolithic.

Recent work by Bocquet-Appel and colleagues (e.g. 2005) takes a broader perspective. Using space-time densities of western European archaeological sites, these researchers attempt to reconstruct meta-population sizes over the course of several chrono-typological phases of the Upper Palaeolithic. They predict a long-term demographic trend of relative stability from the Aurignacian through the Gravettian, and into the last glacial maximum, with a population of 4,000–6,000, followed by a dramatic increase in numbers to approximately 29,000 during the late glacial (Bocquet-Appel et al. 2005, 1664). This work represents an exceptionally valuable contribution to the study of Palaeolithic population dynamics, and the temporal trend predicted is broadly mirrored by the results given below.

THE STRUCTURE OF THE ARCHAEOLOGICAL RECORD

The research surveyed above has assessed group sizes, population densities and land use patterns at scales from the single individual to the meta-population using both qualitative and quantitative methods. However, with the exceptions of Gamble and Steele (1999) at the level of the single site, and Bocquet-Appel and colleagues (2005) at the meta-population scale, none of these various estimates have been related to the underlying archaeology. Furthermore, without exception, the basic biology of the hominins responsible for the material has not been factored into equations that seek to reconstruct land use. Archaeologists need to analyse material, both archaeological and skeletal, at the level at which the 'cognitive group' might operate: I argue here that the relevant scale is neither that of single sites nor continental surveys, but clusters of sites clearly delimited by appropriate geography, chronology and typology. Archaeologists need to approach the issue of scale with as much care as ecologists (e.g. Levin 1992); only then can we begin to examine what might be meaningful groups as represented in the archaeological record.

The issue of scale in archaeology is intimately related to the notion of the site as the focus for excavation; historically, this has often blinded researchers to the importance of regional ecological context. The development of site catchment analysis in the early 1970s was a reaction to this problem, with researchers beginning to examine the wider contexts of individual sites and the extent to which they might have overlapped both temporally and spatially (e.g. Vita-Finzi and Higgs 1970). This framework fed into the 'off-site' approach of the late 1970s and early 1980s, and prompted insights such as that of Dunnell and Dancey, that 'the archaeological record is most usefully conceived as a more or less continuous distribution of artefacts over the land surface, with highly variable density characteristics' (1983, 272). The themes of non-site archaeology are particularly relevant to the Palaeolithic record and to the questions addressed here. That the landscape rather than the site may be the most viable unit of analysis in reconstructions of prehistoric land use is implicit in Isaac's 'scatters and patches' approach (Isaac 1981; Isaac et al. 1981), which recognized that the vast majority of artefacts in the East Turkana region of East Africa occurred outside the densest areas of archaeology that were the focus of collection and excavation (Isaac et al. 1981, 263).

Elsewhere, Foley (1981) considers the effects of ecological variables such as resource distribution and topography on home range size and structure, and argues that regional scale survey is the proper way to capture the essence of settlement systems. He suggests that, in contrast to the traditional approach in which spatial resolution is sacrificed for the benefit of tight stratigraphic sequences from single sites, 'it is equally valid to obtain superior spatial information about prehistoric adaptation at the cost of lessened chronological resolution' (Foley 1981, 9). This inversion of the traditional view is particularly appropriate, he argues, given 'the fundamental importance of spatial patterning in ecology, and the fact that long term trends may be of greater significance to the prehistorian than the understanding of a few short events' (Foley 1981, 9). It is the view promoted here that the examination of spatio-temporally broad datasets is precisely the technique that will bring us closer to an understanding of smaller-scale phenomena. Put simply, patterns emerge at larger scales that would have been impossible to detect in a more focused study; though these patterns may be generic, they provide new lines of enquiry for the study of long-term trends in the record. Below I outline a case study demonstrating how one such trend, that of changes in hominin group size, might be illuminated by such an approach.

A QUANTITATIVE APPROACH TO THE RECORD

The data used in the analyses summarized here are the spatial distributions of archaeological sites grouped by geography (i.e. spatial proximity), dating (i.e. chronological proximity), geology (i.e. stratigraphic
proximity) and lithic typology. The numbers of sites in each group studied here may well be affected by future research efforts; however, as the
model employed corrects for sample sizes during preliminary analyses the
results presented here are robust. The procedure, presented formally in
Grove (2008a, 81–99), involves the following stages:

(1) The location of each individual site in a group is input as (x,y)
coordinates, measured from an arbitrary but consistent origin to
the south-west of the group. From these coordinates the distance
from each site to every other is measured; these distances are then
summed and divided by the number of sites N to derive a measure
of the mean interpoint distance (MID; see Bonetti and Pagano
2005).

(2) The MID forms the radius of a circle which is centred over each
site in turn. The number of sites other than the focal site falling
within each circle is counted; the resulting counts of all circles are
summed and divided by N to arrive at the sites per area (SPA)
count. Estimated range area (RA) is then calculated as $(N \div SPA)$
$\times \pi MID^2$.

(3) Next, estimated population density (PD) for the relevant hominin(s)
(i.e. the species thought to be responsible for the archaeology) is calculated from a regression of population density on body mass
(Damuth 1981). The body mass estimates for the hominins are taken
from McHenry (1996). Group sizes are then calculated as $RA \times PD$.
Where more than one hominin could be responsible for the archaeology, multiple estimates can be produced.

(4) Finally, the RA estimate is fitted to the site distribution from which
it was estimated via Gaussian kernel density estimation (Baxter et
al. 1997) so that the summed area within the outer contour boundary is equal to RA.

This procedure is summarized graphically in Figure 19.2.

The fact that the model requires only distributional data means that it
can be applied to any number of well-studied archaeological regions: provided that individual sites are mapped, and that their contemporaneity
can be established within a suitable archaeo-geological framework, an

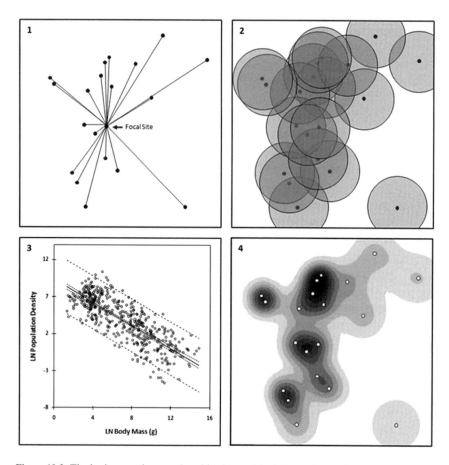

Figure 19.2. The basic procedure employed in the model of Grove (2008a) for the estimation of group size, range area, and land use. (1) The distances from a focal site to each of the other sites is measured; this is repeated for each individual site, whereupon the mean of these inter-site distances is calculated. (2) The mean inter-site distance (*MID*) forms the radius of a circle which is centred over each site in turn. The number of other sites falling within each circle is counted, and the average is taken across circles to form the sites per area count (*SPA*). The estimated range area (*RA*) is then $(N \div SPA) \times \pi MID^2$ where N is the total number of sites. (3) Using a regression of population density on body mass (Damuth 1981), hominin population densities (*PD*) are calculated from the body mass estimates of McHenry (1996). Group sizes are then calculated as simply $RA \times PD$. (4) Finally, the *RA* estimate is fitted to the site distribution via Gaussian kernel density estimation.

analysis at the landscape scale can be undertaken. Output can be directly related to the sites on which the estimates are based: contrary to the 'floating estimates' produced by most previous researchers, reconstructions of land use intensity can be mapped directly onto existing site plans to provide an intuitive picture of ranging patterns. Tests of the model with modern ethnoarchaeological hunter-gatherer data have proven the accuracy of both the group size and range area estimates, with observed values falling within the 95 per cent confidence intervals of predicted values in all cases (Grove 2008a, 2008b). In addition, reconstructed land use intensity contours accord well with ranging patterns described in the primary literature (e.g. Yellen 1977).

The foremost advantage of the method, however, is that it relates directly to the structure of the archaeological record. Much of the land use literature surveyed above stresses the fact that a great deal of archaeological material exists outside the confines of identified sites (e.g. Dunnell & Dancey 1983; Isaac 1981; Isaac et al. 1981). The basic data in most site reports, however, do not allow for the reconstruction of relationships between sites or for the estimation of the 'scatters between the patches'. Kernel density estimation provides direct information about probable clustering and densities of activity (and therefore material) between identified sites, providing estimates of land use that are consistent with our understandings of the spatial distributions of archaeological materials.

In order to provide a trajectory of group size evolution comparable to that resulting from the analyses of Aiello and Dunbar (1993), four thoroughly investigated and well documented datasets were chosen at suitable intervals throughout a time period ranging from 1.75 million years until 14,000 years ago. Each of these datasets represents a series of penecontemporaneous archaeological sites related to one another via lithic technology and common geology. The datasets presented here were selected because they represent spatially and temporally constrained clusters distinct from areas of the surrounding landscape. Though the temporal divisions are necessarily wider as one looks further back into the record, the following case studies can be shown to be broadly comparable in most respects.

Olduvai Gorge

Detailed discussions of the archaeology and palaeoanthropology of the four regions are beyond the scope of this chapter (see Grove 2008a and the primary literature referenced below); however, it is useful at this point to engage in a brief survey of the most salient aspects. Locations, ages, industrial affiliations and key references for the four regions are summarized in Table 19.1. The first area to be considered is that of Olduvai Gorge, perhaps the most extensively investigated repository of Early

Stone Age (ESA) archaeology (e.g. Leakey 1971; Potts 1988). The gorge runs through the Serengeti Plain in northern Tanzania, near the western margin of the Eastern Rift Valley. The sites of interest to the current study are those occurring in Beds I and II: chronological reconstructions suggest that Bed I dates to between 1.87 and 1.75 million years ago, while Bed II was laid down between 1.75 and 1.27 million years ago. In order to restrict the sample, and to control for broad changes in behaviour during this period, the sites of Beds I and II are here divided into those that have produced Oldowan tools and those that have yielded material of Acheulean type. Sites yielding Oldowan and Acheulean material (in fact, most sites) are included in both samples. As many as five hominin species have been linked to the archaeology: *Australopithecus boisei*, *Homo rudolfensis*, *Homo habilis*, *Homo ergaster* and *Homo erectus*. Though these species are regarded as separate here, many researchers would support a *sensu lato* habiline subset that includes a number of specimens (e.g. KNM-ER 1813) previously assigned to *H. rudolfensis*; in addition, most would agree that *H. ergaster* is synonymous with 'early African *H. erectus*'. More importantly for the following discussions, however, is the ordering of body masses, from which it is clear that *H. erectus* and *H. ergaster* are considerably heavier than *H. habilis sensu stricto* and *A. boisei*, with *H. rudolfensis* intermediate depending upon the specimens one admits to the taxon.

The Oldowan, which can be dated to between 2.6 and 1.5 Ma in Africa, is often characterized as an 'expedient technology' aimed at providing hominins with quick access to cutting edges (e.g. Roche et al. 1999). It is further argued by some that the tool forms identified by archaeologists would not have been regarded as distinct types by their hominin makers (e.g. Toth 1985). Suffice to say that most forms are variably reduced cobbles and pebbles, though hammerstones and anvils, light-

Table 19.1. Locations, ages, industrial affiliations and key references for the sites discussed in the text

Area	Latitude	Longitude	Ages (Ma)	Industry	Reference
Olduvai	-2°58'	35°22'	1.500–1.870	Oldowan	Leakey 1971
			1.270–1.500	Acheulean	Leakey 1971
Koobi Fora	3°57'	36°13'	1.390–1.880	KBS / Karari	Isaac & Harris 1997
Boxgrove	50°51'	–0°43'	0.478–0.524	Acheulean	Roberts & Parfitt 1999
Paris Basin	49°19'	2°43'	0.115–0.13	Magdalenian	Audouze 1987

duty scrapers, awls and some smaller polyhedrons indicate a greater flexibility than is often perceived. The Acheulean, characterized by that quintessential *fossil directeur* the hand-axe, is preceded at Olduvai by the Developed Oldowan A (DOA), which dates to between 1.65 and 1.53 million years ago (Kimura 2002; Leakey & Roe 1994). The subsequent Developed Oldowan B (DOB) dates to between 1.53 and 1.20 million years ago, and is thus at least partly contemporary with the Acheulean. The Acheulean itself first appears shortly after 1.5 million years ago at Olduvai and extends past the upper limits of Bed II; however, for present purposes the Olduvai sample is divided into an Oldowan (including DOA) sample, and an Acheulean sample which includes contemporary DOB assemblages and is truncated at 1.27 million years ago.

Koobi Fora

While the Olduvai material is split into two chrono-typological phases in an attempt to detect any shift in group size and land use strategies, the material from the second region surveyed, Koobi Fora, is viewed as a single block in order to examine the possibility of identifying the long periods of stasis often discussed by Palaeolithic archaeologists. The sites considered in this second case study form part of the archaeological record of the Lake Turkana Basin, the Plio-Pleistocene strata of which are collectively known as the Omo Group. Lake Turkana, located to the north-east of Kenya and abutting the border with Ethiopia, has long been a focus of investigation for palaeoanthropologists. The sites analysed are located on the Karari Ridge, the densest area of archaeology in the East Turkana region, and are situated geologically within the KBS and Okote members. Recent dating of these deposits (McDougall & Brown 2006) has shown that the KBS member dates to between approximately 1.88 and 1.64 million years, and the Okote between around 1.64 and 1.39 Ma. The industries of the KBS member and the subsequent Karari industry may be distinct—the tools of the KBS member are probably regional variant of the Oldowan (Isaac and Harris 1997) while the Karari industry, although similar to the DOA in raw material and expedient flaking, is differentiated by the Karari scraper (thought to be a culturally transmitted regional facies; Isaac and Harris 1997). Nevertheless, the sites attributed to the KBS and Karari industries are analysed together in the current sample as a counterpoint to the division created within the Olduvai group.

Boxgrove

The third group of sites is dated to approximately a million years after those from Olduvai and Koobi Fora, and is found in southern Britain. Whilst still culturally Acheulean, the Lower Palaeolithic of Boxgrove and its environs allows assessment of the changes that occur between the earliest appearance of the industry in Africa and the much later European component. The quarry at Amey's Eartham Pit in Boxgrove, West Sussex, lies some 12 km north of the current shoreline of the English Channel and is the most spectacular of a series of contemporaneous sites located geologically along the Goodwood-Slindon raised beach (Roberts 1986; Roberts et al. 1997), including major finds from the Lavant area as well as from the geological type site at Slindon, which have been dated on the basis of mammalian biostratigraphy to OIS13, a temperate period equivalent to the end of the British Cromerian (Dutch Cromerian IV) and lasting almost 50,000 years from 524 to 478 ka. In particular, the stratigraphic level of interest here is Unit 4c. Based on comparisons with the IJsselmer Polder soil and a pedological sequence, MacPhail argues that 'the character of Unit 4c as a whole implies that it represents only a short period of soil ripening and human occupation, perhaps as little as 10–20 years' (1999, 130). Thus Boxgrove and the Lower Palaeolithic of the Sussex Downs more generally gives us an ideal opportunity to examine a narrow temporal window onto hominin life during the formation of a geographically widely identified palaeosol. In terms of the hominins responsible for these sites, Boxgrove has yielded two teeth and a tibia of *Homo heidelbergensis*, the only species to have been as far north as Britain during the relevant period.

The Paris Basin

Finally, the fourth case study employed here examines a series of sites attributed to the Upper Magdalenian of the Paris Basin. The sites in question date to between 13 and 11.5 ka, and include the remarkably well preserved archaeological assemblages of Pincevent and Verberie. The sites employed here are more widely spaced than those considered during earlier periods, but are clearly related via their chronology and lithic records. It is possible that, during this period, prehistoric hunters and gatherers were simply more mobile than at any previous phase in the Palaeolithic, as they tracked caribou herds on their annual migrations (e.g. Enloe 2001). The hominin material from these sites is unequivocally that of *Homo sapiens*.

DISCUSSION: ARCHAEOLOGY AND THE
EVOLUTION OF GROUP SIZE

The results of the analyses are first discussed with regard to the general temporal trajectory; following this, certain more specific points of interest are highlighted. The group sizes predicted by Grove (2008a), based on the procedure explained above and shown schematically in Figure 19.2, are graphed against age in Figure 19.3 (solid line). As can be seen, the general trend is one of group size increase, which begins slowly and gathers considerable pace as it approaches the Upper Palaeolithic. It should be noted that, though all sites contribute equally to the LSR (least squares regression) trajectory described, Koobi Fora sits slightly above the line, with Boxgrove slightly below it. The former finding could be due to the fact that Koobi Fora is regarded here as a monolithic rather than a phased sample, whilst the latter finding could be due to the effect of the very large group sizes predicted for the Paris Basin sample; a trajectory that omits the Paris Basin sample is shown by the dotted line in Figure 19.3. This second trajectory implies a much slower increase in group size over the period surveyed, with Magdalenian group sizes an order of magnitude smaller than the Paris Basin dataset suggests. A possible reason for this contradiction lies in the high levels of mobility practised by Magdalenian hunter-gatherers during the hunting of migratory herds. Put simply, a group utilizing a series of sites sequentially during a seasonal round would look very similar archaeologically to a group that was large enough to occupy all those sites simultaneously. There is, in addition, considerable archaeological support for high seasonal mobility in the Magdalenian based on the presence of antler from different (and exclusive) stages of the annual cycle at Pincevent, Verberie and Ville-Saint-Jacques (Enloe & David 1997), and from the transport of materials within the Paris Basin. The exotic flint at Etiolles was sourced from at least four separate locations (Olive & Taborin 2002), while Mauger (1994) has identified flint from 80 km away. Taborin (1993) reports that shells used as ornaments were sometimes transported over distances as far as 400 km during this period, though the extent to which this reflects mobility as opposed to trade is unknown.

That Boxgrove sits below the line is of particular interest with respect to the social brain hypothesis and particularly the group size trajectory predicted by Aiello and Dunbar (1993), which suggests that the period represented here by Boxgrove, at about half a million years ago, marks something of a threshold in the evolution of group size; a threshold

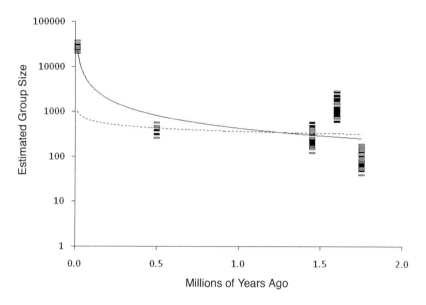

Figure 19.3. Group sizes suggested by the distribution of archaeological sites in the four regions surveyed, based on Grove (2008a). Estimates are based on the procedure outlined in Figure 19.2, where the estimated group size of a particular species during a given spatio-temporal window is a product of that species' body mass and population density combined with the spatial extent and density of archaeological sites. The solid and dashed lines show the predicted group size trajectories through time when the Paris Basin estimates are included and excluded, respectively. Separate data points for each date are due to the calculation of up to 36 estimates per date based on various permutations of (a) the hominin presumed responsible for the record and (b) the 95 per cent confidence intervals of both the body mass estimation and population density estimation regressions. Trajectories are fitted to averages per date in both cases.

which, furthermore, has been associated with the origins of language via the 'vocal grooming' hypothesis (e.g. Dunbar 2003). The current study, however, suggests that Boxgrove pre-dates the major shift in group size, which occurs at some as yet unspecified point prior to the Magdalenian. The trajectories of Figure 19.3 are informative on this point, as both suggest late thresholds perhaps coincident with the speciation of modern *Homo sapiens* at approximately 200 ka. This matter cannot be resolved by the current analyses, but the notion of a Middle Stone Age origin for behavioural modernity, encompassing the widespread appearance of symbolism, art and language, is attested by a growing body of African archaeological evidence (McBrearty & Brooks 2000). Perhaps the most informative way of advancing this research therefore would be to prioritize the examination of case studies dating to approximately a quarter of

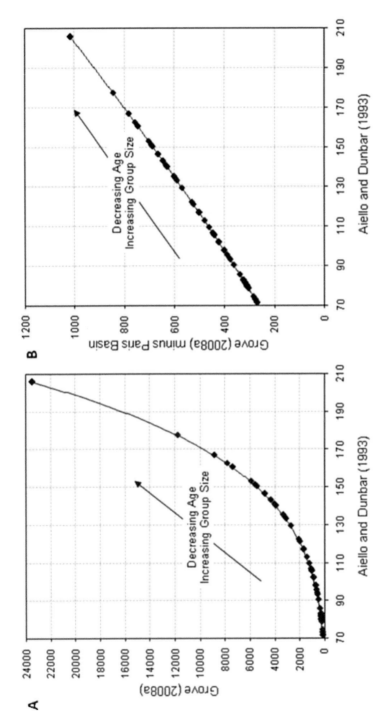

Figure 19.4. Comparison between the group sizes predicted by Aiello and Dunbar (1993) and Grove (2008a). Each point represents a particular age for which equations derived from the two datasets are applied; where possible, these dates are those identified for the specimens included in the Aiello and Dunbar (1993) sample. (A) shows the comparison with the Paris Basin sample included, (B) with it excluded. This difference shifts the relationship from a power law to a linear ratio; see text for further discussion.

a million years ago, thus bisecting the Boxgrove and Paris Basin results and, importantly, pre-dating the proposed date of speciation.

When compared to the group sizes estimated by Aiello and Dunbar (1993), those presented here follow a similar trajectory in terms of scale, but are consistently considerably larger. This comparison is made explicit in Figure 19.4a, where it is shown that the average estimate produced in the study of Grove (2008a) is equivalent to the average estimate of Aiello and Dunbar (1993) raised to the fourth power. Thus, while the absolute differences between the trajectories are small during earlier periods, they become considerably larger as we approach the present. Interestingly, this scaling relationship shifts from a power law to a linear ratio when the Paris Basin sample is omitted (Figure 19.4b), raising questions about the demographic shift evidenced in the late Upper Palaeolithic (Bocquet-Appel et al. 2005).

With reference to previous work on hunter-gatherer social organization and demography (e.g. Birdsell 1958), Gamble (1998) has defined groups of approximately 5, 20, 100–400 and 2,000–2,500 individuals as intimate, effective, extended and global networks respectively. The estimates presented here for all groups prior to the Upper Palaeolithic sit within or just above the level of the extended network, which itself encompasses the 150 persons comprising the modern human cognitive group (Aiello & Dunbar 1993). The importance of these values lies in their relevance to the 'stretching of social systems across space and time' (Gamble 1998, 442) identified via numerous lines of archaeological evidence to have occurred during the chronological progression of the Palaeolithic. Gamble (1998) envisages the emergence of a social landscape between 100,000 and 60,000 years ago, catalysed by the development and elaboration of the extended network and indexed by the appearance of abundant symbolic resources and greater evidence for wide-ranging transport of lithics. It may therefore be the case that the archaeological landscape surveyed during the Upper Magdalenian is of a quite different character from that manifest at Boxgrove and during earlier periods.

The mechanism behind this difference is of central importance to the evolution of human social structure. In particular, one must ask whether the intimate, effective and extended networks of the Lower Palaeolithic were each extended so as to encompass a greater spatial and demographic reach, or whether, by contrast, the global network was created as a novel social tier, leaving the pre-existing lower tiers unchanged. The nested structure of human social systems has been subject to study in both hunter-gatherer and Western populations (Hamilton et al. 2007; Zhou et al. 2005), with the finding that group sizes conform to a discrete, self-similar hierarchy. These results suggest a basic structuring principle in human populations whereby groups of preferred size are organized in a geometric series, and further suggest that, in the context of the current results, upper tiers of the hierarchy are formed by the periodic aggregation of lower-level tiers. Such aggregations occur on seasonal and annual scales among hunter-gatherers today, and may have been a signature of societal development over evolutionary time. The hypothesis that modern periodic population dynamics recapitulate a phylogenetic pattern characterized by the addition of outer grouping tiers over the course of hominin evolution is one that requires considerable further development and examination, but is consistent with the analyses presented in the current chapter.

The social brain hypothesis establishes a series of nested group sizes that correspond at least qualitatively to those presented by Gamble (1998), and demonstrate a close coherence with those that emerge time and again from the ethnographic and archaeological literature of hunter-gatherer societies (see Barnard ch. 12 this volume). Though precedence is often given to 'Dunbar's Number' of 150, the hypothesis suggests levels of 5, 15, 50, 150, 500 and so on (see Roberts ch. 6 this volume). Of this series, the 'active network' of 150 and the 'megaband' of 500 are of particular relevance to the current research, and highlight an interesting difference between the results based on primatological relationships and those emerging from the archaeology. While Dunbar's early development of the hypothesis (1992, 1993) focused on primatological analogues that ultimately gave rise to the prediction of a group size of 150 for *Homo sapiens* (Aiello & Dunbar 1993), the current study finds group sizes that are consistently larger. Thus it appears that, during the Lower Palaeolithic, the groups of archaeological sites surveyed correspond to those utilized by the megaband rather than the active network. This discrepancy between the primatological data at the core of the hypothesis and the archaeological data that best inform on the evolution of hominin grouping patterns clearly suggests that, by the time of the first appearance of our genus, hominin groups had already added a supplementary tier of social grouping beyond that found in extant primates.

The incremental addition of grouping tiers combined with general increases in population size and density to produce a marked demographic shift by the time of the Upper Palaeolithic. This finding is commensurate not only with Gamble's (1998) scenario concerning the emergence of the global network but also with research suggesting that the movement of lithic raw materials had increased substantially by the time of the Upper Palaeolithic (Féblot-Augustins 1997). It was noted above that the population estimates produced here for the Paris Basin sample could be at least partly the result of greater mobility practised by the reindeer hunters of this period. While it is always difficult to distinguish archaeologically between mobility and trade as causes of raw material movement, the proliferation of long-distance material transfers evidenced during the Upper Palaeolithic has been interpreted by Marwick (2003) as indicative of the flow of both materials and information through extensive interpersonal networks that pervade the landscape by this time. Population increases coupled with greater mobility would undoubtedly have enhanced the ability of hunter-gatherer groups to amass valuable ecological and social information.

The inter-group knowledge flow and increasingly elaborate social environment provided by the development of the global network emerged as a result of, and concomitantly acted as a stimulus to, the socio-cognitive evolution of *Homo sapiens*. The importance of sophisticated local socialization processes during ontogeny (Grove & Coward 2008) was paralleled by the increasingly distributed nature of the global social environment from which an individual's relations were drawn. Via the method outlined above, the archaeological evidence—too often neglected in discussions of human cognitive evolution—can be employed in the reconstruction of prehistoric group sizes and social interactions. Archaeology provides the only source of data with sufficient time depth to examine the behavioural implications of the social brain hypothesis from an evolutionary perspective; it is thus vital that such studies are extended.

Note. The models discussed in this chapter were developed during the course of my PhD research; I would like to thank Clive Gamble for his insightful and encouraging supervision. Fiona Coward, Clive Gamble and Robin Dunbar provided comments on an earlier draft of this chapter. This research is funded by the British Academy Centenary Research Project, 'Lucy to Language: The Archaeology of the Social Brain'.

REFERENCES

Aiello, L. C. & Dunbar, R. I. M. (1993). Neocortex size, group-size, and the evolution of language. *Current Anthropology* 34: 184–193.
Anton, S. C., Leonard, W. R. & Robertson, M. L. (2002). An ecomorphological model of the initial hominid dispersal from Africa. *Journal of Human Evolution* 43: 773–785.

Audouze, F. (1987). The Paris Basin in Magdalenian times. In O. Soffer (ed.) *The Pleistocene old world: regional perspectives*, pp. 183–199. London: Plenum Press.

Baxter, M. J., Beardah, C. C. & Wright, R. V. S. (1997). Some archaeological applications of kernel density estimates. *Journal of Archaeological Science* 24: 347–354.

Binford, L. R. (1981). *Bones: ancient men and modern myths*. New York: Academic Press.

Binford, L. R. (1984). *Faunal remains from Klasies river mouth*. New York: Academic Press.

Birdsell, J. (1958). On population structure in generalized hunting and collecting populations. *Evolution* 12: 189–205.

Boaz, N. T. (1970). Early hominid population densities—new estimates. *Science* 206: 592–595.

Bocquet-Appel, J. P., Demars, P. Y., Noiret, L. & D. Dobrowsky (2005). Estimates of Upper Palaeolithic meta-population size in Europe from archaeological data. *Journal of Archaeological Science* 32: 1656–1668.

Bonetti, M. & Pagano, M. (2005). The interpoint distance distribution as a descriptor of point patterns, with an application to spatial disease clustering. *Statistics in Medicine* 24: 753–773.

Damuth, J. (1981). Population-density and body size in mammals. *Nature* 290: 699–700.

Dunbar, R. I. M. (1992). Neocortex size as a constraint on group-size in primates. *Journal of Human Evolution* 22: 469–493.

Dunbar, R. I. M. (1993). Coevolution of neocortical size, group size and language in humans. *Behavioral and Brain Sciences* 16: 681–735.

Dunbar, R. I. M. (2003). The social brain: mind, language, and society in evolutionary perspective. *Annual Review of Anthropology* 32: 163–181.

Dunnell, R. C. & Dancey, W. S. (1983). The siteless survey: a regional scale data collection strategy. *Advances in Archaeological Method and Theory* 6: 267–287.

Enloe, J. G. (2001). Magdalenian. In P. M. Peregrine & M. Ember (eds) *Encyclopedia of prehistory*, vol. 4: *Europe*, pp. 179–190. London: Kluwer Academic.

Enloe, J. G. & David, F. (1997). Rangifer herd behaviour: seasonality of hunting in the Magdalenian of the Paris Basin. In L. J. Jackson & P. Thacker (eds) *Caribou and reindeer hunters of the northern hemisphere*, pp. 47–63. Aldershot: Avebury Press.

Féblot-Augustins, J. (1997). *La circulation des matières premières au Paléolithique*. Liège: Études et Recherches Archéologiques de l'Université de Liège 75.

Foley, R. A. (1981). A model of regional archaeological structure. *Proceedings of the Prehistoric Society* 47: 1–17.

Gamble, C. S. (1998). Palaeolithic society and the release from proximity: a network approach to intimate relations. *World Archaeology* 29: 426–449.

Gamble, C. S. & Steele, J. (1999). Hominid ranging patterns and dietary strategies. In: H. Ullrich (ed.) *Hominid evolution: lifestyles and survival strategies*, pp. 396–409. Gelsenkirchen: Editions Archaea.

Grove, M. (2008a). The evolution of hominin group size and land use: an archaeological perspective. Unpublished PhD thesis, University of London.

Grove, M. (2008b). Estimating hunter-gatherer group size via spatio-allometric analysis. *PaleoAnthropology* 2008: A10.

Grove, M. & Coward, F. (2008). From individual neurons to social brains. *Cambridge Archaeological Journal* 18: 387–400.

Hamilton, M.W., Milne, B. T., Walker, R. S., Burger, O. & Brown, J. H. (2007). The complex structure of hunter-gatherer social networks. *Proceedings of the Royal Society B* 274: 2195–2202.

Isaac, G. L. (1971). The diet of early man: aspects of archaeological evidence from Lower and Middle Pleistocene sites in East Africa. *World Archaeology* 2: 278–299.

Isaac, G. L. (1978). The food-sharing behaviour of proto-human hominids. In B. Isaac (ed.) *The archaeology of human origins*, pp. 289–311. Cambridge: Cambridge University Press.

Isaac, G. L. (1981). Stone Age visiting cards. In I. Hodder, G. L. Isaac & N. Hammond (eds) *Pattern of the past*, pp. 131–155. Cambridge: Cambridge University Press.

Isaac, G. L. & Harris, J. W. K. (1978). Archaeology. In M. G. Leakey & R. E. Leakey (ed.) *Koobi Fora Research Project*, vol. 1: *The fossil hominids and an introduction to their context*. Oxford: Clarendon Press.

Isaac, G. L. & Harris, J. W. K. (1997). The stone artefact assemblages: a comparative study. In G. L. Isaac (ed.) *Koobi Fora Research Project*, vol. 5: *Plio-Pleistocene archaeology*, pp. 262–362. Oxford: Clarendon Press.

Isaac, G. L., Harris, J. W. K. & Marshall, F. (1981). Small is informative: the application of the study of mini-sites and least-effort criteria in the interpretation of the Early Pleistocene archaeological record at Koobi Fora, Kenya. In B. Isaac (ed.) *The archaeology of human origins*, pp. 258–267. Cambridge: Cambridge University Press.

Kimura, Y. (2002). Examining time trends in the Oldowan technology of Beds I and II, Olduvai Gorge. *Journal of Human Evolution* 43: 291–321.

Leakey, M. D. (1971). *Olduvai Gorge*, vol. 3: *Excavations in Beds I and II, 1960–1963*. Cambridge: Cambridge University Press.

Leakey, M. D. & Roe, D. A. (1994). *Olduvai Gorge*, vol. 5: *Excavations in Beds III, IV, and the Masek Beds*. Cambridge: Cambridge University Press.

LeBlanc, S. (1971). An addition to Naroll's suggested floor area and settlement population relationship. *American Antiquity* 36: 210–211.

Lee, R. B. & DeVore, I. (eds) (1968). *Man the hunter*. New York: Aldine.

Lee, R. B. & DeVore, I. (eds) (1976). *Kalahari hunter-gatherers: studies of the !Kung San and their neighbors*. Cambridge, MA: Harvard University Press.

Levin, S. A. (1992). The problem of pattern and scale in ecology. *Ecology* 72: 1943–1967.

McBrearty, S. & Brooks, A. S. (2000). The revolution that wasn't: a new interpretation of the origin of modern human behavior. *Journal of Human Evolution* 39: 453–563.

McDougall, I. & Brown, F. H. (2006). Precise $^{40}Ar/^{39}Ar$ geochronology for the upper Koobi Fora formation, Lake Turkana, northern Kenya. *Journal of the Geological Society, London* 163: 205–220.

McHenry, H. M. (1996). Sexual dimorphism in fossil hominids and its socioecological implications. In J. Steele & S. Shennan (eds) *The archaeology of human ancestry: power, sex, and tradition*, pp. 91–109. London: Routledge.

MacPhail, R. I. (1999). Sediment micromorphology. In M. B. Roberts & S. A. Parfitt (eds) *Boxgrove: a Middle Pleistocene hominid site at Eartham Quarry, Boxgrove, West Sussex*, pp. 118–149. London: English Heritage.

Martin, R. D. (1981). On extinct hominid population densities. *Journal of Human Evolution* 10: 427–428.

Marwick, B. (2003). Pleistocene exchange networks as evidence for the evolution of language. *Cambridge Archaeological Journal* 13: 67–81.

Mauger, M. (1994). L'approvisionnement en materiaux silicieux au Paléolithique Supérieur. In Y. Taborin (ed.) *Environments et habitats Magdaléniens dans le centre du Bassin Parisien*, pp. 78–93. Paris: Editions de la Maison des Sciences de l'Homme.

Naroll, R. (1962). Floor area and settlement population. *American Antiquity* 27: 587–589.

Nordbeck, S. (1971). Urban allometric growth. *Geographical Analysis B* 53: 54–67.

Olive, M. & Taborin, Y. (2002). Etiolles: a blade production site? In L. E. Fisher & B. V. Eriksen (eds) *Lithic raw material economies in late glacial and early postglacial Europe*, pp. 101–116. Oxford: British Archaeological Reports.

Potts, R. B. (1988). *Early hominid activities at Olduvai*. New York: Aldine de Gruyter.

Roberts, M. B. (1986). Excavation of the Lower Palaeolithic site at Amey's Eartham Pit, Boxgrove, West Sussex: a preliminary report. *Proceedings of the Prehistoric Society* 52: 215–245.

Roberts, M. B. & Parfitt, S. A. (1999). Boxgrove: A Middle Pleistocene hominid site at Eartham Quarry, Boxgrove, West Sussex. London: English Heritage.

Roberts, M. B., Parfitt, S. A., Pope, M. I. & Wenban-Smith, F. F. (1997). Boxgrove, West Sussex: rescue excavations of a Lower Palaeolithic landsurface (Boxgrove Project B, 1989–91). *Proceedings of the Prehistoric Society* 63: 308–358.

Roche, H., Delagnes, A., Brugal, J.-P., Feibel, C., Kibunjia, M., Mourrell, V. et al. (1999). Early hominin stone tool production and technical skill 2.34 million years ago in West Turkana, Kenya. *Nature* 399: 57–60.

Taborin, Y. (1993). *La parure en coquillage de Paléolithique*. Gallia Préhistoire Supplement 29. Paris: Editions CNRS.

Toth, N. (1985). The Oldowan reassessed: a close look at Early Stone Age artefacts. *Journal of Archaeological Science* 12: 101–120.

Vita-Finzi, C., & Higgs, E. S. (1970). Prehistoric economy in the Mount Carmel area of Palestine: site catchment analysis. *Proceedings of the Prehistoric Society* 36: 1–37.

Wiessner, P. (1974). A functional estimate of population from floor area. *American Antiquity* 39: 343–350.

Yellen, J. E. (1977). *Archaeological approaches to the present: models for reconstructing the past*. New York: Academic Press.

Zhou, W.-X., Sornette, D., Hill, R. A. & Dunbar, R. I. M. (2005). Discrete hierarchical organization of social group sizes. *Proceedings of the Royal Society B* 272: 439–444.

20

Fragmenting Hominins and the Presencing of Early Palaeolithic Social Worlds

JOHN CHAPMAN & BISSERKA GAYDARSKA

INTRODUCTION: FROM RUBBISH TO MEANING

IF ANYTHING CHARACTERIZES archaeological remains, it is their fragmentary nature. Whether the fragment in question is the fragment of a pot, a fragment of a house or a part (fragment) of a graveyard, it ultimately leads to the reconstruction of a fragment of our past. It is a surprise, then, that for a very long time that fragments constituted 'rubbish' in archaeology, probably because of 'the commonplace that archaeology is concerned with the rubbish of past generations' (Thomas 1999, 62). This perspective drastically curtailed the potential of archaeologists to construct interesting narratives based on fragments.

Three converging debates in archaeology and sociology set the agenda of a new research perspective—that of the fragmentation premise. The first debate occurred in sociology in the 1970s and was concerned with the cultural definition of rubbish. Here, waste management was closely related to cultural order and the consistent labour of division required to regulate matter that was out of place (Munro 1997). The other two discussions took place within archaeology and have established the basis for most mainstream research in the discipline into the 21st century. The debate over the particularities of site formation started earlier and enjoyed long and exhaustive attention. Encapsulated in a sentence, taphonomic modification and object dispersion are central to our understanding of the archaeological record—not as 'a living assemblage' (e.g. left as it was used in the past) but as shaped by the results of deliberate practices and post-depositional modifications (Schiffer 1987). The other key discourse in archaeology with crucial implications for the fragmentation premise was the post-processual insight into the active role of material

Proceedings of the British Academy **158**, 413–447. © The British Academy 2010.

culture—e.g. grave goods do not *reflect* status but rather *negotiate* status (Hodder 1982).

This post-processual mode saw the first attempts to study the meaning of fragments, rather than simply accept them as rubbish. A good example is Talalay's recognition of the unbalanced selection of right and left figurine leg fragments in the Greek Neolithic (1993). Following up this trend, the 5th Annual Meeting of the European Association of Archaeologists hosted a session on 'Fragmentation'. The papers demonstrated that deliberate fragmentation of objects and re-use 'after the break' was a characteristic of many prehistoric and early historic societies in Eurasia, over a much longer timescale, and over a much wider area, than had previously been thought.

An extended summary of these early attempts to find the social meaning of fragments in archaeology was Chapman's monograph *Fragmentation in archaeology* (2000). Based mostly on materials from the Balkan Neolithic and Copper Age, the book sought to 'make sense' of the numerous patterns of fragmentation found in site assemblages by first formulating five possible reasons for the presence of fragments in the archaeological record (2000, 23–7); and, second, trying to explain why and how deliberate fragmentation is a socially anchored practice (2000, 37–58). While accidental breakage is not to be excluded, experimental work has proved that such an explanation is not universally applicable. Objects are buried because they are broken (Garfinkel 1994), ritual 'killing' of objects occurs (Hamilakis 1998) and fragments are dispersed to ensure fertility (Bausch 1994). Although well attested in the archaeological record, such behaviours received little attention before their recognition as deliberate social practices (Chapman 2000). The innovative explanation of fragmentation added to the list of social practices was *enchainment*—a concept more readily accepted and internalized in social anthropology than in archaeology (see Strathern 1988).[1] Personal enchainment through gift exchange was argued to be valid also for the exchange of fragmentary objects. A fragment may stand for the complete object in one place and thus presence the persons and places of the object's origins and later biography in other places. This is an example of people interrelating through fragment enchainment.

---

[1] 'Enchainment' is related to, but must be differentiated from, 'fractality'—the quality of repeated organizational similarities at different scales (Lapidus & van Frankenhuisen, 2004; Sornette 2000; Vicsek 2001). Here, enchained relations can be constructed at three different fractal scales—the fragment, the complete object and the set of objects.

Once deliberate fragmentation was established as a regular prehistoric and later practice and the full range of artefacts from a completely excavated site were recovered, then the basic question for every fragmentarist arose—where are the missing fragments? To answer this question and to address some of the criticisms of the first fragmentation book, a series of museum and archival studies were undertaken that evolved into the second fragmentation book—*Parts and wholes* (Chapman & Gaydarska 2006).

The book is centred around site-based re-fitting studies undertaken on two classes of material usually considered as having a specific meaning or high value—fired clay figurines and *Spondylus* shell ornaments. As many published and accessible re-fitting studies from around the world as possible were also included in the book in an attempt to define practices of disposal/discard and meaningful fragment re-use on the basis of the patterns of the most widespread fragment dispersal and re-fitting. Despite a variety of research aims and final conclusions, all the re-fitting studies supported the fragmentation premise, which is characterized by deliberate fragmentation and fragment curation as well as the practical use of fragments, including children's play with fragments. The main arguments for the fragmentation premise, and its implications, are summarized in the following two sections, before turning to a new research application.

THE FRAGMENTATION PREMISE

A few terminological clarifications relating to site formation and the type of contexts of discovery in archaeology are necessary before we move to the main points of the fragmentation premise. We start with the classic example of the so-called *closed find contexts*—burial pits. Another type of *closed context* is the burnt house. These are contexts that are believed to suffer little or no later intervention and therefore appear as they were left in the past.

The next forms of context are the *semi-opened contexts*, usually associated with unburnt house debris, pits with documented stages of infilling and middens. The semi-opened archaeological structures are prone to later deliberate or unconscious disturbance, during which whole or fragmented objects can be removed or added to the initial assemblage.

The last type of context is the *open contexts*, represented by the open settlement space or any other open surface in the past. Any whole object or object fragment left on the surface outside a building could have been moved there from another context.

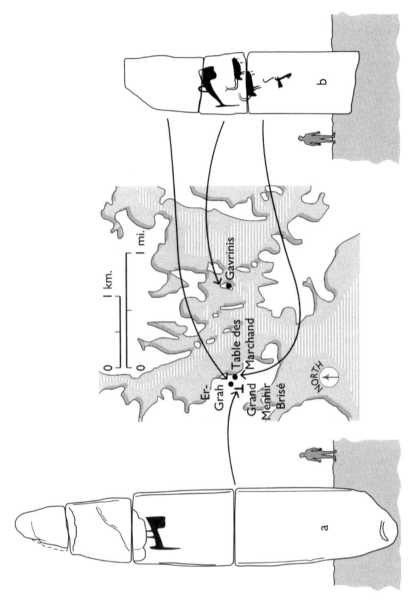

Figure 20.1. Decorated megalithic slabs broken and re-used, Breton Neolithic (source: Scarre 1998, upper figure, p. 62)

Table 20.1. Inter-site re-fits

Sites	Date	Material	Inter-site distances
Achtal (4 caves)	Gravettian	flint	5 km
Gyrinos Lake (6 sites)	Mesolithic–Neolithic	flint	6 km
Aldenhovener Platte (2 sites)	LBK	flint	0.5–3 km
Locmariaquer (3 sites)	Neolithic	decorated menhir	5 km
Trent valley (2 sites)	Late Bronze Age	bronze sword	5 km
Velsen fort (4 sites)	Early Roman	Samian bowls	3–8 km

The arguments that we advance for the reality of deliberate fragmentation and frequent re-use of fragments are sensitive to context and based upon four kinds of data: (1) re-fits between fragments of the same object found at different sites; (2) re-fits between fragments of the same object found in different contexts within the same site; (3) orphan fragments (i.e. parts of an object whose other parts are missing) from settlements with total excavation and good recovery methods; and (4) orphan fragments from closed contexts.

In seven of the cases outlined in Chapman and Gaydarska (2006), there is physical matching of different fragments of the same broken object found on different sites (from 2 to 6 fragments; Table 20.1). The most striking case in this group is the examples of decorated megalithic slabs from the Breton Neolithic, whose engraved patterns were broken across the image, with one part built into one monument and the other half used to construct a second tomb—the largest example of fragment re-fitting yet identified in prehistoric Eurasia and one of the most revealing for enchained relations between people, places and objects (L'Helgouach & Le Roux 1986; Figure 20.1). The longest distance currently known to separate fragments of the same object is 63 km, with waste flakes found at a habitation site re-fitting with a quartz cobble at a separate workshop site in the Chuckwalla Valley, southern California (Singer 1984).

The most numerous cases (n = 23) outlined concern re-fits of fragments found within the same site (Table 20.2, Figure 20.2). Secure examples linking mortuary and/or burnt house contexts are still relatively rare, but are important for demonstrating the incidence of deliberate fragmentation and the re-use of fragments at the site level. It is also highly probable that the far larger number of cases of re-fitting fragments linking semi-closed contexts also supports deliberate fragmentation practices

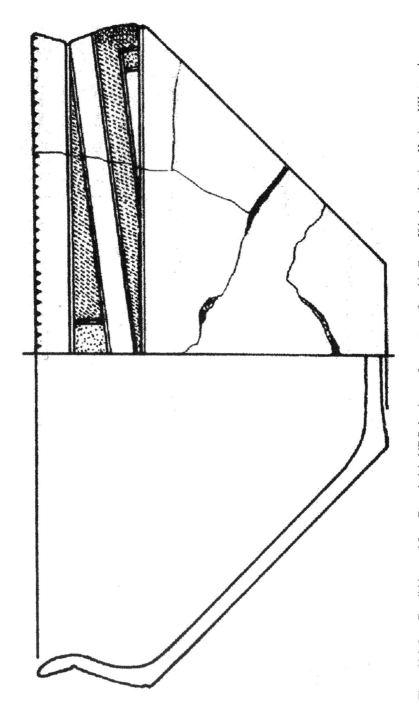

Figure 20.2. Late Eneolithic vessel from Durankulak, NE Bulgaria: one fragment was found in Grave 584, the other in a Horizon VII stone house on the nearby tell (source: Todorova et al., 2002, pp. 59–60 and Tabl. 99/11)

Table 20.2. Intra-site re-fits from closed and semi-closed contexts

Sites	Date	Material	Type of context
Endröd 119	Early Neolithic	pottery	S (pits and unburnt houses)
Ovcharovo-Gorata	Middle Neolithic	figurines and altars	S (pits)
Dimini	Late Neolithic	shell rings	S-O (unburnt house—open area)
Durankulak	Late Copper Age	pottery	C (house—grave)
Shlyakovsky	Late Copper Age	flint	C (grave—grave)
Dolnoslav	Final Copper Age	figurines	C-C (burnt houses)
			C-S (house—midden)
			C-O (house—open area)
Gubakút	LBK	pottery	S (pits)
Frimmersdorf 122	LBK	pottery	S (pits)
Molino Casarotto	Middle Neolithic	pottery	S (unburnt houses)
Rocca di Rivoli	Late Neolithic	pottery	S (pits)
Windmill Hill	Earlier Neolithic	pottery	S (ditch levels)
Kilverstone	Earlier Neolithic	pottery/flints	S (pits)
Hekelingen	Late Neolithic	flint	S (unburnt houses)
Barnhouse	Late Neolithic	pottery	S (unburnt houses and pits)
Chalain Site 2C	Final Neolithic	pottery	S (unburnt houses)
Shakadô	Middle Jomon	figurines	C (sealed ritual pits)
Phylakopi	Late Bronze Age	pottery and figurines	S (rooms in shrines)
Itford Hill	Middle Bronze Age	pottery	C-S (grave—unburnt house)
Runnymede Bridge	Late Bronze Age	pottery	S-S, S-O (mostly between open areas)
Speckhau cemetery	Early Iron Age	pottery	C (contexts in tumuli)
Nørre Fjand	Early Iron Age	pottery	C (burnt houses)
Wyszogród Site 2A	Early Medieval	pottery	S (pits)
Awatovi	Western Pueblo	pottery	S (rooms in houses)

Key to types of context: C—closed; S—semi-closed; O—open.

rather than children's play or other less structured mechanisms of fragment dispersion, because the fragments were often found in deep, sealed layers of different pits.

The study of parts missing from settlements that have been totally excavated is almost entirely dominated by lithic re-fitting. Data on the operational chain (*chaîne opératoire* [Leroi-Gourhan 1964], defined as a way of defining the stages in making a tool, from the collection of raw material to the finished object) have been used to estimate the quantities of blades detached from cores discarded in one place and exported to other places (Torrence 1982). For ceramics and other non-lithic finds, the identification of fragments with no re-fitting parts is commonly explained by poor preservation, rubbish left lying on the surface, sherd destruction for re-use as temper in pottery, etc. While varying regional climatic conditions and the degree of surface exposure of the artefacts should not be underestimated, the widely varying contexts of the data (Table 20.3) show that it would be unwise to identify post-depositional climatic factors as the main variable causing orphan fragments. It begins to look probable that one of the factors in the diminution of these assemblages was the deliberate removal of sherds from the site, whether locally or further away. An alternative practice would involve bringing sherds onto these sites from vessels already broken elsewhere. One of the most serious problems for re-fitting of sherds and Balkan figurines is determining the direction of movement of the fragments. However, whatever the direction of movement of the enchained fragment, the important point to be underlined is the movement of fragments between sites. Thus, the orphan fragment argument complements the cases of inter-site fragment re-fitting even though it may be impossible to identify both places of deposition precisely.

The last category of fragments to consider is the orphan fragments found in closed contexts. Everything said about the movement of orphan fragments from settlements, with their wide range of sometimes problematic contexts, can be stated more definitively for the closed contexts boasting the deposition of once-whole but now incomplete objects. Table 20.4 represents just a sample of the wide range of especially (but not only) mortuary contexts that have been investigated. These examples provide

Table 20.3. Orphan sherds from settlement contexts

Sites	Date	Material	Type of context
Gyrinos Lake	Mesolithic / Neolithic	flint	S, O
Endröd 119	Early Neolithic	pottery	S
Dimini	Late Neolithic	shell ring	C, S, O
Parța tell I	Late Neolithic	pottery	C
Ovcharovo	Copper Age	figurines	C, S, O
Goljamo Delchevo	Copper Age	figurines	C, S, O
Vinitsa	Copper Age	figurines	C, S, O
Sedlare	Late Copper Age	figurines	C, S, O
Dolnoslav	Final Copper Age	figurines	C, S, O
Rocca di Rivoli	Late Neolithic	pottery	S
Kilverstone	Earlier Neolithic	pottery/flints	S
Tremough	Late Neolithic/ Early Bronze Age	pottery	S, O
Runnymede Bridge	Late Bronze Age	pottery	S, O
Tremough	Romano Cornish	pottery	S, O
AZ I:1:17 (Anasazi)	AD 11th	pottery	S, O
Shoofly Village, AZ	AD 12th–13th	pottery	S, O
Sonora Site 205	Hokoham	pottery	sherds brought onto site
Little Egypt, Georgia	AD 16th 17th	pottery	S, O

Key to types of context: C—closed; S—semi-closed; O—open.

Table 20.4. Orphan fragments from closed (C) and semi-closed (S) contexts

Sites	Date	Material	Type of context
Durankulak cemetery	Late Neolithic – Late Copper Age	shell rings figurines pottery	C (grave)
Varna cemetery	Late Copper Age	shell rings pottery	C (grave)
Tiszapolgár-Basatanya	Early–Middle Copper Age	pottery	C (graves)
Nissehøj	Middle Neolithic	pottery	S (courtyard outside megalith)
Knowth	Neolithic	decorated stones	C (burial mound)
Lockington	Late Neolithic / Early Bronze Age	pottery	C (grave)
Mušja Jama	Late Bronze Age	metalwork	C (karst sink-hole)
Trent Valley	Late Bronze Age	bronze sword	S (hilltop deposits)
Speckhau cemetery	Early Iron Age	pottery	C (contexts in tumuli)

Key to types of context: C—closed; S—semi-closed; O—open.

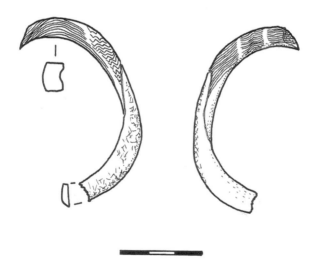

Figure 20.3. Orphan fragment of *Spondylus* shell ring, Varna Eneolithic cemetery (drawn by Vessela Yaneva)

strong evidence for the widespread nature of enchained relations between the mortuary domain and the world of the living in European prehistory (Figure 20.3). The two cases of metalwork deposits are also indicative of wider relations across the landscape, perhaps proving the norm in times/places where so-called 'scrap-metal' hoards have been deposited.

THE IMPLICATIONS OF THE FRAGMENTATION PREMISE

The implications of the fragmentation premise are many and varied (Chapman & Gaydarska 2006, note 14),but probably the most important concern the notions of *enchainment* and *personhood*. The dynamic nominalist approach has been proposed to understand the construction of identity through self-categorization (Hacking 1995). In this approach, agency and structure come together in the formation of identities, which may be described as the process of self-description through categorization. This process leads to the emergence of new kinds of persons as they are materialized. This perspective builds on Gamble's understanding of the relation between the body, which is primary, and material culture, which is secondary and derives symbolic meaning from corporeal metaphors (Gamble 2007). It adds a layer of co-evolution to Gamble's precedence of the body over material culture, as bodies that have made new forms of material culture are themselves thereby transformed into new bodies through the acquisition of new corporal skills and competences.

One aspect of personhood whose existence follows from the fragmentation premise is fractal personhood, in which a person emerges out of other people, places and things, materializing relations of enchainment with these other entities through broken as well as complete objects. We have seen, for example, how fragments of the same object linked the newly dead and the world of the living as often as enchainment maintained links between households and settlements. Conceptualizing the fragments of broken things as non-human dividuals helps us to understand the relationship between individuals (viz., complete objects) and dividuals (LiPuma 1998). In this way, the 'individual' aspect of personhood stood for the sum of all of the parts of the person's social identity or, as Binford (1971) put it, the 'social persona'. Enchained relations connect the distributed elements of a social persona, as well as the places and persons to which it is related. Studies of a variety of material forms indicate four important aspects of personhood—personhood and houses, personhood and settlements, personhood and the dead, and personhood and new roles and specializations.

The everyday practices of living in houses and visiting other houses led to a wide variety of relations, some of which were materialized and made visible through deposition. Thus, for example, the inter-household dispersion of re-fitting fragments of fired clay figurines at the Bulgarian Copper Age tell of Dolnoslav helps us draw a picture of households where persons are making whole figurines which embody different stages of their life course. These demonstrate a greater likelihood of figurine wear, re-use and fragmentation with increasing age (Figure 20.4). In a fractal perspective, figurines were born into different households, emerging out of the houses and their occupants. The accumulation of figurine collections in and by each household told the story of the persons of that household and perhaps, following Biehl (2003), addressed an additional narrative of the household's own biography. In turn, this materialization of persons created different kinds of person through their embodiment in different forms and through the highly contrasting kinds of fragmentation affecting different figurines.

The most important enchained relations between persons living in separate households were mediated by re-fitting figurine fragments deposited in different houses; the three examples known from Dolnoslav, for example, exhibited three different principles of opposition. The fragmentation of pieces that could be re-fitted later emerged out of these enchained relations between households.

There was a complex relationship between community structure and fractal aspects of personhood, often mediated by the household. The fractal perspective suggests that (in)dividual persons emerged out of face-to-face contacts and exchanges within the community, just as fractal

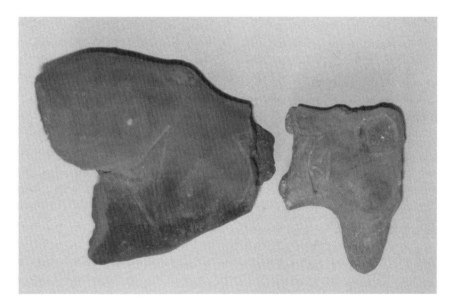

Figure 20.4. Re-fitting figurine fragments, Dolnoslav Eneolithic tell (photograph by Bisserka Gaydarska)

objects emerged out of the quotidian enchainment of (in)dividuals. The relative importance of the house and the overall community depended initially on its settlement context. For an extended family living in an isolated homestead, the house was the central focus of identity as symbol and practice—far more so than for a household in a village community. In the former, there were tensions between the potential to create the household's particular local set of material culture and the need to exchange appropriate objects betokening personal identities and membership of the breeding network linking the household to another 30 or 40 homesteads. The spatial dispersal of labour into enchained homesteads constrained the intensified production of relations-and-things. In the village, the multiplication of identical elements (house, oven, storage area, sleeping platform) gave the settlement a coherence that reinforced the identities of each separate household. It also framed the enchained relations within and between households in a consistent way, supporting communally accepted principles of personhood and identity in the wider landscape.

The mortuary arena stimulated each household, in the light of their fractal relations with the newly dead, to make decisions about which objects to bring to the grave and which to leave at home. Much of the variability in the incidence of grave goods may well have related to these practices, as potential grave goods evoked the memories of past people, places and things, and participated in their history and ancestral qualities as well as their places of origin and routes to the cemetery. While fragments of locally produced ceramics may well have materialized very local histories and everyday enchained links, exotic marine shell fragments were more likely to have recapitulated long-distance relationships and the histories of entire corporate groups.

Personhood was developed not only in contexts of houses, settlements and cemeteries, but also in connection with major changes in community lifeways. The emergence of farming in Eurasia comprised perhaps the most important changes in the last 10 millennia (Price 2000). New types of person were created in these developments, in particular the 'farmer' and the 'herder', but also the 'potter', the 'polished stone tool-maker' and perhaps the 'brewer'. These new types of person co-emerged fractally with new foodstuffs and objects, such as flour, bread, lamb chops, barley beer, pottery and axes—the one could not have occurred without the other. Notions of personhood would have been influenced by the wide range of new, enchained relations, not least gendered relations, which were based upon these identities as well as their interplay with traditional types of person—'hunter', 'shellfish-collector', 'flint-knapper' and 'leather-worker'. The communal values of the new products went hand in hand with the status of their creators. It is probable that, while those dwelling in dispersed homesteads would have included some of these new classes of people, meeting others seasonally, settled villagers would have included the full range of types of persons, with everyday contacts for most people. The discovery of the value of the secondary products of animals (Sherratt 1997) would have ushered in new episodes of person-creation, with 'dairy producers' making milk, cheese and yoghurt, and 'ploughmen' harnessing animal traction, alongside the diversification of traditional persons such as weavers (now making woollen textiles) and carpenters (now shaping wooden wheels, planks and complex joints for carts). The values assigned to the new things transformed the traditional system of communal values, itself confirming new statuses for new types of person.

Fractal personhood thus embodies the full range of enchained relationships, creating a person from the formative contributions of things, places and other persons. It is noteworthy that such a form of personhood is not uniformly related to deliberate object fragmentation, which is absent in Melanesia and South India, for example. However, such a form of personhood has been demonstrated in many times/places in later European prehistory.

But what of early human evolution in the Palaeolithic? Here, archaeological finds are far less complex than the pottery, figurines, polished stone ornaments and shell jewellery of the farming period, often being limited to stone tools and the by-products of their making, as well as animal bones with traces of modification by hominins. In the following sections, the concepts of fragmentation, enchainment and presencing are used as the basis for exploring the hitherto under-theorized relations between the earliest hominins, their stone tools and their cultural practices.

FRAGMENTATION, ENCHAINMENT AND PRESENCING—PERSPECTIVES ON HOMINID EVOLUTION

David Bohm is perhaps best known for his profound statement of ontological holism in *Wholeness and the implicate order* (1980). Here, he outlines the basis for 'undivided wholeness in flowing movement', as best exemplified by a vortex in a running stream. However, and despite the holism central to his work, he realized that there is not and cannot be any escape from fragmentation since, ironically, it is the one thing in our lives which is universal. Bohm identifies the concept of fragmentation as very deep and pervasive in human consciousness. For Bohm, to divide up is to simplify—to make manageable the totality of the world and our experience of it. The innocent beginning of the process is to regard conceptual divisions as a useful way of thinking about things. The problems arise when those fragments of consciousness take flight and become independent entities with their own separate existence. The habit of seeing and experiencing the world as composed of fragments can lead to a way of thinking based upon such fragments. The response of seeking to break up the experiences of the world to correspond with such a way of thinking can clearly lead to the proof of the correctness of such a fragmentary worldview (Bohm 1980, 3–4). The Golden Age of wholeness stands as a desired absence on which to look back and contemplate how good things once were. Without it, there is only, *pace* Munro (1997), the endless labour of division.

Bohm's perspectives on human consciousness can also shed light on things, since breakage, loss and absence would have been part and parcel of Palaeolithic lives. Archaeologists have developed the *chaîne opératoire* as a way of defining the stages in making a tool, from the collection of raw material to the finished object. This works best with, say, flint tools made using a reduction sequence, where fragments of different types are detached at each operational stage from a series of ever smaller 'wholes' (Mellars 1996). Thus, in the Early Palaeolithic examples, our term 'fragmentation' carries with it a sense of 'deliberate' action only insofar as the reduction sequence is purposive—and not necessarily the sense of 'deliberate' re-use of fragments produced in the reduction sequence.

Such reduction sequences for stone and bone tool production would have produced whole objects (tools) and many fragments (*débitage*). Everyone would have become used to seeing fragments of once-whole things lying around their living area. The opportunistic use of broken objects became part of a way of life—a re-use of things that was in fact an extension of their biographies. Discarded blunt knives were re-used as scrapers, wooden sticks were used as scoops or to dig out pits. Moreover, broken or damaged hand-axes were re-shaped to produce a slimmed-down, shorter working version (McPherron 2000). These were the first steps in the realization that parts of things could be useful and could be used as separate entities in their own right. This was even more clear in the case of the meat removed for consumption by scavenging or butchery.

The utility of fragments also confirmed the idea that whole and part could somehow be related and that the object now in pieces had once been whole. Away from their own home and visiting a place where tribal lore had it that others once lived there, people would have seen fragments of unknown antiquity and identity that attracted their attention because they were already accustomed to the re-use of fragments in their own lives. The thought that these fragments could be useful may also have been supplemented with the notion that these fragments once belonged to someone else—that there was anOther identity somehow implicated in the fragments. In the sense of Peircean semiotics (Jones 2007; Peirce 1958 [1904]), the association between the part and the whole was an index; the experience of the one presenced the other.

The presencing of past persons through the re-use of fragmentary material culture was, in itself, a large step that had enormous and surely unintended consequences for future social practices. To the extent that people in the past made variable uses of objects and places from their own past (Bradley 2002),[2] those people would have developed an appreciation of both the practical and the symbolic potential of broken things. The growing role of fragments in past lifeways would have altered people's perceptions of wholeness and divisibility, not only in the sense of wholeness being effective and useful (who needs a broken hand-axe?) but also by an acceptance of both parts and wholes as separate entities, reciprocally indexing each other. Under certain circumstances, perhaps characterized by changing views about the nature of relations between persons, the well-known utilitarian idea of fragments being connected to past whole objects could have been linked to another concept—that fragments could have been linked to past persons—to produce a metaphorical link between the relationships among object parts and whole objects, and among persons and their communities. Two forms of logic are important here: relational logic, in which the part somehow stood for the whole object, and rational logic, where the fragment grew out of the whole object. Both forms of logic were probably important, in varying degrees, in various Palaeolithic communities; each form of logic could have led to the further step of linking persons and objects in the creation of things out of people, and also as people in their own right.

---

[2] However, there are some prehistorians, such as Stephen Aldhouse-Green (pers. comm.), who would deny the antiquity of a 'sense of the past' before 250,000 BP.

Moreover, the social group itself may well have undergone seasonal changes in composition (fission-fusion) and the length of the separation of people would also have been critical to the extent of their use of discarded objects, a notion that will be discussed further below. The increasing recognition of not only the usefulness but also the power of fragments led to an acceptance of worldviews in which fragments took their place as one class of entity amongst many.

As it stands, this sketch is based upon *post hoc* logic and a generalized account of an undated sequence of conjectural changes. But is it possible to connect this possible set of relationships between human consciousness, social practice and the material world to the *longue durée* of the Palaeolithic? Covering a period extending from in excess of 2.5 million years ago to 500,000 years ago in Africa, this exploration of early fragmentation seeks to do just this—to identify areas in hominid evolution in which the concepts of fragmentation, enchainment and presencing can make a useful contribution to that fledgling species—social archaeology in the Palaeolithic. There are two specific aims: to investigate the question, raised by Bohm's research, of the possible co-evolution of the fragmentation of consciousness and of objects; and to identify ways of overcoming the false dichotomy between the presence/absence of symbolic representations in the Palaeolithic.

This approach takes a bottom-up, interactional look at hominin social life by considering social relations and social structure as properties that emerge through personal negotiation and performance (Gamble & Gittins 2004; Hinde 1976). We seek to go further than Ingold's (1993) principle that techniques of making are embedded in people's experience of shaping things by arguing that, in addition, persons were embedded in the objects that they made by virtue of the objects' entanglement in interpersonal relations (Strathern 1998). We do this by using the concepts of 'enchainment' and 'presencing' (Chapman 2000: 30–40).

In Melanesian ethnography, enchainment is 'a condition of all relations based on the gift' (Strathern 1988: 161). Thus, giving a gift enchains the gift-giver to the beneficiary, as well as enchaining the object to both persons. Enchainment is thus a key practice by which material culture and social relations constitute and re-constitute personhood. Presencing is concerned to bring the absent person, place or object into focus in a specific social context. An example of presencing is the knapped tool that refers to an absent place—the raw material source—which a member of the group had visited. To the extent that the phenomenon of presencing was already part of primate behaviour (pers. comm., R. I. M. Dunbar), early hominins were building on a primate legacy in establishing relations across the landscape. The difference between hominin and non-human animal behaviour was that the presencing between individuals and resources was reciprocal: if the member of a human group member was absent on a foraging trip, the stone tool could presence the person, whereas this does not happen with chimpanzee tools.

The most serious potential obstacle to understanding the relationships between persons and tools in the remote past is the common attitude among specialists in human evolution that meaning and symbolism are an add-on to the more basic functional, economic and secular uses of tools (Henshilwood & Marean 2003). The idea that tools have no necessary implicit communicative functions is used to support the distinction—central to much Palaeolithic research—between modern humans with symbolic behaviour and pre-modern hominids without. In supporting this argument, Wadley (2001, 207) admits that 'artifacts are not automatically imbued with symbolism: that happens only when they are used to define or mediate social relations'. But our point is exactly this—that the processes of the creation of tools out of persons do indeed define and mediate social relations from the earliest times when objects are used— i.e. some 2.7 million years ago (Figure 20.5). The making of tools cannot be other than a practice which links human individuals into a spatial network of material acquisition and transformation, a temporal pattern of regular action (perhaps a tradition) and a social process of the objectification of persons through the production of tools (Miller 1987). Such relationships between persons and tools are supported by Byers' argument (1999) that both primate and early hominin tools were not only expressive framing devices but also action-cues for the communication of intentions and desires, to which we would add material metaphors that established relationships.[3] The integration of these views leads to the conclusion that external symbolic storage on a simple level goes back to the origins of tool-making (see below for discussion of Merlin Donald's model). This notion will be the focus of the second half of our chapter. Let us approach the question of possible co-evolution from the viewpoint of objects before turning to social groups in their landscapes and, finally, consciousness.

---

[3] The dichotomy between symbolic and non-symbolic is also undermined by the use of Peircean semiotics rather than the Saussurean version which rests on such a distinction (Knappett 2005).

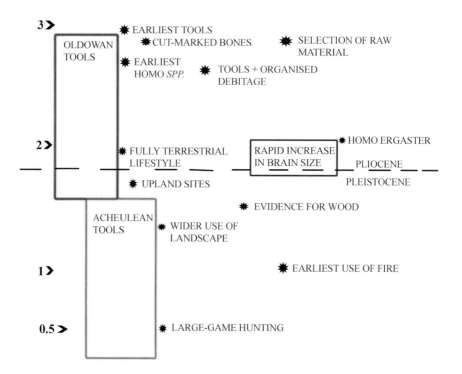

Figure 20.5. Time-line for the Early Palaeolithic (drawn by Bisserka Gaydarska)

OBJECTS

The australopithecines

Mithen (1996) has defined a central paradox about Early Palaeolithic hominin lifeways: while the archaeological evidence suggests small groups with minimal social structure, the fossil record and the palaeo-ecological data suggest the potential evolution of a greater degree of complexity and variability. Dunbar (e.g. 1993) emphasizes that a key aspect of the long-term behavioural basis of early humans was living in face-to-face, small bands who communicated with each other in initially limited ways (Buckley & Steele 2002) and cooperated in all social activities (Key & Aiello 1999). Tomasello (1999) makes the key point that early learning was not just *from* another group member but *through* that group member, which helped to reinforce shared identity.

On a small, local scale, the material world after 2.7 million years ago was implicated in the formation of group and personal identity through repeated visits to the same raw material source, the carrying of stone, animal products, gathered food and firewood to other places, and the embodiment of the necessary skills to make tools or cut animal flesh or wood. Early Oldowan flake and core tools (Figure 20.6) are characterized by a reductive technique with basic flaking revealing simple spatial relations of knapping (Wynn 2002).

Nevertheless, if one hominin could make a flake tool while another could not, a performative advantage was set up that could enable the removal of meat from a carcass. The consumers of that meat were connected to the tool-using 'butcher' in a social as well as a material relationship. This person also became part of a chain of presencing linked to the absent kill-site and its hunters, as well as any absent members of the consuming family.

Lithic transport across the landscape was related to the production of fragments from lumps, nodules or blocks (Stout et al. 2005). The sources of whole nodules—so far restricted to 1 km away from the knapping site (Marwick 2003)—were noted and related through presencing to the useful parts of the nodule themselves, even when these parts were discarded in another, always nearby, place. The return to the same favoured raw material source reinforced the relationship between resource (stone), individual (person) and place, most particularly for those directly involved in the movement and use of raw materials.

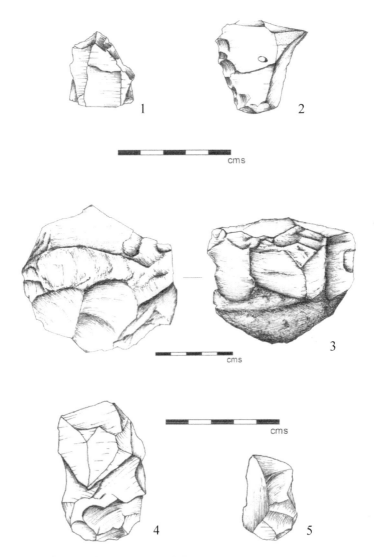

Figure 20.6. Oldowan tools: scrapers (1–2), bifacial core (3), pre-determined flakes (4–5) (source: de la Torre et al. 2003, Figs 5, 11, 13)

Thus, early forms of the relationships between persons, places and things were developed in ways that broke down the difference between utilitarian, communicative and symbolic functions. This account under-lines the key point that the occurrence of relationships between resource, person and place leads, in the particular social structures and ecological contexts of the Lower Palaeolithic, to the creation and use of metaphor-

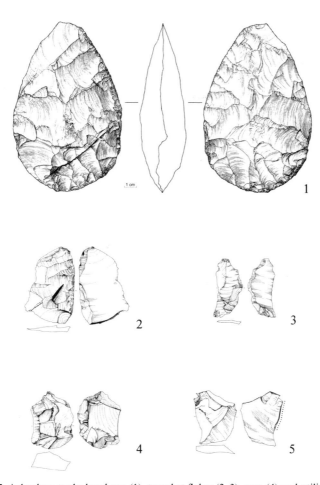

Figure 20.7. Acheulean tools: hand-axe (1), tranchet flakes (2–3), core (4) and utilized flake (5) (source: Roberts et al. 1997: Figs 26, 29)

ical and symbolic understandings of the practices and situations. The increasing intensity of production and use of material culture invariably led to the creation of more and more fragments. It is unlikely that their ubiquity went unnoticed and unexploited for very long.

What light does fragmentation shed on Mithen's Early Palaeolithic paradox? The perspective developed here suggests that, interestingly, the lamented absence of early complexity is an illusion; it cannot be detected through excavation but it can be theorized in terms of the enchained relationships between persons, places and things. The emergence of relations between persons in different face-to-face groups increased the potential for previously undeveloped social complexities by providing a material means for the maintenance of social relations beyond the face-to-face. It is worth considering that this form of australopithecine social relationships was co-present with the earliest tools.

The first species of *Homo*

A suite of crucial changes in hominin evolution came about beginning ca. 2 million years ago, with the emergence of the first species of the *Homo* genus (*Homo habilis/rudolfensis*). This species is characterized by a larger brain size than before, fully bipedal mobility and a fully terrestrial lifestyle (Aiello 1996). Aiello links the new species' adaptation to open-country environments with an increase in group size spurred on by the need for defence against predators. Cachel and Harris (1998) have detected more complex ranging and foraging behaviours than found in earlier dwelling practices, noting in addition an expansion to upland settlements such as Gadeb in the Ethiopian Highlands. Marwick (2003) notes that the first known instance of hominins moving lithics more than 1 km is dated to ca. 1.9 million years ago while over the period 1.9–1.6 million years ago, the maximum distance of lithic transport increased to 13 km—still within a group's capabilities of direct procurement. Marwick proposes that this distance may well equate to the minimum home range of these early Oldowan-tool-producing hominins.

These disparate lines of evidence converge on the conclusion that there were important changes towards more complex hominin sociality over this long period of time. These changes would have taken the form of larger face-to-face social groups (Rodseth et al. 1991), wider social networks stretching over greater distances across the landscape (Cachel & Harris 1998) and the extension of kinship categories to describe the wider networks (Barnard 1999).

Gamble (1998) has used network analysis to indicate ways in which social relations could have been 'stretched' across time and space. It would appear from the Oldowan data that there may well have been limited releases from face-to-face proximity in effective networks at a much earlier date. This suggests that Oldowan enchainment was based upon the movement of tools between sites and raw material transport from source to site. Equally, the high degree of fragmentation involved in Oldowan knapping suggests systematic understanding of the relationship between complete nodules and their fragments.

Some time after ca. 1.2 million years ago, there was an increase in the maximum distance that *Homo erectus* populations in East Africa were moving lithics for the production of Acheulean tools, from 15 km to 100 km (Marwick 2003), if not further in the case of African obsidian (C. Gamble pers. comm.). For Marwick, there were two main implications of this finding: the skills of hominid groups in the acquisition of information about larger areas than previously, and the ability to exploit much wider landscapes than previously, perhaps signalling the emergence of proto-language for improved face-to-face negotiation. It is also likely that exchange of lithics and perhaps other materials was also predicated on such developments (I. Morley pers. comm.). These longer trips were also surely exploited for other purposes, such as the collection of information on other resources, foraging and hunting.

A concomitant of this wider-ranging lithic transport is a far wider range of absent places, things and persons who have nonetheless been incorporated into hominid social networks. It may be supposed that the scale of spatial interaction envisaged here is consistent with the emergence of Gamble's (1998) extended network. It is hard to imagine that such a growth in social network size could be achieved without new forms of categorization for people in each form of network, including a higher proportion of non-kin than previously. Nettle (1999) has suggested that improvements in language skills would have helped to maintain generalized reciprocity in far larger social networks than face-to-face contacts. It is clear that network-building is an important social task: the dangers of social fragmentation to hunter-gatherer communities have been addressed by Skeates (2005), who suggests that enchainment emphasizes the importance of contacts between increasingly separate groups. In this more extended world, how could group members transcend distance and overcome absence?

Davidson (1991) has discussed the displacement of objects in both time and space, suggesting that reference can be made to an absent object as a memory of a former time. However, it is not only objects but also people and places that can be presenced (the mirror-image of displacement). The formation of materially rooted enchained links between people and places is a means of maintaining, through cultural memory, the solidarity of the group during absences. To the extent that group identity was linked to utilized places, whether for the production, exchange or consumption of resources (e.g. the feasting attested at Olduvai), individuals would have been more likely to return to claim their membership of the group, as well as the memories attached to that group and its movements through the landscape. There is emerging evidence of special deposition of objects, such as the later example of the Acheulean hand-axes at Boxgrove, as a way of reinforcing the special nature of the relationship between groups and places, thereby also presencing group members in other places (Hallos 2005; Pope et al. 2007).

In summary, the action-cues of early tools led to a performance-based understanding of the relationship between persons and tools, which incorporated fragmentation of raw materials, animal carcasses and wood at an early stage. Increases in hominid social group size, combined with the increased artefact–agent space (*pace* Lane & Maxfield 1997) across the landscape, led to the emergence of enchainment between persons and objects as a second practice complementary to, and as important as, that of fragmentation in its creation and perpetuation of links between the social and the material. The third key symbolic development—presencing on a wide scale—was crucial in spanning the gaps in space and absences in time in expanded networks. But what of consciousness?

COGNITIVE DEVELOPMENTS

Let us now turn to the second aspect of the object–consciousness co-evolutionary scenario. In the literature on human cognition, there are many stimulating discussions that identify key steps in cognitive evolution, whether the transition to conceptual thinking (Lowe 1998), the extension of intentionality from conspecifics to things (Tomasello 1999), the use of spatial relations to structure time (Boroditsky 2000) and the emergence of the self as a mental construct (Bower 2005; Metzinger 2003). While all of these developents are potentially vital to our understanding of the evolution of mind, the authors have made little attempt to relate these concepts to any kind of archaeological timescale, nor to integrate their thinking with a Bohmian fragmentation perspective. The main exceptions to these strictures are Merlin Donald and Steve Mithen, both of whom have created stadial models of the evolution of the human mind. Before turning to the insights of Donald and Mithen, we shall first investigate the extent to which Bohm's three-stage model of the evolution of consciousness (1980), which he does not relate to archaeological data, supports the co-evolution of materiality and cognition.

As we have read, Bohm postulates a somewhat different three-stage process: (1) fragments of consciousness take flight and become independ-

ent entities with their own separate existence, leading to: (2) a way of seeing and experiencing the world as composed of fragments, and in turn: (3)
a way of thinking based upon such fragments. In terms of the capacities
of early hominin conceptualization before the emergence of stone tools,
a partial understanding of the environment would be expected given the
very local patterns of movement; nonetheless, fragments of consciousness
(Bohm's first stage) would have needed to represent the segments of the
world observed in nature and in culture for any sense of dwelling in a
local place.

Bohm's second stage is more readily recognizable in early hominin
practices such as the fabrication of stone and wooden tools. While there
are always complete objects (nodules, lava flows, trees), the conversion of
these complete things into useful, workable objects normally implies the
importance of fragments, if not necessarily their priority over complete
things. The example of hand-axe production reminds us that an estimated
range of 50–200 flakes (*débitage*) was created for every single core-tool.
But, in comparison with the original flint nodule, the hand-axe is just as
much a fragment as a waste flake! Until the development of additive technology, as in the composite tools appearing in the late Middle Pleistocene
(McBrearty & Brooks 2000), a very high proportion of all tools were
fragments of something greater. How probable was it that lithic knappers
did not come to appreciate this practical and ontological fact through
their daily embedded practice?

The process of basing one's thought processes on fragments (Bohm's
third stage) is at once revolutionary and full of fascinating implications
for the relationships between objects and objects, as much as between
objects and humans, as well as humans and humans. Three long-term,
repeated aspects of the Early Palaeolithic *habitus* are important for cognitive developments—the opportunities for greater feedback in links
between objects and cognition, the question of larger artefact–agent
spaces in the landscape and the relation of fragmentation to the fission-
fusion mobility pattern.

There is a sense that the vast majority of satisfying and useful 'products'
in the Early Palaeolithic were fragments derived from greater wholes—
whether venison steaks, flake tools, pointed sticks or nuts, honey and
berries. It is possible to argue that this visually obvious part of the daily
habitus was perhaps so obvious that it provoked the group to no special
comment, as did many aspects of the *habitus* (Bourdieu 1977). However,
the ubiquity of fragments could equally have provided a clue for thinking
about the world as full of fragments—treating them as entities in their

own right while retaining their links to a 'parent body', whether of flint or antelope. The notion of tools as a metaphorical extension of persons would then be seen as the substitution of one 'parent body'—the natural—for another—the personal. However, just as small tools were fragments of larger tools, which were in turn parts of large nodules, persons were parts of larger social entities, whether bands or communities. This leads to a consideration of the wider spatial context of hominin networks.

The extension of social networks after 1.2 million years ago to cover distances of up to 100 km or more led to a different form of spatial fragmentation. Some tool fragments came from perhaps unimaginably far away and offered the potential to be conceptualized as exotic objects which presenced social groups beyond normal network contacts. It is clear that exotic tools opened a window onto a more expansive social world—but it was also a more fragmented social world, with more boundaries to cross, fewer kinsfolk to contact but, equally, few opportunities to meet those new people. The existence of a wider social world led to the possibility that this world was conceptualized through material symbols, foremost among them being the exotic fragments. How does this picture of wider social networks relate to dwelling?

To the extent that the hominins that made up early cooperative groups stayed together for most of the time, the notion of the fragmentation of the group would not have been significant. However, interpersonal rivalry or hostility could lead to fission and the loss of any member of an intimate network of 5–7 persons would have been serious to the group. It is probable that tools made by the departed member remained in use in the group as a source of presencing, while their favourite places in the landscape were linked to the absent individual in group memory. The increase in hominid group sizes after 2 million years ago led to a more complex sociality which would have included higher dispute rates as much as a greater potential for cooperative action (Johnson 1982). It is well known that one classic hunter-gatherer strategy for avoiding conflict is to move away; the implication of this strategy for group fragmentation, however, has not been discussed.

A less dramatic form of group fragmentation is represented by the seasonal fission and fusion of groups reliant on more or less clustered food resources through the annual cycle; this was of greater importance than conflict-based fission because this division was permanently built into the temporal structure of the group. But, unlike the irreversible reduction of a knappping sequence, seasonal fission-fusion was cyclical, with the eternal return to a state of nucleation, interspersed by less social if less conflict-ridden episodes of dispersion across the landscape. The cyclical model of seasonal settlement provides a major challenge to Bohm's idea that mental models were dominated by fragments. It is not that processes of division are excluded or indeed unimportant—rather that the wholeness that represents the group ideal is repeatedly re-created and then dissolved. There is much anthropological, and some Palaeolithic, evidence of groups who look forward to nucleation time as the most sociable of times in their year (Yellen 1977). In this sense, practices of seasonal fission and fusion incorporated the undivided whole into the annual cycle as a counterpoint to group division. This may well have become the spatial basis for changing relations between parts and wholes, which could be viewed in two complementary ways: either as fragmentation and re-joining of a social whole constituted by the larger group or as the aggregation and dispersal of numerous smaller wholes (I. Morley pers. comm.).

In summary, David Bohm's three-stage model of cognitive development based upon fragmentation shows a good fit with most of the Early Palaeolithic data, with the exception of the cyclical pattern of fission-fusion in dwelling practice. His first stage is consistent with primate cognition, while the making of stone tools through reduction sequences and from resources separate from dwelling areas introduces the necessary and sufficient conditions for his second stage. The third stage probably arose out of the feedback from the ubiquity of stone tool and other fragments in everyday life, reinforced by the symbolic significance of exotic tool fragments. But the cyclical fission-fusion cycle of dwelling fits uneasily with Bohm's model and requires further study for any possible integration. How do these insights compare with the cognitive evolutionary schemes of Donald and Mithen?

In his neurocognitive approach, Donald (1991) posits four main stages in cognitive evolution, separated by three major changes in physical type. Prior to the earliest hominins, the episodic stage refers to reactive primate cognition, with their representative style tied to environmental events which stimulate a narrow range of expressive outputs. The evolution of early hominins is related to the mimetic stage, which culminates in the abilities of *Homo erectus* individuals to rehearse, evaluate and refine their own actions. Through this development, it was conscious perception that supervised all bodily actions in an ability which Donald terms 'non-verbal action modelling', or mimesis. The evolution of oral–mythic culture and speech over several hundred thousand years led to the third stage, culminating in the speciation of modern *Homo sapiens*. Here, mythic archetypes and allegories created an oral, public version of reality with direct influence over the form of human thought and convention. In this stage, modern *sapiens* populations created new levels of culture through their introduction of a vast array of new representations and external storage media. It was with the emergence of writing and other state-controlled forms of external symbolic storage that the fourth, theoretic stage developed in later pre- and proto-history.

Mithen's deep awareness of the cognitive literature stimulated a theory of mind that relates concepts of hard-wired, multiple, content-rich types of modular intelligence to archaeological findings (1996). Mithen's research is an outgrowth of Fodor's (1983) concept of modular intelligence, Gardner's (1983) notion of interacting, multiple intelligences and Cosmides and Tooby's model of hard-wired, multiple, content-rich types of intelligence with one specialized module for making quick decisions (Barkow et al. 1992). The result is a three-stage model of human cognitive development, in which the minds of the australopithecines and *Homo habilis* are dominated by general intelligence (stage I); the minds of *Homo erectus* and the Neanderthals are the product of general intelligence supplemented by multiple specialized intelligences, such as the social, the natural historical, the technical and the linguistic, working in isolation from each other (stage II); and the minds of modern humans consist of multiple specialized intelligences working together, centrally inegrated yet with a flow of knowledge and ideas between domains (stage III). While the lack of domain integration prevented earlier developments, it was the cognitive fluidity of stage III modern humans that enabled the cultural explosion of the period 60,000–30,000 BC (Mithen 1996). How do the alternative models of Donald and Mithen relate to Bohm's ideas about the fragmentation of consciousness?

The first two stages of Donald's model are the stages most closely related to Bohm's scheme—the primate episodic stage and the mimetic stage of early hominins. One of the defining characteristics of the first, primate stage—complex episodic event-perceptions—is consistent with Bohm's first stage of fragments of consciousness taking flight to become independent entities with their own separate existence. Donald states that the process of enculturation, leading to the collective mind typifying humans living in symbol-using cultures, 'must have started very slowly, presumably with very gradual increments to a primate knowledge-base' (Donald 1998, 12). In Donald's list of 15 primate cognitive functions that, he argues, underwent radical transformations in the mimetic stage, two are particularly relevant to the Bohmian scheme—(15) the integration of material culture into the process of explicit knowledge representation, and (12) autobiographical memory (Donald 1998, 13). The combination of hominins whose past actions were accessible to themselves and each other was as basic to the creation of enchained relations as the emerging role of material representations was significant for fragmentation practices. Together, these two developments enabled the appreciation of personal, family and group 'pasts', as well as the ability to use objects as symbols of other objects and persons (Lowe 1998). Thus, Donald's insights provide a useful cognitive framework for the development of Bohm's second stage of hominids who see and experience the world as composed of fragments— the tools that are physical fragments of larger identities and which are, at the same time, examples of external storage of information about rela- tions between persons, places and things. The third stage in Bohm's model postulates a more abstract level, with hominins developing a way of thinking based upon such fragments. This is not consonant with the key advances of Donald's linguistic-mythic stage but resembles rather the potential of the 'collective mind' for understanding the material realities of a fragmented world—as Donald puts it, recoded knowledge driven by public representations (1998, 13). These public representations—the Oldowan and Acheulean tools of the Early and Middle Palaeolithic— framed everyday action for hominin groups, symbolizing an increasingly wide suite of socio-spatial concepts.

Equally, the relationship of Bohm's scheme to Mithen's model of modular minds is one of temporal priority. Early hominins with the gen- eralized intelligence of Mithen's stage I would have developed the capac- ity to see and experience the world as composed of both wholes and fragments, as well as formulating ways of thinking based upon such wholes and fragments, related to both social groups and the material world. The development of early forms of metaphorical thinking, per- mitting things and places to be conceptualized as people, would have been aided by the ways in which fragments were thought of in relation to wholes. In Bohmian terms, to divide up for the sake of simplification—to make manageable the totality of the world and our experience of it—is indeed complementary to the concept of modular minds that forms the basis of Mithen's model.

In summary, the three cognitive approaches of Bohm, Donald and Mithen are not mutually exclusive; rather, they offer useful connections to further our understanding of the earliest stages of hominin evolution. These results support the idea of the co-evolution of cognition and objects. Moreover, the removal of the rigid distinction between the pres- ence/absence of symbolic behaviour allows the definition of a more nuanced set of relationships between material culture and persons from 2.5 million years ago. The development of strategies of tool-making led then to the recognition of the importance of fragmentation and the relationships between complete and partial objects. These practices led to the capacity to see and experience the world as composed of both wholes and fragments, as well as formulating ways of thinking based upon such wholes and fragments. It was only later, ca. 2 million years ago, that enchained relations based on material culture emerged with the development of larger social groups interacting across wider landscapes, gaining the potential for greater social complexity that parallels the slow evolution ca. 1.7 million years ago of visually distinctive Acheulean tool types.

In summary, the artificially created 'absence' of symbolic culture before the evolution of anatomically modern humans ca. 160,000 years BP can be filled in through the use of concepts such as fragmentation, enchainment and presencing—all of which can be used in the construction of a bottom-up picture of social relations negotiated between persons and groups and with the full participation of the material culture that enmeshed early hominid social relations. These practices indicate that early hominin social relations, including the use of symbolism, analogy and metaphor, will have had embryonic, if not relatively developed and complex, forms well before the appearance of the so-called suite of behaviours associated with modern humans in Europe.

CONCLUSIONS

In this chapter, we have introduced the fragmentation premise—the idea that the deliberate breakage of a complete object and the re-use of the resultant fragments as new and separate objects 'after the break' was a common practice in the past. Despite its initial implausibility, this premise has much to commend it and we present four kinds of supporting archaeological evidence. We also summarize the main implications of the fragmentation premise for the study of enchained social relations and of the creation and development of personhood in the past. To the extent that the boundaries of the human body can be considered permeable and open to the influences of other persons, things and places, personhood can be conceptualized as 'fractal', with objects emerging out of persons rather than being in contra-distinction to them, and broken objects considered as non-human dividuals. Enchained relations connect the distributed elements of a person's social identity using material culture.

These concepts of fragmentation, enchainment and presencing are used to think through some of the earliest manufactured objects in the world—the hominin tools of the period 2.5–0.5 million years ago. In contrast to the standard separation of symbolic behaviour by anatomically modern humans after 200,000 years ago from non-symbolic behaviour by early pre-*sapiens* populations, we propose a scenario in which the use of tools and the movement of lithic resources over the landscape led to the emergence of enchained social relations, consonant with increases in brain size following 2 million years ago. We support the notion of the co-evolution of fragmentation in both consciousness and in objects, using Mithen's model of cognitive evolution and Donald's model of external symbolic storage as cognitive scaffolding in this project.

Note. Many thanks to members of the 'Social Brain' research group, and especially Clive Gamble, for their kind invitation to present at the British Academy conference. We are also very grateful to Clive Gamble, Robin Dunbar, Stephen Aldhouse-Green, Rob Hosfield, Iain Morley and Freddie Foulds for their valuable comments on our first venture into uncharted Palaeolithic waters. We acknowledge with thanks Vessela Yaneva's illstration of the Varna shell ring (Figure 20.3). We thank Chris Scarre for providing Figure 20.1, Henrieta Todorova for Figure 20.2, I. de la Torre for Figure 20.6 and the Prehistoric Society and Julie Gardiner for Figure 20.7.

REFERENCES

Aiello, L. C. (1996). Terrestriality, bipedalism and the origin of language. In: W. G. Runciman, J. Maynard Smith & R. I. M. Dunbar (eds) *Evolution of social behaviour patterns in primates and man*, pp. 269–289. Proceedings of the British Academy 88. London and Oxford: Oxford University Press for the British Academy.

Barkow, J. H., Cosmides, L. & Tooby, J. (eds) (1992). *The adapted mind: evolutionary psychology and the generation of culture*. Oxford: Oxford University Press.

Barnard, A. (1999). Modern hunter-gatherers and early symbolic culture. In: R. Dunbar, C. Knight & C. Power (eds) *The evolution of culture: an interdisciplinary view*, pp. 50–70. Edinburgh: Edinburgh University Press.

Bausch, I. (1994). Clay figurines and ritual in the Middle Jomon period: a case study of the Shakado site in the Kofu Basin. Unpublished MA dissertation, University of Leiden.

Biehl, P. (2003). *Studien zur Symbolgut des Neolithikums und der Kupferzeit in Südosteuropa*. Bonn: Habelt.

Binford, L. R. (1971). Mortuary practices: their study and their potential. In: J. Brown (ed.) *Approaches to the social dimensions of mortuary practices*, pp. 6–29. Washington, DC: Memoir of the Society for American Archaeology 25.

Bohm, D. (1980). *Wholeness and the implicate order*. London: Routledge & Kegan Paul.

Boroditsky, L. (2000). Metaphoric structuring: understanding time through spatial metaphors. *Cognition* 75: 1–28.

Bourdieu, P. (1977). *Outline of a theory of practice*. Cambridge: Cambridge University Press.

Bower, J. R. F. (2005). On 'Modern behaviour and the evolution of human intelligence'. *Current Anthropology* 46(1): 121–122.

Bradley, R. (2002). *The past in prehistoric societies*. London: Routledge.

Buckley, C. & Steele, J. (2002). Evolutionary ecology of spoken language: co-evolutionary hypotheses are testable. *World Archaeology* 34: 26–46.

Byers, S. (1999). Communication and material culture: Pleistocene tools as action cues. *Cambridge Archaeological Journal* 9(1): 23–41.

Cachel, S. & Harris, J. W. K. (1998). The lifeways of *Homo erectus* inferred from archaeology and evolutionary ecology: a perspective from East Africa. In: M. D. Petraglia & R. Korisettar (eds) *Early human behaviour in global context: the rise and diversity of the Lower Palaeolithic record*, pp. 108–132. London: Routledge.

Chapman, J. (2000). *Fragmentation in archaeology: people, places and broken objects in the prehistory of South Eastern Europe*. London: Routledge.

Chapman, J. & Gaydarska, B. (2006). *Parts and wholes: fragmentation in prehistoric context*. Oxford: Oxbow Books.

Davidson, I. (1991). The archaeology of language origins—a review. *Antiquity* 65: 39–48.

Donald, M. (1991). *Origins of the modern mind: three stages in the evolution of culture and cognition*. Cambridge, MA: Harvard University Press.

Donald, M. (1998). Hominid enculturation and cognitive evolution. In: C. Renfrew & C. Scarre (eds) *Cognitive storage and material culture: the archaeology of symbolic storage*, pp. 7–18. Cambridge: McDonald Institute.

Dunbar, R. I. M. (1993) Coevolution of neocortical size, group size and language in humans. *Behavioral and Brain Sciences* 16: 681–735.

Fodor, J. A. (1983). *The modularity of mind: an essay on faculty psychology*. Cambridge, MA: MIT Press.

Gamble, C. S. (1998). Palaeolithic society and the release from proximity: a network approach to intimate relations. *World Archaeology* 29: 426–449.

Gamble, C. S. (2007). *Origins and revolutions: human identity in earliest prehistory*. Cambridge: Cambridge University Press.

Gamble, C. S. & Gittins, E. K. (2004). Social archaeology and origins research: a Palaeolithic perspective. In: L. Meskell & R. Preucel (eds) *A companion to social archaeology*, pp. 96–118. Oxford: Blackwell.

Gardner, H. (1983). *Frames of mind: the theory of multiple intelligences*. New York: Basic Books.

Garfinkel, Y. (1994). Ritual burial of cultic objects: the earliest evidence. *Cambridge Archaeological Journal* 4(2): 159–188.

Hacking, I. (1995). Three parables. In: R. B. Goodman (ed.) *Pragmatism: a contemporary reader*, pp. 237–249. London: Routledge.

Hallos, J. (2005). '15 minutes of fame': exploring the temporal dimension of Middle Pleistocene lithic technology. *Journal of Human Evolution* 49: 155–179.

Hamilakis, Y. (1998). Eating the dead: mortuary feasting and the politics of memory in the Aegean Bronze Age societies. In: K. Branigan (ed.) *Cemetery and society in the Aegean Bronze Age*, pp. 115–131. Sheffield: Sheffield Academic Press.

L'Helgouach, J. & Le Roux, C.-T. (1986). Morphologie et chronologie des grandes architectures de l'Ouest de la France. In: J.-P. Demoule & J. Guilaine (eds) *Le Néolithique de la France*, pp. 181–191. Paris: Picard.

Henshilwood, C. S. & Marean, C. W. (2003). The origin of modern human behaviour: critique of the models and their test implications. *Current Anthropology* 38: 627–651.

Hinde, R. A. (1976). Interactions, relationships and social structure. *Man* 11: 1–17.

Hodder, I. (1982). *Symbols in action: ethnoarchaeological studies of material culture*. Cambridge: Cambridge University Press.

Ingold, T. (1993). Tool-use, sociality and intelligence. In: K. R. Gibson & T. Ingold (eds) *Tools, language and cognition in human evolution*, pp. 429–445. Cambridge: Cambridge University Press.

Johnson, G. A. (1982). Organisational structure and scalar stress. In: C. Renfrew, M. J. Rowlands & B. A. Segraves (eds) *Theory and explanation in archaeology*, pp. 389–421. London: Academic Press.

Jones, A. (2007). *Memory and material culture*. Cambridge: Cambridge University Press.

Key, C. A. & Aiello, L. C. (1999). The evolution of social organisation. In: R. Dunbar, C. Knight & C. Power (eds) *The evolution of culture: an interdisciplinary view*, pp. 15–33. Edinburgh: Edinburgh University Press.

Knappett, C. (2005). *Thinking through material culture: an interdisciplinary perspective*. Pittsburgh, PA: University of Philadelphia Press.

Lane, D. A. & R. Maxfield (1997). Foresight, complexity and strategy. In: W. B. Arthur, S. N. Durlauf & D. A. Lane (eds) *The economy as an evolving complex system 2*, ch. 4. Reading, MA: Addison-Wesley.

Lapidus, M. L. & van Frankenhuisen, M. (eds) (2004). *Fractal geometry and applications* Providence, RI: American Mathematical Society.

Leroi-Gourhan, A. (1964). *Le geste et la parole, 1: technique et langue*. Paris: Albin Michel.

LiPuma, E. (1998). Modernity and forms of personhood in Melanesia. In: M. Lambek & A. Strathern (eds) *Bodies and persons: comparative views from Africa and Melanesia*, pp. 53–79. Cambridge: Cambridge University Press.

Lowe, E. J. (1998). Personal experience and belief: the significance of external symbolic storage for the emergence of modern human cognition. In: C. Renfrew & C. Scarre (eds) *Cognitive storage and material culture: the archaeology of symbolic storage*, pp. 89–96. Cambridge: McDonald Institute.

McBrearty, S. & Brooks, A. S. (2000). The revolution that wasn't: a new interpretation of the origin of modern humans. *Journal of Human Evolution* 39: 453–563.

McPherron, S. P. (2000). Handaxes as a measure of the mental capabilities of early hominids. *Journal of Archaeological Science* 27: 655–663.

Marwick, B. (2003). Pleistocene exchange networks as evidence for the evolution of language. *Cambridge Archaeological Journal* 13(1): 67–81.

Mellars, P. (1996). *The Neanderthal legacy: an archaeological perspective from western Europe*. Princeton, NJ: Princeton University Press.

Metzinger, T. (2003). *Being no-one: the self-model theory of subjectivity*. Cambridge, MA: MIT Press.

Miller, D. (1987). *Material culture and mass consumption*. Oxford: Blackwell.

Mithen, S. (1996). *The prehistory of the mind*. London: Thames & Hudson.

Munro, R. (1997). Ideas of difference: stability, social spaces and the labour of division. In: K. Hetherington & R. Munro (eds) *Ideas of difference*, pp. 3–24. Oxford: Blackwell.

Nettle, D. (1999). Language variation and the evolution of societies. In: R. Dunbar, C. Knight & C. Power (eds) *The evolution of culture: an interdisciplinary view*, pp. 214–227. Edinburgh: Edinburgh University Press.

Peirce, C. S. (1958 [1904]). *Values in a universe of chance: selected writings of Charles S. Peirce 1839–1914*. New York: Doubleday Anchor.

Pope, M., Russel, K. & Watson, K. (2007). Biface form and structured behaviour in the Acheulean. *Lithics* 27: 1–14.

Price, T. D. (ed.) (2000). *Europe's first farmers*. Cambridge: Cambridge University Press.

Roberts, M. B., Parfitt, S. A., Pope, M. I. & Wenban-Smith, F. F. (1997). Boxgrove, West Sussex: rescue excavations of a Lower Palaeolithic landsurface (Boxgrove Project B, 1989–91). *Proceedings of the Prehistoric Society* 63: 303–358.

Rodseth, L., Wrangham, R. W., Harrigan, A. & Smuts, B. B. (1991). The human community as a primate society. *Current Anthropology* 32: 221–254.

Scarre, C. (1998). *Exploring prehistoric Europe*. New York: Oxford University Press.

Schiffer, M. B. (1987). *Formation processes of the archaeological record*. Albuquerque: University of New Mexico Press.

Sherratt, A. (1997). *Economy and society in prehistoric Europe: changing perspectives*. Edinburgh: Edinburgh University Press.

Singer, C. A. (1984). The 63-kilometer fit. In: J. E. Ericson & B. A. Purdy (eds) *Prehistoric quarries and lithic production*, pp. 35–48. Cambridge: Cambridge University Press.

Skeates, R. (2005). *Visual culture and archaeology*. London: Duckworth.

Sornette, D. (2000). *Critical phenomena in natural sciences: chaos, fractals, self-organisation and disorder: concepts and tools*. Berlin: Springer

Strathern, M. (1988). *The gender of the gift*. Berkeley: University of California Press.

Strathern, M. (1998). Social relations, and the idea of externality. In: C. Renfrew & C. Scarre (eds) *Cognitive storage and material culture: the archaeology of symbolic storage*, pp. 135–147. Cambridge: McDonald Institute.

Stout, D., Quade, J., Semaw, S., Rogers, M. J. & Levin, N. E. (2005). Raw material selectivity of the earliest stone toolmakers at Gona, Afar, Ethiopia. *Journal of Human Evolution* 48: 365–380.

Talalay, L. (1993). *Deities, dolls and devices: neolithic figurines from Franchthi Cave*. (Excavations at Franchthi Cave Fascicule 9). Bloomington: University of Indiana Press.

Thomas, J. (1999). *Understanding the Neolithic*. London: Routledge.

Todorova, H., Dimov, T., Bojadžiev, J., Vajsov, I., Dimitrov, K. & Avramova, M. (2002). Katalog der prähistorischen Gräber von Durankulak. In: H. Todorova (ed.) *Durankulak Band II. Die prähistorischen Gräberfelder. Teil II*. Berlin/Sofia: DAI/Anubis.

Tomasello, M. (1999). *The cultural origins of human cognition*. Cambridge, MA: Harvard University Press.

de la Torre, I., Mora, R., Domínguez-Rodrigo, L., de Luque, L. & Alcalá, L. (2003). The Oldowan industry of Peninj and its bearing on the reconstruction of the technological skills of Lower Pleistocene hominids. *Journal of Human Evolution* 44: 203–224.

Torrence, R. (1982). The obsidian quarries and their use. In: C. Renfrew & J. M. Wagstaff (eds) *An island polity: the archaeology of exploitation on Melos*, pp. 193–221. Cambridge: Cambridge University Press.

Vicsek, T. (ed.) (2001). *Fluctuations and scaling in biology*. Oxford: Oxford University Press.

Wadley, L. (2001). What is cultural modernity? A general view and a South African perspective from Rose Cottage Cave. *Cambridge Archaeological Journal* 11: 201–221.

Wynn, T. (2002). Archaeology and cognitive evolution. *Behavioral and Brain Sciences* 25: 389–403.

Yellen, J. E. (1977). *Archaeological approaches to the present*. New York: Academic Press.

21

Small Worlds, Material Culture and Ancient Near Eastern Social Networks

FIONA COWARD

In Ersilia, to establish the relationships that sustain the city's life, the inhabitants stretch strings from the corners of the houses, white or black or grey or black-and-white according to whether they mark a relationship of blood, of trade, authority, agency. When the strings become so numerous that you can no longer pass among them, the inhabitants leave: the houses are dismantled; only the strings and their supports remain. (Italo Calvino, *Invisible Cities*, p. 62)

A WEALTH OF EVIDENCE from primatology indicates that highly complex social relationships are part of our primate heritage (see e.g. refs in Lehmann et al. ch. 4 this volume). Nevertheless, human culture remains distinctive in terms of its sheer temporal and geographical scale. Research into how and when this 'scaling up' of human social relations occurred is largely divided between two opposing chronologies. Work focusing on the biological and neurological substrates for sociality in primates, humans and in the hominin fossil record has suggested that many of the relevant palaeoanthropological developments seem to occur after 500,000 years ago, being tentatively associated with (particularly late populations of) *Homo erectus* sensu lato (review in Grove and Coward 2008). This would see all modern human cognitive capacities in place at the evolution of genetically and anatomically modern *Homo sapiens*, possibly up to 200,000 years ago but certainly before 50,000 BP (see e.g. Klein 1999 for review), a logical and persuasive position given that modern humans across the globe display the same cognitive capacities and are remarkably genetically homogeneous (see references in Lahr & Foley 1998, 142).

However, such an early chronology is at odds with one based on material culture change, which identifies the impressive developments of post-anatomically modern human prehistory (notably the Middle–Upper Palaeolithic transition and/or the so-called 'Neolithic Revolution') as the definitive break-point(s) in the journey from 'hominin brain' to 'human

Proceedings of the British Academy **158**, 449–479. © The British Academy 2010.

mind'. The tension between these early and late chronologies has created what Renfrew has called the 'sapient paradox' (e.g. 2007; Renfrew et al. 2008).

It is certainly true that group size—a central factor in the early chronology's constellation of cognitive evolution—underwent perhaps its biggest increase not during hominin evolution *per se*, but well after the appearance of modern humans, as the first permanent villages developed in the Near East during the Epipalaeolithic and early Neolithic (ca. 12,000–8,000 radiocarbon years ago; e.g. Kuijt & Goring-Morris 2002). These developments are thought to form part of an 'explosion' of material culture that proponents of a late chronology argue represents a definitive break with the mobile hunter-gatherer lifeway *Homo sapiens* had pursued for over 100,000 years beforehand. These changes are claimed to be dramatic enough to represent a radical new form of social life, and perhaps even of cognition and/or language (Humphrey 2007): a new 'symbolic material culture' stage of cognitive evolution to add to Donald's scheme of cognitive evolution (1991) held to be 'characteristic of early agrarian societies with permanent settlement, monuments and valuables' (Renfrew 1998), i.e. firmly aligned with the appearance of Neolithic cultures (see also e.g. Runciman 2005; Watkins 2004, 105).

Some problems associated with this late chronology have been discussed elsewhere (e.g. Coward & Gamble 2008, in press; Gamble 1999). However, the real problem with both the early and the late chronologies is their reliance on 'flick of the switch' metaphors: the identification of a moment when hominin brains become human minds. Origin points- and revolutions-focused explanations have a long history and an enduring cultural appeal (e.g. Gamble 2007); however, it has more recently been argued that the development of distinctively 'human' cognitive capacities was a much more gradual and long-term process (Coward & Gamble 2008).

MATERIAL CULTURE IN COGNITIVE EVOLUTION

The lack of direct evidence for hominin brains and the relative paucity of the fossil record make the role of material culture in the process of cognitive evolution one of the most pressing issues for research. Many animal species use material objects for various purposes, and all great apes can use and indeed make tools in captivity (see e.g. reviews in Berthelet & Chavaillon 1993). Even in the wild the tool kits of some great apes are so group-specific and persistent over time that they can justifiably be termed 'material cultures' (e.g. McGrew 1992; van Schaik et al. 2003). It would seem, then, that the cognitive capacities for learning and behavioural flexibility are part of our primate heritage. However, as yet even the best primate stone tool knapper—the chimpanzee Kanzi—has never produced anything as complex even as mode 1 technology (the Oldowan, the very first recognizable stone tool industry known from 2.6 Ma; Schick & Toth 1995, 139; Schick et al. 1999). By the time mode 2 technology appears in the archaeological record in the shape of the Acheulean handaxe (associated with *Homo erectus*), the high standard of technical—and perhaps not incidentally, aesthetic—skill involved, together with the persistence of the technology for more than a million years across much of the Old World makes it clear that the scale of material engagement even at this early stage of hominization is beyond that available to other primate species.

The specific cognitive mechanisms necessary for manufacturing these different forms of stone tool remain a topic for much debate (e.g. Coolidge & Wynn 2005). However, research is now beginning to focus on the social implications of the cumulative cultural transmission they imply, including the role of teaching and pedagogy (e.g. Coward 2008; Matsuzawa 2007; Thornton & Raihani 2008; Tomasello 1999) and the contribution of derived forms of theory of mind which allow the appreciation of goals rather than simply actions (e.g. Gallese 2006).

However, perhaps the distinguishing characteristic of human material engagement is the extent to which the objects which humans manufacture and use are integrated into our social relations. The idea of distributed personhood—the notion that personhood is neither discrete nor bounded and synonymous with a body, but spills out through one's relationships with others such that it makes more sense to speak of 'dividuals' than 'individuals'—has become more widely accepted recently (Bird-David 1999; Jones 2004; Marriott 1976; Strathern 1988, 1998; Thomas 2002, e.g. 34). In this paradigm, the accumulation, fragmentation and movement of things acts to enchain people across time and space (Chapman 2000; Coward & Gamble 2008; Gamble ch. 2 this volume): the classic ethnographic examples are those of the Melanesian Kula ring (Malinowski 1920, 1922) and the Ju/'hoansi (Kalahari) *hxaro* exchange system (e.g. Layton & O'Hara ch. 5 this volume), where the circulation of objects links people together across space and over time. During this process the objects themselves acquire biographies and identities of their own (Gosden & Marshall 1999; Hoskins 1998) and become incorporated into our social lives in very similar ways to our fellow humans as different ('more than human'; Whatmore 2002, 161) kinds of nodes in our very heterogeneous social networks. Such practices date to very early in the process of hominization: there is evidence for the purposeful movement of material objects even in the very earliest sites from the Lower Pleistocene in Africa (Coward & Gamble in press; references in Roberts ch. 6 this volume; Schick & Toth 1995, 213). Over the course of hominization, such practices become *part of* cognition and social interaction rather than merely aids or prompts (Coward & Gamble 2008)—the defining characteristic of *extended*, rather than merely *embedded*, cognition (Rowlands ch. 16 this volume).

MATERIAL CULTURE AND NETWORKS

Viewed from such a perspective, the archaeological record is not a passive by-product of social relationships: rather, it *is* social relationships (Barrett, 2000 [1988]; Gamble 1999, 2007; Knappett 2005). The patterning of material culture is a direct result of the social relationships between individuals and groups in which these objects were caught up.

Archaeologists have long been comfortable dealing with populations, assemblages and distributions, with diffusion viewed in terms of the spread of traits across a homogeneous population and geography, analogous to the transmission of disease (e.g. Ammerman & Cavalli-Sforza 1973). Such approaches have more recently been complemented by consideration of 'mosaic' patterns of social and material culture change across space and over time (see e.g. Asouti 2006; Clark 2001; Douglas-Price 2000; Simek 2001, 201). As long ago as 1952 Hägerstrand's Monte Carlo simulations demonstrated the significance of contextual factors for processes of diffusion, emphasizing for example how communication and the regularity and quality of interpersonal contact channel the spread of traits (cited in McGlade & McGlade 1989). Research since has highlighted the simple fact that the spread and timing of traits is situation-specific and highly contextual (see review and references in McGlade & McGlade 1989, 285–287; also Coward & Grove submitted). In short, it is simply not possible to address the distribution of material culture (or, indeed, disease; see e.g. Lindenbaum 1978) without tackling the individual relationships that lie at the heart of the processes governing their spread. To this end, Dodds and Watts (2005) have recently suggested that a natural progression would be to consider diffusion models for a *networked* population of individuals, echoing Katherine Wright's recent call for a focus on networks rather than regions or cultures in archaeology (2008).

The burgeoning literature on the structure, properties and significance of social networks has a great deal to offer archaeology. A network perspective provides a much more realistic picture, not only of *objective* sociality, but also potentially of individuals' *subjective* experience of their worlds. Hägerstrand's time-geography, for example, described human activity as a web of individual paths in time-space:

> This space-time region contains the social system and is the setting of everyday life. As time flows, organisms and objects of different life-space describe paths which together form a large and complex web, where paths are born, move around (some more, some less) and die, combining all the time into different constellations. (in Carlstein 1982, 40)

Furthermore, individual paths are not isolated: what Hägerstrand calls 'stations' (sites, dwellings, resources, etc.) form 'pillars' in time-space, while there may be 'channels' of transport and communication etc. which serve to link individual paths together in space-time. The illustrations in Carlstein (1982, Figures 2.1–2.7, pp. 40–4) are simply networks viewed from a three-dimensional perspective that, although unfamiliar, serve to remind us of our embeddedness in the social and physical world: not a two-dimensional quantitative 'surface to be occupied' but 'a world to be inhabited' and experienced in terms of movement along paths and tracks (Ingold 2000, 155). One of the strengths of such a network perspective is that it allows—in fact, *demands*—a heterogeneous way of thinking about social relations. Humans, animals, plant species, things and places are all tangled up in the same network, as in Actor-Network Theory (see e.g. Latour 1996; Law 1999; Whatmore 2002, 2006). The world is always shared with others whose paths meet, avoid, branch off from, run parallel to or merge with one another over the course of their lives: 'Putting together all the trails of all the different beings that have inhabited a country—human, animal and plant, ordinary and extraordinary—the result would be a dense mass of intersecting pathways' (Ingold 2000, 144).

The classic anthropological example is that of Australian Aboriginal groups, who perceive the entire country in terms of networks of places linked by paths of movement (e.g. Munn 1973, 215): however, such network (or relational, or rhizomatic) modes of thought are not solely applicable to hunter-gatherers in contrast to the 'genealogical' (substantive, objective, etc.) cognitive style of agriculturalists (Deleuze & Guattari 1988, 18). As Ingold has argued, the latter arises out of the former and

exists alongside and complementary to it in the particular context of agricultural groups (Ingold 2000, 133–134), while Actor-Network Theory is
consistently and successfully applied to modern Western societies (e.g.
Jacobs 2006; Latour 1996).

Another strength of a network approach is that the networks being
investigated are simultaneously bottom-up and top-down. Individual
actors are part of the network and so are influenced by their associations
with other nodes—but at the same time the network is created by them,
so it can never be static or completely deterministic (Callon 1987). There
is thus no tension between the structuring role of large-scale cultural and
geographical patterning and decision-making and performance on the
part of the individual; indeed, as Latour (1999, 18) has pointed out, the
idea is to bypass the whole structure/agency debate altogether, as actors
and networks become two faces of the same phenomenon.

PREHISTORIC SOCIAL NETWORKS

Studies of prehistoric social networks are not entirely new; however, they
have mainly been applied to island contexts so far—the Pacific islands
were studied by Irwin (1983), Hunt (1988) and Hage and Harary (1996),
and the Bronze Age Aegean archipelago by Broodbank (2000) and Evans
et al. (in press). These studies have certainly demonstrated the robustness
of the methodology and its potential in prehistoric contexts—but all of
these examples have focused primarily on the *geographical* aspect of these
island networks. However, the entanglement of social interaction and
material culture into a heterogeneous relational network means that
similar methodologies can be used to investigate the material components
of prehistoric networks and inform on how the wider networks of
interaction of which they are a part change over time.

The datasets

The datasets discussed here are based on a database initially compiled by
Sue Colledge as part of the AHRB-funded project 'The Origin and
Spread of Neolithic Plant Economies in the Near East and Europe'
(Colledge et al. 2004)[1] and significantly extended by the author. The data-
base contains 780 individual levels from 591 sites dated to the

---

[1] http://ads.ahds.ac.uk/catalogue/collections/blurbs/452.cfm

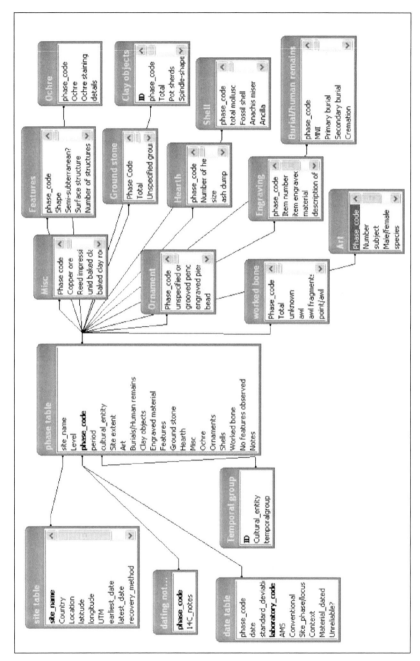

Figure 21.1. Structure of the database

Epipalaeolithic and Early Neolithic (PPNA and PPNB [Pre-Pottery Neolithic A and B]) from the Near East (including Israel, Jordan, Saudi Arabia, Egypt [the Sinai Peninsula], Iran, Iraq and south-eastern Turkey [south of the Taurus Mountains]). These tables are linked to a database of ^{14}C dates for sites in the Near East as well as to tables recording the finds recovered from those sites. Seven different varieties of material culture are recorded: art (defined as representations of various forms); burial data; items engraved with (non-representational) designs of various kinds; structural and architectural features; ground stone; hearths; lithics; ochre; ornaments and jewellery; shells and worked bone (Figure 21.1). Some artefacts are recorded in more than one table—for example, engraved grooved polishers are recorded in both the ground stone and the engraved items tables.

Data were gleaned from the widest possible variety of sources. Where possible original definitive reports were used, but many sites have been reported to date only in interim reports (more recent reports being prioritized over earlier). A number of region- and theme-specific reviews were also extremely useful, including those by Bar-Yosef (1970); Aurenche (1981a, 1981b, 1981c); Wright (1992a, 1992b); Hours et al. (1994); Sayej (2004); Kozlowski and Aurenche (2005), as well as online databases such as the TAY project[2], CANEW[3] and the CONTEXT radiocarbon database (Böhner & Schyle 2002–2006).[4]

In the analyses presented here only sites with radiocarbon dates were included; dates were calibrated using OxCal v4,[5] with all dates in this chapter being calibrated in years BC. Dated sites were divided into datasets of non-mutually-exclusive 1,000-year intervals from 21,000 to 6,000 cal. BC on the basis of the range of dates within 1 standard deviation from the mean calibrated date; most sites therefore appear in more than one consecutive interval. For example, a date of 8658+/-101 BP from Jericho II (P-381) is calibrated to between 8170 and 7524 at 68 per cent probability and therefore appears in both the 9–8 kyrs cal. BC and 8–7 kyrs cal. BC time intervals.

Dates were not audited, although those explicitly considered problematic by excavators were removed from the analysis, as were dates with errors of more than 1,000 radiocarbon years which would otherwise have dominated the datasets. Only two sites stood out as problematic during

[2] http://www.tayproject.org/enghome.html
[3] http://www.canew.org/
[4] http://context-database.uni-koeln.de/site.php
[5] http://c14.arch.ox.ac.uk/embed.php?File=oxcal.html

the compilation of these datasets: Nemrik 9, believed to date to the PPNA, has a total of 81 radiocarbon dates ranging from >40,000 (Gd-5237) to 3990+/-510 cal. BC (Gd-4194), thus covering most of the time periods analysed here. However, the dates cluster around 10,500 BP, and the excavators consider it probable that the site dates to between 10,500 BP (~10,800–10,165 cal. BC) and 8,400 BP (~7,592–7,195 cal. BC; Kozlowski 1989, 25–26), and therefore Nemrik appears in these analyses only in intervals between 11 and 7 kyrs cal. BC. The second site, Salibiya IX, has yielded two dates of 20,050+/-230 and 12,470+/-620 cal. BC, and is variously assigned to either the Khiamian (PPNA) and/or the Late Natufian or a mixture between the two. Given these uncertainties, the site was not included in these initial analyses. The sites included in each dataset are listed in Table 21.1.

One final concern was that higher levels of mobility earlier in the record might create 'noise' in these datasets (Chapman pers. comm.); therefore, sites yielding solely lithic material culture were excluded from these initial analyses. Obviously, however, this is an issue that will be investigated more closely in future.

For analysis by social network techniques (using UCINET 6; Borgatti et al. 2002), datasets need to be in the format of an adjacency matrix with as many rows/columns as there are actors in the dataset under investigation. In social network analysis 'actors' need not be individuals but are discrete social units at a variety of levels of analysis ranging from the individual to the corporate and national: in this analysis, discrete levels of sites from the Epipalaeolithic and early Neolithic Near East at which various kinds of material culture have been recovered become nodes in the networks. Scores in the cells of the matrix record information about the relational ties between each pair of sites; the range and variety of ties that may be investigated is extensive but routinely includes transfers of material resources (see e.g. Wasserman & Faust 1994, 18 for further discussion).

In this study, the material culture inventories from the sites/levels in each 1,000-year time-slice were used as material proxies for social interactions between those sites. In the case of a single discrete and transportable object, such as a particular kind of ground stone implement—a pestle in Figures 21.2a and 21.2b—the object might have been directly physically transferred between sites through processes of transport, trade, exchange, etc. More generally, the idea behind the practices associated with different objects may have been shared purely in the sense of being held in common: two sites with even rather different specific forms of ground stone still clearly share the kinds of practice that are associated

Table 21.1. The datasets

Kyrs cal. BC	No. sites	Sites
>21	4	Ohalo II; Rakefet Cave XIII; Uwaynid 18 upper; Wadi Hammeh 26
21–20	6	Haon II level 3; Nahal Oren Terrace VIII, IX (Noy); Ohalo II; Rakefet Cave XIII; Uwaynid 18 upper; Wadi Hammeh 26
20–19	5	Haon II level 3; Nahal Oren Terrace VIII, IX (Noy); Ohalo II; Rakefet Cave; Wadi Hasa 1065 B-E
19–18	6	Haon II level 3; Nahal Oren Terrace VIII, IX (Noy); Ohalo II; Wadi Hammeh 31; Wadi Hasa 1065 B-E; Wadi Jilat upper phase A
18–17	13	Ein Gev I levels 3 & 4; Haon II level 3; Hamifgash IV; Kharaneh IV D; Mdamagh; Nahal Oren Terrace VIII, IX (Noy); Ohalo II; Rakefet Cave XIII; Urkhan e-Rubb IIa; Wadi Hammeh 31; Wadi Hasa 1065 B-E; Wadi Jilat 6 Upper phase A
17–16	11	Ein Gev I levels 3 & 4; Ishkaft Palegawra lower; Kharaneh IV D; Mdamagh; Mushabi XIV 1; Mushabi XVII; Nahal Oren Terrace VIII, IX (Noy); Urkhan e-Rubb IIa; Wadi Jilat 10; Wadi Jilat 6 Upper phase A
16–15	7	Ishkaft Palegawra lower; Kharaneh IV D; Mdamagh; Mushabi XIV 1; Mushabi XVII; Urkan e-Rubb IIa; Wadi Jilat 10
15–14	17	Ain Mallaha III, IV; Beidha natufian; El Wad B2; Ishkaft Palegawra lower; Wadi Judayid J2 C; Mdamagh; Mushabi I; Mushabi XIV 1; Mushabi XVII; Neve David; Nahal Zin D5; Urkan e-Rubb IIa; Wadi Jilat 10; Wadi Jilat 22 C & E; Wadi Jilat 8
14–13	18	Ain Mallaha III, IV; Beidha natufian; El Wad B2; Hayonim Cave B; Ishkaft Palegawra lower; Wadi Judayid J2 C; Mdamagh; Mushabi I; Mushabi V; Mushabi XIV 1; Mushabi XVI; Mushabi XVII; Neve David; Nahal Zin D5; Salibiya I; Wadi Jilat 10; Wadi Jilat 22 E; Wadi Jilat 8
13–12	17	'Ain Ghazal MPPNB; Ain Mallaha III, IV; Beidha natufian; El Wad B2; Hayonim Cave B; Hayonim Terrace B, C/D; Wadi Judayid J2 C; Mushabi V; Mushabi XIV 1; Mushabi XVI; Neve David; Nahal Sekher 23; Qermez Dere; Salibiya I; Tor Hamar A-E1; Wadi Hammeh 27; Wadi Jilat 10
12–11	22	'Ain Ghazal MPPNB; Tell Abu Hureyra 1; Ain Mallaha III, IV; Beidha natufian; El Wad B2; Hayonim Cave B; Hayonim Terrace B, C/D; Ishkaft Palegawra lower; Jarmo aceramic JI8–6, JAIII, IV, V; Wadi Judayid J2 C; Jericho Natufian; Kebara Cave B; Nahal Sekher 23; Qermez Dere; Rakefet Cave Natufian; Rosh Horesha; Saflulim; Salibiya I; Shinera IV; Wadi Hammeh 27; Zawi Chemi Shanidar B
11–10	45	'Ain Ghazal MPPNB; Tell Abu Hureyra 1; Ali Kosh (Ali Kosh, Bus Mordeh); Abu Madi 1 5–12; Ain Mallaha Ic & III/IV; Beidha natufian; Çayönü Ia (round buildings); Dhra PPNA; Dja'de; El Wad B1 & 2; Ganj Dareh Tepe E; Gilgal I; Hallan Çemi Tepesi; Hayonim Terrace B, C/D; Jarmo aceramic JI8–6, JAIII, IV, V; Wadi Judayid J2 C; Jericho Natufian; Kebara Cave B; Munhata; M'lefaat; Maaleh Ramon East; Maaleh Ramon West; Tell Mureybet IA & IB & II & III; Nemrik; Neve David; Netiv Hagdud; Nahal Oren Terrace V/VI (Noy); Qermez Dere; Rakefet Cave Natufian; Ramat Harif; Rosh Horesha; Saflulim; Salibiya I; Shanidar B1; Shunera IV; Wadi Shu'eib; Zawi Chemi Shanidar B

Table 21.1. *Continued.*

Kyrs cal. BC	No. sites	Sites
10–9	53	'Ain Ghazal MPPNB; Tell Abu Hureyra 1 & 2A; Ali Kosh (Ali Kosh, Bus Mordeh); Abu Madi 1 5–12 & 1–4; Ain Mallaha Iab & Ic & III/IV; Abu Salem; Beidha natufian; Çayönü Ia (round buildings); Cafer Höyük III; Dhra PPNA; Dja'de; El Wad B1; Ganj Dareh Tepe D-A & E; Gesher; Gilgal I; Hallan Çemi Tepesi; Halula I/II levels 1–20; Hayonim Terrace B, C/D; Iraq ed Dubb II; Jerf el Ahmar I/W, -1/-II/E; Jericho I & II & Natufian; Munhata; M'lefaat; Maaleh Ramon West; Tell Mureybet IA & II & III & IV; Nemrik; Nevali Çori; Netiv Hagdud; Nahal Hemar; Nahal Oren Terrace V/VI (Noy); Qermez Dere; Ramat Harif; Rosh Horesha; Shunera IV; Tepe Abdul Hosein; Wadi Shu'eib; Zahrat adh-Dhra; Zawi Chemi Shanidar B
9–8	59	'Ain Ghazal MPPNB; Tell Abu Hureyra 1 & 2A; Ali Kosh (Ali Kosh, Bus Mordeh); Abu Madi 1 5–12 & 1–4; Ain Mallaha Iab & Ic & III/IV; Asiab; Tell Aswad IA & IB & II; Beidha Neolithic; Çayönü Ia (round buildings) & IB (grill/channel buildings) & IC (cobble-paved buildings); Cafer Höyük I & II & III; Dhra PPNA; Dja'de; El Aoui Safa; El Kowm II; Ghwair 1; Ganj Dareh Tepe D-A & E; Gesher; Gilgal I; Tell Ghoraifé IA; Gritille A-D; Göbekli Tepe; Hallan Çemi Tepesi; Horvat Galil; Halula I/II levels 1–20; Jarmo acermaic JI8, JAIII/IV/V; Jerf el Ahmar VII-oE, IV-III/W & I/W, -1/-II/E; Jericho I & II; Munhata; M'lefaat; Motza; Tell Mureybet III & IV; Nemrik; Nevali Çori; Nahal Divshon; Netiv Hagdud; Nahal Hemar; Nahal Oren Terrace V/VI (Noy); Qermez Dere; Shunera IV; Tepe Abdul Hosein; Tepe Guran D-V; Wadi Jilat 26; Wadi Jilat 7 II; Wadi Shu'eib; Yiftah'el; Zahrat adh-Dhra
8–7	63	Ain Abu Nekheileh; 'Ain Ghazal LPPNB & MPPNB; Tell Abu Hureyra 1 & 2A & 2B; Ali Kosh (Ali Kosh, Bus Mordeh); Akarçay Tepe all PPNB; Asiab; Tell Aswad IB & II; Azraq 31; Beidha Neolithic; Bouqras; Çayönü Ia (round buildings) & IB (grill/channel buildings) & IC (cobble-paved buildings); Cafer Höyük I & II & III; Dja'de; El Kowm II; Er-Rahib; Es-Siffiya; Ghwair 1; Ganj Dareh Tepe D-A & E; Tell Ghoraifé IA & II; Gritille A-D; Göbekli Tepe; Horvat Galil; Halula I/II levels 1–20; Jarmo acermaic JI8, JAIII/IV/V; Jericho I & II; Kfar HaHoresh; Munhata; Motza; Tell Mureybet IV; Magzalia; Nemrik; Nevali Çori; Nahal Divshon; Nahal Hemar; Nahal Issaron C; Qdeir 1; Tell Ramad I; Tell Ras Shamra Vc1–3; Tepe Abdul Hosein; Tell Damishliyya 1–7; Tell es-Sinn; Tepe Guran D-V; Wadi Jilat 26; Wadi Jilat 7 II; Wadi Shu'eib; Yiftah'el
7–6	37	Ain Abu Nekheileh; 'Ain Ghazal MPPNB; Tell Abu Hureyra 2A & 2B; Ali Kosh (Ali Kosh, Bus Mordeh); Bouqras; Çayönü Id (cell plan/large room buildings); Cafer Höyük I; El Kowm I lower & II; Er-Rahib; Es-Siffiya; Ganj Dareh Tepe D-A; Tell Ghoraifé IA & II; Gritille A-D; Halula I/II levels 1–20; Jarmo acermaic JI8, JAIII/IV/V; Khirbet Hammam; Kfar HaHoresh; Laboureh A1, bottom of B; Munhata; Motza; Nahal Divshon; Nahal Hemar; Nahal Issaron C; Qdeir 1; Tell Ramad I; Tell Ras Shamra Vc1–3; Tepe Abdul Hosein; Tell Damishliyya 1–7; Tell es-Sinn; Tepe Guran D-V; Tell Sabi Abyad II; Tell Seker al-Aheimar; Wadi Shu'eib

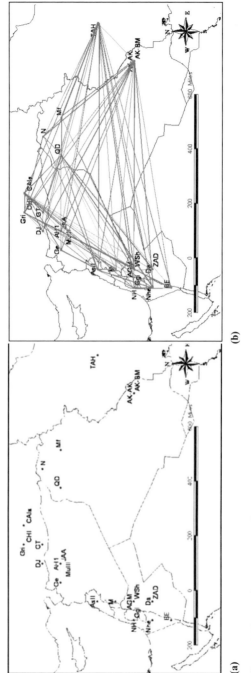

Figures 21.2(a) and **(b)**. Presence of pestles in sites dated 9,000–8,000 cal. BC: sites as nodes, co-occurrence of material culture as ties

with that kind of technology, specifically subsistence strategies prioritizing the grinding of vegetable foods.

The distribution of particular forms of material culture between sites thus becomes a material reflection of some form of social relationship (in its widest sense) between those sites. Further, the range of different forms become the heterogeneous relationships connecting sites into multiple, heterogeneous interlinked networks. For example, the co-occurrence of ground stone pestles at different sites is recorded as a relation between those sites (regardless, in this analysis, of the *number* of pestles found), as is the co-occurrence of dentalium beads, female figurines, internal hearths, etc. The result is a matrix in which the total number of different forms of material culture shared between each pair of sites is treated as the strength of the relationship between them.

This use of valued relations is potentially somewhat problematic in that many formal methods of social network analysis are defined primarily for binary or dichotomous relations, where a relation is either present or absent. However, given the sheer quantity of different forms of material culture that formed part of this study, when dichotomized many of the social networks studied here simply collapsed to form maximally connected ('complete') networks where virtually all nodes were connected to virtually all others. Many applications of social network analysis to anthropological and archaeological situations avoid this problem by connecting nodes only to a specified number of their closest neighbours (often three; see e.g. Broodbank 2000, 180; Hunt 1988, 137; Irwin 1983, 35–36), and this will certainly be a feature of future analyses. However, for the purposes of the current chapter it was deemed important to maximize the data, and relations are therefore valued: the specific implications of this are discussed in more detail at the appropriate points below.

Results

Mean distances between sites in each dataset generally increase over time (Figure 21.3; distance is measured here as geodesic distance, which simply equates to the value of the relations in the shortest path between every pair of sites). At the same time, the proportion of sites connected directly declines (Figure 21.3; values range 0–1). However, a permutation-based ANOVA (see Hanneman & Riddle 2005 for discussion of why standard statistical tests should not be applied to network data, in which individual observations are not necessarily independent) found these variations between datasets were not statistically significant (10,000 permutations, 15 degrees of freedom: f-statistic 1.1640; r^2 0.045; p = 0.0863). This increase in distance may well be a function of the general increase in the size of the datasets over time (see Table 21.1).

A corollary of this increase in distance is that individual sites become differentially connected over time. In general, the more ties an actor/site has, the more power they (may) have; autonomy makes an actor less dependent on any specific other actor, and hence more powerful. The number/value of an individual actor/site's ties (degree centrality) is thus a good measure of their 'centrality' in a network and hence (potentially) their power, and the variability in that measure over the network is a measure of how uniformly (or otherwise) power is distributed between sites. Network centralization measures (UCINET 6's routine for computing network centralization had to be adapted for valued data)[6] track this variability by expressing the degree of variability in degree centrality outlined above as a percentage of the maximum possible variability in a network of the same size[7] (Hanneman & Riddle 2005; Wasserman & Faust 1994). As Figure 21.3b demonstrates, the trend in measures of network centralization is generally upward from 16,000–15,000 cal. BC (the middle/late Epipalaeolithic, specifically late Kebaran/early Geometric Kebaran).

At the same time, however, the mean strength of the ties between sites (Figure 21.3c) increases over time. A permutation-based ANOVA revealed highly significant statistical differences among the datasets (10,000 permutations, 15 degrees of freedom: f-statistic = 22.9658, r^2 = 0.484, p = 0.0001). *Post hoc* permutation-based t-tests (all at 10,000 permutations) using the 7–6 kyr cal. BC dataset as the dependent variable demonstrated that there were no significant differences between this dataset and those dating 12–7 kyrs cal. BC: tested against the 13–12 kyrs cal. BC p = 0.0446 and against all preceding datasets p = 0.0001.

Overall density of networks—the proportion of the maximum possible strength of ties that is realized—also, generally speaking, increases between 21,000 and 6,000 cal. BC (Figure 21.3d): a permutation-based ANOVA was highly significant (10,000 permutations, 15 degrees of freedom: f-statistic = 11.9362; r^2 = 0.328; p = 0.0001). *Post hoc* permutation-based t-tests (all at 10,000 permutations) found no significant differences

---

[6] $((r(g-1))-r)(g-1)$ where g = number of actors; r = number of relations.
[7] That of a 'star graph' whose degree centrality is given by $(g-1)(g-2)$ where 'g' is the number of actors in the network.

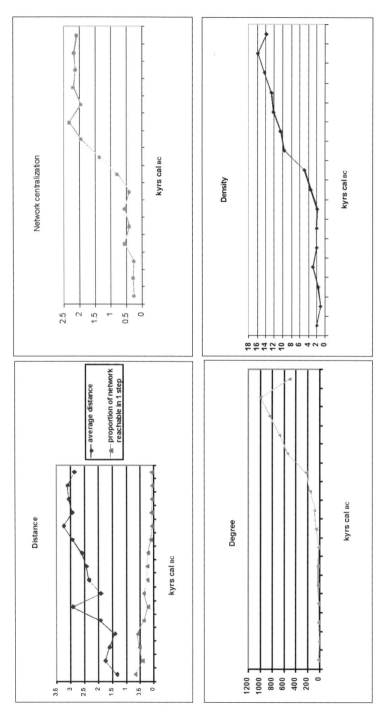

Figure 21.3 (a) Distance, **(b)** Network centralization, **(c)** Degree, **(d)** Density

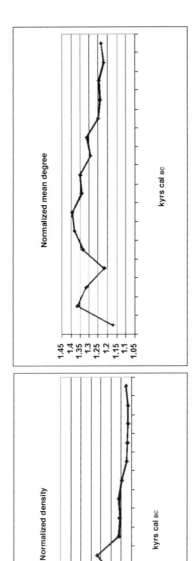

Figures 21.4 (a) and **(b)**. Declining network density and degree when normalized for the number of contributing forms of material culture

between the 7–6 kyrs cal. BC datasets and those dating 11–7 kyrs cal. BC but significant differences with those dating to before 11 kyrs cal. BC (10–9 kyrs, p = 0.0444; 13–12 kyrs cal BC, p = 0.0134; 14–13 kyrs cal. BC, p = 0.0002; all preceding datasets p = 0.0001).

The cause of this increase would appear to be the sheer diversity of forms of material of the later sites: when normalized for the number of different kinds of material culture contributing (using UCINET's 'marginal' normalizing routine), the later datasets are indeed generally less dense and the strength of ties (degree) declines over time (Figures 21.4a and 21.4b).

DISCUSSION

The material component of social networks will of course only ever give a partial view of the wider social networks in which they are embedded: in addition to the perennial issues of differential preservation of different kinds of object, variable investigation, excavation and publication in different countries and regions, etc., there may be many forms of relationship between groups, sites and individuals that do not have material correlates. Furthermore, the data presented here are restricted to the minority of sites that have been robustly dated, resulting in some very small datasets (particularly early on in the sequence).

In addition, a wide variety of different kinds of correspondences in material culture are treated together here which may in reality hide a similarly disparate repertoire of behavioural strategies, such as the physical trade of individual items; the movement of individuals with particular kinds of knowledge relating to manufacturing and technological traditions (perhaps through marriage networks); the spread of ideas, motifs, etc. independent of any physical movement of items or people, and so on. Each of these practices may be associated with rather different kinds of networks and/or forms of material culture with their own distinctive properties, costs and benefits. However, it seems unlikely that such a fine-grained teasing apart of the individual factors involved in prehistoric material culture networks will ever be completely possible. The uncertainties in dating (each dataset here covers 1,000 years and thus many generations), coupled with the aforementioned sampling issues necessitates a broad view of the problem; clearly the networks presented here potentially subsume many more specialized sub-networks within them. However, that in itself will contribute to the patterns of increasing fragmentation, within-network distinctiveness and variability that are demonstrated here.

In short, the material networks investigated here represent *minimum* or maximally parsimonious starting points for investigating how the social networks of the Near East develop over the course of the Epipalaeolithic and early Neolithic. This makes it all the more interesting that several statistically significant trends have emerged: over time networks grow in size and become more dense, the mean strength of ties between sites (degree) becomes stronger while variability in the distribution of those ties (network centralization) increases, and connectivity between sites (distance) declines (although this last is not statistically significant).

There are therefore some very interesting comparisons to be made between the patterns demonstrated by these networks and those known from modern human and primate social networks; in general, larger social groups are less dense than smaller (see references in Hanneman & Riddle 2005; Lehmann et al. ch. 4 this volume; Wasserman & Faust 1994).

The constraints on network size discussed by Roberts (ch. 6 this volume) may be significant here, and include:

(1) Cognitive constraints on keeping track of dynamic patterns of interactions with different others (furthermore, increasingly *individualized* others with more divergent behaviours; Read ch. 10 this volume) as well as their interactions with one another, and

(2) time and energy constraints: relationships require continual maintenance if they are not to 'decay'. Competing demands on time and emotional intensity inevitably means that, as the number of individuals in each hierarchical level (support, sympathy, band or active network) of the network increases, the level of emotional intimacy and frequency/intensity of interaction necessarily decreases.

As a result, it would seem that there may be an absolute limit to the number of friends and acquaintances any individual can maintain at different hierarchical layers. Various means of off-setting these costs and constraints have been suggested, most famously the expansion of the neocortex documented among primates and humans, which it would seem has allowed us to steadily increase the size of our social groups over time to the observed level of ~150 ('Dunbar's number'; Aiello & Dunbar 1993;

Dunbar 1993, 1996, 2003). However, many modern humans live in much greater aggregations than this: indeed, since 2008 humans as a species have been a majority city-living species (UNFPA 2007). At the same time, however, it would seem that Dunbar's number has remained a highly significant building block for the social groups of historical Western humans and even *Homo urbanus* (e.g. Dunbar 1993, Tables 1 and 2 684–686). Nor is there any evidence for further enlargement of the neocortex among city-dwellers, or of an increased ability to deal cognitively with ever-higher levels of intentionality.

In short, some additional strategies must be off-setting these costs and maximizing the benefits of networks. Other chapters in this volume have discussed some of these, including:

(1) Categorical modes of thought, which simplify the cognitive load of social surveillance (see e.g. Read ch. 10 this volume regarding kin systems).

(2) Specialized roles and individualization: e.g. Roberts (ch. 6 this volume) discusses the role of 'kinkeepers' in acting as hubs for social surveillance of extended kin and the dissemination of relevant information to interested parties, thus lightening the demands on their time. Interestingly, 'kinkeepers' tend to be older females; there is some evidence to suggest that males and females maintain slightly different roles within social networks that reflect the different costs and benefits applicable to the different sexes but that also complement each other in terms of maintaining more extended social networks. Of course, more than gender distinguishes between individuals along more continua than gender; age and personality differences and increasing individualization (Read ch. 10 this volume) may also contribute to the complexity of overall social networks through greater variability between individual ego-networks (see e.g. Coward & Grove submitted).

(3) Extended cognition: Rowlands (2003, e.g. 166, and ch. 16 this volume) has argued that in 'off-loading' some aspects of cognition to the external world individuals can lighten their personal cognitive loads (the 'Barking Dog' principle; see Gamble ch. 2 this volume). Language may be one such strategy, allowing the enhanced sharing of ideas and information (see discussion in Gamble ch. 2 this volume). The *structure* of the networks of which individual relationships are a part may also lighten the cognitive load of maintaining them, as the positioning of any one dyadic relationship between

two individuals may be variably held in place by its entanglement in the other relationships surrounding it (Roberts ch. 6 this volume).

The use of material culture is also highly pertinent here: as discussed above, the incorporation of non-human *things* into social networks allows for their other-than-human qualities—notably, in the case of material culture, the qualities of *durability, persistence* and *divisibility* (from humans; from other associated items of material culture and in and of themselves through practices of fragmentation; Chapman 2000, see Gamble 1998, ch. 2 this volume)—to be co-opted (or exapted) for the purposes of constructing and maintaining ever-greater social networks. As argued above, the use of material culture in this way would seem to date back to very early in the process of hominization (see also Gamble and Roberts chs 2 and 6 this volume, and *contra* the arguments for a late advent of material engagement discussed earlier).

All of these strategies would seem to be relevant for the analysis presented here: as noted above, the main reason that these Epipalaeolithic and early Neolithic networks increase in density over time is the sheer number of different forms of material culture contributing to those networks. When networks are normalized to compensate for this, density behaves as would be expected by decreasing as networks increase in size over time. Off-loading the cognitive costs of maintaining large social networks by extending social networks to include material culture may therefore be a crucial factor in the shift to village life that occurred during the Epipalaeolithic and early Neolithic of the Near East.

Ethnographic evidence suggests that in small-scale mobile societies, social networks tend to be open and ephemeral, with patterns of social interaction primarily organized around kinship and close physical proximity: 'Within a small group of individuals such as a hunter-gatherer residential groups . . . there are fairly direct and unambiguous links between each individual' (Whitelaw 1991, 182). Daily hunter-gatherer life generally occurs in full view, with most time spent within range of intimate and personal distance of one another (Wilson 1988). Knowledge of one another is therefore multiplex, personal and biographical, and the social networks involved are what Hillier and Hanson refer to as 'dense encounter sets' (1984, 27): interactions occur repeatedly between the same individuals, who by virtue of their common enmeshment within the same matrix of relationships, will share (at least to some degree) a common way of life (Lofland 1973).

Of course, even in larger and/or less mobile groups there will be groups of kin or individuals whose closeness results in frequent intimate and personal interactions and mutual knowledge. However, these clusters of strongly related individuals must maintain relations with other such clusters in their wider community unless the group as a whole is to fission—an option that obviously becomes less feasible almost by definition as groups become more sedentary. Furthermore, as groups increase in size, it is inevitable that any one individual will encounter any other less frequently; larger societies are inherently less dense 'encounter sets' than smaller (Hillier & Hanson 1984, 27), with concomitant increases in the cognitive, temporal and energetic costs outlined above. Sociologists have noted that one strategy which may off-set some of these costs by reducing the potential 'overload' of information is the simplification of some relationships (Lofland 1973; Milgram 1977). Of course, there is always the potential to invest more in any relationship, but in large-scale societies any individual can only afford to have 'weak ties' with the majority of people he/she interacts with: categorical rather than biographical relationships (Granovetter 1973, 1983; Lofland 1973; Milgram 1977; see also Read ch. 10 this volume). It is these weak ties that are crucial for maintaining the links between dense kin- and proximity-based groups and that make the difference between fission or growth of social groups—however, alongside the cognitive ability to deal with categorical relationships discussed above, weak ties also require some cognitive mechanism for adjustment to the fracturing of co-presence and personal knowing (Lofland 1973; Whitelaw 1991, 158).

One such mechanism, and perhaps the most important for explaining how the networks of the Epipalaeolithic and early Neolithic can become larger, more fragmented and yet simultaneously denser, is the increasing incorporation into these networks of material culture. In small, dense groups the intimate and personal relations between strongly associated individuals means that they 'share, to some degree, a particular understanding of the world' (DeMarrais et al. 1996; see also Coser 1975, 254; Douglas 1973, 78). As a result, communication codes in a variety of modes may be more restricted, such that 'more meanings are implicit and taken for granted as the speakers are so familiar with one another' (Bernstein cited in Coser 1975, 254). However, while such dense and complex relations of course continue to exist in larger groups, they do so alongside more simplified interactions, and the individuals participating in these do not have intimate personal knowledge of one another by which to judge their embodied performances. Communication in these more fragmented networks requires *elaborated* forms of communication (Bernstein cited in Granovetter 1973, 1983). In these situations, there is generally a greater emphasis on spatial and environmental cues to define what Goffman (1959) calls 'settings' through the elaboration of material culture, effectively 'distributing' the information required for social cognition and effective performance in the physical and material world (Lofland 1973, 82–83; Rapoport 1981, 30, 1990, 16; Sanders 1990, 71)— hence the general association of greater degrees of formal segregation and organization of space in larger societies and particularly among sedentary agriculturalists, despite some exceptions such as the Mongols (Kent 1990; see also Donley-Reid 1990; Rapoport 1969; Whitelaw 1991, 1994, 238). Perhaps, then, the changing material culture networks of the Epipalaeolithic and early Neolithic described above represent a gradual shift from 'the tribal human confronting, with fear and suspicion, the infrequent stranger ... [to] ... the cosmopolitan human confronting, with ease and ability, the constant stranger' (Lofland 1973, xi).

However, it is important to note that the two organizing principles— kin and restricted communication/material culture codes and weakly linked acquaintances and elaborated codes—are not mutually exclusive but are present to some degree in all modern human societies. For example, among Central Australian Aboriginal groups, the emphasis between the two forms of integration varies both by season (relating to differences in resource structure and mobility) and, more fundamentally, by sex, with women more inclined to form close clusters and men to act as 'weak links' between these (Hillier & Hanson 1984, 236; see also Postmes et al. 2005). Interestingly, this pattern has also been noted among primate groups (e.g. Kudo & Dunbar 2001; see also Roberts' notes on 'kinkeepers', ch. 6 this volume). As Lofland concludes: '*The cosmopolitan did not lose the capacity for knowing other personally. But he gained the capacity for knowing others only categorically*' (1973, 177, italics in original; see also Read ch. 10 this volume).

In short, then, we should be cautious about heralding the changes in social networks suggested by the analysis presented here as revolutionary. They are more likely to relate to a shift of emphasis in the kinds of social strategies pursued and the kinds of resource utilized by individuals— adding those associated with weaker, categorical social relations to the repertoire of resources used in multiplex and personal relationships that are part of our primate heritage or that had developed during the process of hominization (Coward & Gamble 2008).

In fact, very similar patterns have been documented in primate social networks. Lehmann et al. (ch. 4 this volume) describe primate social networks becoming increasingly more fragmented (less dense and less well-connected) among species with larger neocortices (which is of course in turn highly correlated with group size; Aiello & Dunbar 1993; Dunbar 1992, 1993); Lehmann et al. (this volume) suggest that low levels of density and connectivity and greater fragmentation (more, more distinctive grooming 'clans' or densely clustered subgroups) can be used as an operational definition of social complexity. Furthermore, they find that it is neocortex size, rather than group size *per se*, which is more strongly related to density; primates with bigger brains tend to be those species who are better at finding cognitive strategies for linking up small, dense kin-based clusters with 'weak links'. Layton and O'Hara (ch. 5 this volume) further discuss some of the ecological characteristics that distinguish humans from other primates, suggesting that greater reliance on meat-eating among humans necessitates much lower population densities: larger group sizes, but spread over much greater areas. They suggest that this would have required mechanisms for sustaining reduced frequency of direct interaction with acquaintances than is the case for primates.

The overall direction of these developments, therefore, appears to be towards the so-called 'small-world' phenomenon, where path length (the distance between any two nodes) is small and 'clustering' (the tendency of the 'nodes' to form small, dense groups) is high; the formation of such networks is governed by the probability of nodes being connected outside of their immediate group—i.e. by the proportion of 'weak' connections between dense groups (Buchanan 2002; Newman 2000, 2001; Watts 2003; Watts & Strogatz 1998). The result of this process—where highly connected individuals enjoy the so-called 'six degrees of separation' effect—is such a robust and efficient structure for a dynamic network that it has been identified in real-world situations ranging from power grids to ecological foodwebs to the neural network of the nematode worm *Caenorhabditis elegans* and, famously, the structure of the worldwide web (see e.g. Buchanan 2002; Watts 2003 for discussion and references). Among humans—and primates more generally—the benefits of moving towards such a 'small-world' social organization may be its efficiency in terms of time and energy (as well as cognitive effort), and its structural flexibility, simultaneously allowing for small groups of close (supportive) others and broader circles of overlapping but individualized (thus reducing competition) more distant others who allow navigation of the wider social world. These wider social networks may have fulfilled a variety of functions, perhaps most importantly reducing risk by tapping into a wider range of natural and social resources through trade, marriage, etc.

CONCLUSION

The analyses presented here demonstrate some interesting trends in the material culture component of social networks over the course of the Epipalaeolithic and early Neolithic of the Near East between 21,000 and 6,000 years cal. BC. Mean tie strength between sites increases over time and becomes more variable, connectivity decreases and overall density of networks increases. Interestingly, however, when networks are normalized for the variety of different forms of material culture contributing to them, density actually decreases over this period.

These developments echo those documented among primates more generally, as well as among modern human groups, and appear to represent new strategies for off-setting the increased costs associated with maintaining relationships among larger groups living first at lower population densities in the case of mobile hunter-gatherers (Layton & O'Hara ch. 5 this volume) and more recently at higher densities. Off-loading demanding cognitive tasks through such strategies as language (almost certainly in place by the speciation of *Homo sapiens*, *contra* Humphrey 2007) and the incorporation of material culture into social relations has allowed human social relationships to become ever more extended in space and time. However, there is nothing deterministic about this process: the specific format of social network varies locally between and even within different groups. The tension between early and late chronologies is therefore a blind alley. As Mellars pointed out in reference to the Neanderthal/modern human debate: 'There seems to be an irresistible urge to polarize scientific debate into extreme positions. The truth is rarely that simple' (1996, 8).

While there may certainly be inflections in the general trend in particular times and places (the so-called 'creative explosion' of the Last Glacial Maximum in Europe, the early Neolithic of the Near East?) the trajectory of hominization appears to be towards greater social complexity measured in terms of the increasing ability to forge and maintain weak links between the small tightly bonded groups that are our primate heritage.

Note. Thanks to Sue Colledge, Stephen Shennan and other members of the Centre for the Evolution of Cultural Diversity, UCL, for allowing me to (ab)use their database; the members of the 'Lucy to Language' project, especially Clive Gamble and Matt Grove; contributors to the British Academy 'Social Brain, Distributed Mind' conference; fellow members of the Royal Holloway University of London Centres for Quaternary Research and Social and Cultural Geography; Ian Clark for help with Excel; two anonymous reviewers for extremely helpful comments on a first draft.

REFERENCES

Aiello, L. & Dunbar, R. (1993). Neocortex size, group size and the evolution of language. *Current Anthropology* 34: 184–193.

Ammerman, A. J. & Cavalli-Sforza, L. L. (1973). A population model for the diffusion of early farming in Europe. In: C. Renfrew (ed.) *The explanation of culture change*, pp. 343–357. London: Duckworth.

Asouti, E. (2006). Beyond the Pre-Pottery Neolithic B interaction sphere. *Journal of World Prehistory* 20: 87–126.

Aurenche, O. (1981a). *La maison orientale: l'architecture du Proche Orient des origines au milieu du quatrième millénaire, tome 1: Texte.* Paris: Institut français d'archéologie du Proche Orient.

Aurenche, O. (1981b). *La maison orientale: l'architecture du Proche Orient ancien des origines au milieu du quatrième millénaire, tome 2: Documents.* Paris: Institut français d'archéologie du Proche Orient.

Aurenche, O. (1981c). *La maison orientale: l'architecture du Proche Orient ancien des origines au milieu du quatrième millénaire, yome 3: tableaux et cartes.* Paris: Institut français d'archéologie du Proche Orient.

Barrett, J. C. (2000 [1988]). Fields of discourse: reconstituting a social archaeology. In: J. Thomas (ed.) *Interpretive archaeology*, pp. 23–32. London: Leicester University Press.

Bar-Yosef, O. (1970). The Epi-Palaeolithic cultures of Palestine. PhD thesis, Israel: The Hebrew University.

Berthelet, A. & Chavaillon, J. (eds) (1993). *The use of tools by human and non-human primates.* Oxford: Oxford University Press.

Bird-David, N. (1999). Animism revisited: personhood, environment and relational epistemology. *Current Anthropology* 40 (Supplement): 67–90.

Böhner, U. & Schyle, D. (2002–2006). Radiocarbon CONTEXT database. doi: 10.1594/GFZ.CONTEXT.Ed1

Borgatti, S. P., Everett, M. G. & Freeman, L. C. (2002). Ucinet for Windows: software for social network analysis. Harvard, MA: Analytic Technologies.

Broodbank, C. (2000). *An island archaeology of the early Cyclades.* Cambridge: Cambridge University Press.

Buchanan, M. (2002). *Small world: uncovering nature's hidden networks.* London: Phoenix.

Callon, M. (1987). Society in the making: the study of technology as a tool for socio-logical analysis. In: W. J. Bijker, T. P. Hughes & T. Pinch (eds) *The social construction of technological systems*, pp. 83–103. Cambridge, MA: MIT Press.

Calvino, I. (1974). *Invisible cities*. London: Picador.

Carlstein, T. (1982). *Time resources, society and ecology*. London: George Allen & Unwin.

Chapman, J., 2000. *Fragmentation in archaeology: people, places and broken objects in the prehistory of south eastern Europe*. London: Routledge.

Clark, G. A. (2001). Discussion: The logic of inference in transition research. In: M. A. Hays & P. T. Thacker (eds) *Questioning the answers: re-solving fundamental problems of the Early Upper Palaeolithic*, p. 39. BAR International series 1005. Oxford: Archaeopress.

Colledge, S., Conolly, J. & Shennan, S. (2004). Archaeobotanical evidence for the spread of farming in the eastern Mediterranean. *Current Anthropology* 45 (Supplement August–October): S35–S58.

Coolidge, F. L. & Wynn, T. (2005). Working memory, its executive functions, and the emergence of modern thinking. *Cambridge Archaeological Journal* 15(1): 5–26.

Coser, R. (1975). The complexity of roles as seedbed of individual autonomy. In: L. Coser (ed.) *The idea of social structure: essays in honor of Robert Merton*, pp. 237–262. New York: Harcourt Brace Jovanovich.

Coward, F. (2008). Standing on the shoulders of giants. *Science* 319: 1493–1494.

Coward, F. & Gamble, C. (2008). Big brains, small worlds: material culture and human evolution. *Philosophical Transactions of the Royal Society Series B* 363: 1969–1979.

Coward, F. & Gamble, C. (in press). Materiality and metaphor in earliest prehistory. In: C. Renfrew & L. Malafouris (eds) *The cognitive life of things*. McDonald Institute Monograph. Oxford: Oxbow Books.

Coward, F. & Grove, M. (submitted). Beyond the tools: social innovation and hominin evolution.

Deleuze, G. & Guattari, F. (1988). *A thousand plateaus: capitalism and schizophrenia*, trans. B. Massumi. London: Athlone Press.

DeMarrais, E., Castillo, L. J. & Earle, T. (1996). Ideology, materialization, and power strategies. *Current Anthropology* 37(1): 15–31.

Dodds, P. S. & Watts, D. J. (2005). A generalized model of social and biological contagion. *Journal of Theoretical Biology* 232: 587–604.

Donald, M. (1991). *Origins of the modern mind: three stages in the evolution of culture and cognition*. Cambridge, MA: Harvard University Press.

Donley-Reid, L. W. (1990). A structuring structure: the Swahili house. In: S. Kent (ed.) *Domestic architecture and the use of space: an interdisciplinary cross-cultural study*, pp. 114–127. Cambridge: Cambridge University Press

Douglas, M. (1973). *Natural symbols*. Harmondsworth: Pelican Books.

Douglas-Price, T. (ed.) (2000). *Europe's first farmers*. Cambridge: Cambridge University Press.

Dunbar, R. I. M. (1992). Neocortex size as a constraint on group size in primates. *Journal of Human Evolution* 20: 469–493.

Dunbar, R. I. M. (1993). Coevolution of neocortical size, group size and language in humans. *Behavioral and Brain Sciences* 16: 681–735.

Dunbar, R. I. M. (1996). *Grooming, gossip and the evolution of language.* London: Faber & Faber.

Dunbar, R. I. M. (2003). The social brain: mind, language and society in evolutionary perspective. *Annual Review of Anthropology* 32: 163–181.

Evans, T., Knappett, C. & Rivers, R. (in press). Using statistical physics to understand relational space: a case study from Mediterranean prehistory. In D. Lane, D. Pumain, S. van der Leeuw & G. West (eds) *Complexity perspectives on innovation and social change.* Berlin: Springer.

Gallese, V. (2006). Embodied simulation: from mirror neuron systems to interpersonal relations. In G. Bock & J. Goode (eds) *Empathy and fairness*, pp. 3–19. Chichester: Wiley.

Gamble, C. (1998). Palaeolithic society and the release from proximity: a network approach to intimate relations. *World Archaeology* 29(3: special issue on Intimate Relations): 426–449.

Gamble, C. (1999). *The Palaeolithic societies of Europe.* Cambridge: Cambridge University Press.

Gamble, C. (2007). *Origins and revolutions: human identity in earliest prehistory.* Cambridge: Cambridge University Press.

Goffman, E. (1959). *The presentation of self in everyday life.* London: Penguin.

Gosden, C. & Marshall, Y. (1999). The cultural biography of objects. *World Archaeology* 31(2): 169–178.

Granovetter, M. S. (1973). The strength of weak ties. *American Journal of Sociology* 78(6): 1360–1380.

Granovetter, M. S. (1983). The strength of weak ties: a network theory revisited. *Sociological Theory* 1: 201–233.

Grove, M. & Coward, F. (2008). From individual neurons to social brains. *Cambridge Archaeological Journal* 18(3): 387–400.

Hage, P. & Harary, F. (1996). *Island networks: communication, kinship and classification structures in Oceania.* Cambridge: Cambridge University Press.

Hanneman, R. A. & Riddle, M. (2005). *Introduction to social network methods.* Riverside, CA: University of California, Riverside.

Hillier, B. & Hanson, J. (1984). *The social logic of space.* Cambridge: Cambridge University Press.

Hoskins, J. (1998). *Biographical objects: how things tell the stories of people's lives.* London: Routledge.

Hours, F., Aurenche, O., Cauvin, J., Cauvin, M.-C., Copeland, L. & Sanlaville, P. (1994). *Atlas des sites du Proche Orient (14000–5700 BP), vol. I: Texte.* Paris: Maison de L'Orient Méditerranéen.

Humphrey, N. (2007). Discussion held at 'The Sapient Mind' conference: archaeology meets neuroscience. McDonald Institute for Archaeological Research, Cambridge, 14–16 September.

Hunt, T. L. (1988). Graph theoretic network models for Lapita exchange: a trial application. In: P. V. Kirch & T. L. Hunt (eds) *Archaeology of the Lapita cultural complex: a critical review*, pp. 135–155. Seattle: Thomas Burke Memorial Washington State Museum Research Reports no. 5.

Ingold, T. (2000). *The perception of the environment: essays in livelihood, dwelling and skill*. London: Routledge.

Irwin, G. J. (1983). Chieftainship, kula and trade in Massim prehistory. In: J. W. Leach & E. Leach (eds) *The Kula: new perspectives on Massim exchange*, pp. 29–72. Cambridge: Cambridge University Press.

Jacobs, J. M. (2006). A geography of big things. *Cultural Geographies* 13: 1–27.

Jones, A. (2004). *Materialising memory: colour, remembrance and the Neolithic/Bronze Age transition*. In: E. DeMarrais, C. Gosden & C. Renfrew (eds) *Rethinking materiality: the engagement of mind with the material world*, pp. 167–178. McDonald Institute Monographs. Oxford: Oxbow Books.

Kent, S. (1990). A cross-cultural study of segmentation, architecture and the use of space. In: S. Kent (ed.) *Domestic architecture and the use of space: an interdisciplinary cross-cultural study*, pp. 127–152. Cambridge: Cambridge University Press

Klein, R. G. (1999). *The human career: human biological and cultural origins*, 2nd edn. Chicago: University of Chicago Press.

Knappett, C. (2005). *Thinking through material culture: an interdisciplinary perspective*. Philadelphia: Pennsylvania University Press.

Kozlowski, S. K. (1989). Nemrik 9: a PPN Neolithic site in northern Iraq. *Paléorient* 15(1): 347–353.

Kozlowski, S. K. & Aurenche, O. (2005). *Territories, boundaries and cultures in the Neolithic Near East*. BAR International Series 1362. Oxford: Archaeopress.

Kudo, H. & Dunbar, R. I. M. (2001). Neocortex size and social network size in primates. *Animal Behavior* 61.

Kuijt, I. & Goring-Morris, N. (2002). Foraging, farming, and social complexity in the Pre-Pottery Neolithic of the southern Levant: a review and synthesis. *Journal of World Prehistory* 16(4): 361–440.

Lahr, M. M. & Foley, R. (1998). Towards a theory of modern human origins: geography, demography and diversity in recent human evolution. *Yearbook of Physical Anthropology* 41: 137–176.

Latour, B. (1996). *Aramis, or For the love of technology*. Cambridge, MA: Harvard University Press.

Latour, B. (1999). On recalling ANT. In: J. Law & J. Hassard (eds) *Actor network theory and after*, pp. 15–25. Oxford/Keele: Blackwell Publishers/The Sociological Review.

Law, J. (1999). After ANT: complexity, naming and topology. In: J. Law & J. Hassard (eds) *Actor network theory and after*, pp. 1–14. Oxford/Keele: Blackwell Publishers/The Sociological Review.

Lindenbaum, S. (1978). *Kuru sorcery: disease and danger in the New Guinea highlands*. London: McGraw-Hill.

Lofland, L. H. (1973). *A world of strangers: order and action in urban public space*. New York: Basic Books.

McGlade, J. & J. M. McGlade (1989). Modelling the innovative component of social change. In: S. E. van der Leeuw & R. Torrence (eds) *What's new? A closer look at the process of innovation*, pp. 281–299. London: Unwin Hyman

McGrew, W. C. (1992). *Chimpanzee material culture: implications for human evolution*. Cambridge: Cambridge University Press.

Malinowski, B. (1920). Kula: the circulating exchange of valuables in the archipela-goes of eastern New Guinea. *Man* 20: 97–105.

Malinowski, B. (1922). *Argonauts of the western Pacific: an account of native enter-prise and adventure in the archipelagoes of Melanesian New Guinea*. London: George Routledge & Sons, Ltd.

Marriott, M. (1976). Hindu transactions: diversity without dualism. In: B. Kapferer (ed.) *Transaction and meaning: directions in the anthropology of exchange and symbolic behaviour*, pp. 109–142 Philadelphia, PA: Institute for the Study of Human Issues.

Matsuzawa, T. (2007). Comparative cognitive development. *Developmental Science* 1(1): 97–103.

Mellars, P. (1996). *The Neanderthal legacy*. Princeton, NJ: Princeton University Press.

Milgram, S. (1977). *The individual in a social world: essays and experiments*. Reading, MA: Addison-Wesley.

Munn, N. (1973). The spatial presentation of cosmic order in Walbiri iconography. In: J. A. W. Forge (ed.) *Primitive art and society*, pp. 193–220. Oxford: Oxford University Press.

Newman, M. E. J. (2000). Models of the small world. *Journal of Statistical Physics* 101(3/4): 819–841.

Newman, M. E. J. (2001). Scientific collaboration models I: network construction and fundamental results. *Physical Review E* 64(016131): 1–8.

Postmes, T., Spears, R., Lee, A. T. & Novak, R. J. (2005). Individuality and social influence in groups: inductive and deductive routes to group identity. *Journal of Personality and Social Psychology* 89(5): 747–763.

Rapoport, A. (1969). *House form and culture*. Englewood Cliffs, NJ: Prentice Hall.

Rapoport, A. (1981). Identity and environment: a cross-cultural perspective. In: J. S. Duncan (ed.) *Housing and identity: cross-cultural perspectives*, pp. 6–35. London: Croom Helm.

Rapoport, A. (1990). Systems of activities and systems of settings. In: S. Kent (ed.) *Domestic architecture and the use of space: an interdisciplinary cross-cultural study*, pp. 9–20. Cambridge: Cambridge University Press.

Renfrew, C. (1998). Mind and matter: cognitive archaeology and external symbolic storage. In: C. Renfrew & C. Scarre (eds) *Cognition and material culture: the archaeology of symbolic storage*, pp. 1–6. Oxford: Oxbow Books.

Renfrew, C. (2007). *Prehistory*. London: Weidenfeld & Nicolson.

Renfrew, C., Malafouris, L. & Scarre, C. (2008). Neuroscience, evolution and the sapi-ent paradox: the factuality of value and of the sacred. *Philosophical Transactions of the Royal Society of London Series B* 363: 2041–2047.

Rowlands, M. (2003). *Externalism: putting mind and world back together again*. Chesham: Acumen.

Runciman, W. G. (2005). Stone Age sociology. *Journal of the Royal Anthropological Institute* 11: 129–142.

Sanders, D. (1990). Behavioral conventions and archaeology: methods for the analy-sis of ancient architecture. In: S. Kent (ed.) *Domestic architecture and the use of space: an interdisciplinary cross-cultural study*, pp. 43–72. Cambridge: Cambridge University Press.

Sayej, G. J. (2004). *The lithic industries of Zahrat Adh-Dhra' 2 and the Pre-Pottery Neolithic period of the southern Levant*. BAR International Series 1329. Oxford: Archaeopress.

Schick, K. D. & Toth, N. (1995). *Making silent stones speak: human evolution and the dawn of technology*. London: Phoenix.

Schick, K. D., Toth, N., Garufi, G., Savage-Rumbaugh, E. S., Rumbaugh, D. & Sevcik, R. (1999). Continuing investigations into the stone tool-making and tool-using capabilities of a Bonobo (*Pan paniscus*). *Journal of Archaeological Science* 26(7): 821–832.

Simek, J. F. (2001). Discussion: space and time. In: M. A. Hays & P. T. Thacker (eds) *Questioning the answers: re-solving fundamental problems of the Early Upper Palaeolithic*, 199–202. BAR International Series 1005. Oxford: Archaeopress.

Strathern, M. (1988). *The gender of the gift: problems with women and problems with society in Melanesia*. Berkeley: University of California Press.

Strathern, M. (1998). Social relations and the idea of externality. In: C. Renfrew & C. Scarre (eds) *Cognition and material culture*, pp. 135–147. Oxford: Oxbow Books.

Thomas, J. (2002). Archaeology's humanism and the materiality of the body. In Y. Hamilakis, M. Pluciennik & S. Tarlow (eds.) *Thinking through the body: archaeologies of corporeality*, pp. 29–45. New York: Kluwer Academic/Plenum Publishers.

Thornton, A. & Raihani, N. J. (2008). The evolution of teaching. *Animal Behaviour* 75: 1823–1836.

Tomasello, M. (1999). The human adaptation for culture. *Annual Review of Anthropology* 28: 509–29.

UNFPA (2007). *State of world population 2007: unleashing the potential for urban growth*. URL (consulted June 2009): http://www.unfpa.org/swp/2007/english/introduction.html

van Schaik, C. P., Ancrenaz, M., Borgen, G., Galdikas, B., Knott, C. D., Singleton, I. et al. (2003). Orangutan cultures and the evolution of material culture. *Science* 299(5603): 102–105.

Wasserman, S. & Faust, K. (1994). *Social network analysis: methods and applications*. Cambridge: Cambridge University Press.

Watkins, T. (2004). Architecture and 'theatres of memory' in the Neolithic of southwest Asia. In: E. DeMarrais, C. Gosden & C. Renfrew (eds) *Rethinking materiality: the engagement of mind with the material world*, pp. 97–106. McDonald Research Monographs. Oxford: Oxbow Books.

Watts, D. J. (2003). *Six degrees: the science of a connected age*. London: Vintage.

Watts, D. J. & Strogatz, S. H. (1998). Collective dynamics of 'small-world' networks. *Nature* 393: 440–442.

Whatmore, S. (2002). *Hybrid geographies: natures, cultures, spaces*. London: SAGE.

Whatmore, S. (2006). Materialist returns: practising cultural geography in and for a more-than-human world. *Cultural Geographies* 13: 600–609.

Whitelaw, T. (1991). Some dimensions of variability in the social organisation of community space among foragers. In: C. S. Gamble & W. A. Boismier (eds) *Ethnoarchaeological approaches to mobile campsites: hunter-gatherer and pastoralist case studies*, pp. 139–188. Ann Arbor, MI: International Monographs in Prehistory 1.

Whitelaw, T. M. (1994). Order without architecture: functional, social and symbolic dimensions in hunter-gatherer settlement organization. In: M. Parker-Pearson & C. Richards (eds.) *Architecture and order: approaches to social space*, pp. 217–243. London: Routledge.

Wilson, P. (1988). *The domestication of the human species*. New Haven, CT: Yale University Press.

Wright, K. (1992a). A classification system for ground stone tools from the prehistoric Levant. *Paléorient* 18(2): 53–81.

Wright, K. I. (1992b). Ground stone assemblage variations and subsistence strategies in the Levant 22,000–5,500 BP. PhD Thesis, Yale.

Wright, K. (2008). 'Households and networks: Levantine social-political structures in the Pre-Pottery Neolithic and beyond', talk given at the Ancient Levant Conference, Institute of Archaeology, UCL, 16–17 May.

22

Excavating the Prehistoric Mind: The Brain as a Cultural Artefact and Material Culture as Biological Extension

STEVEN MITHEN

THE LAST DECADE has seen a remarkable expansion in research devoted to the evolution of human cognition and language. The number of conferences, seminars, books, journal articles, new theories, old theories rediscovered and theories that should simply never have been, has at times appeared overwhelming. Perhaps more than is the case for any other issue, this has allowed archaeology to contribute to wider inter-disciplinary debates about the nature of humankind and society, rather than merely addressing issues of interest to archaeologists alone. Moreover, it has seen Palaeolithic archaeology emerge as the most theoretically advanced area of the discipline. The British Academy 'Lucy to Language Centenary Project' has played, and continues to play, a key role in this transformation of Palaeolithic archaeology from the study of stones and bones to that of human lives, minds and societies.

Within this burgeoning growth of research into the evolution and nature of human cognition, two approaches have emerged as being particularly attractive to archaeologists: the social brain hypothesis and the distributed mind model of embodied cognition. In one regard, these approaches pull in different directions. The first encourages us to look inside the brain of individuals, requiring us to understand neural circuitry and the role of neurotransmitters in the processes of thought and feeling. The second asks us to view the process of cognition as extending beyond the brain, an emergent phenomenon of groups—some members of which may be distant from each other in time and space—mediated by material culture. Unless we are prepared to forsake a comprehensive understanding of cognitive evolution, these two approaches—and others—must be encompassed into a single unified model of human cognition. This requires a rigorous evaluation of their internal logic, their practical value

Proceedings of the British Academy **158**, 481–503. © The British Academy 2010.

and the extent to which they are consistent with each other; perhaps they will be found to be mutually dependent. Hence the considerable value of the conference that gave rise to this volume, and the contents of the volume itself.

My own contribution will primarily be to describe two areas of my own on-going research, one directly related to the social brain and one to the distributed mind. I am keen to find connections between these approaches and hope that bringing case studies of their application together within one article might help towards that end. First, however, I must reflect on the growth of cognitive archaeology in general and my own particular approach, which has been characterized as the 'cathedral model' for the mind. My own dissatisfaction with aspects of that model has led me to be sympathetic to ideas concerning extended and distributed cognition—and rather less so towards a strong version of the social brain hypothesis.

THE CATHEDRAL MODEL FOR THE MIND

The year 1996 was a notable one for publications relating to the evolution of human cognition; quite independently several books appeared including William Noble and Ian Davidson's *Human evolution, language and mind*, Robin Dunbar's *Grooming, gossip and language*, and my own contribution *The prehistory of the mind*. We must, of course, always remember that these and other publications were following in the footsteps of Merlin Donald's 1991 book *Origins of the modern mind*. Moreover, all of this work was building on that of the three pioneers of cognitive archaeology: Glynn Isaac (1986), Tom Wynn (1979, 1981) and Alexander Marshack (1972). They, in turn, were rehearsing questions originally put forward by the pioneers of archaeology such as John Lubbock (1895).

While these books differed in the specific questions they were addressing, they were united by a desire to use the archaeological and fossil record to address the evolution of the mind. My own work (Mithen 1996) sought to answer a single question: how can we resolve the paradox between the evolution of large, metabolically expensive brains by at least 500,000 years ago and the appearance of the first signs of symbolic culture at a mere 50,000 years ago. Now, a decade later, the earliest unambiguous evidence for symbolic culture is just a whisker older, at 70,000 years ago and most clearly evident at Blombos cave in South Africa (Henshilwood et al. 2002). The question I sought to address in *The pre-*

history of the mind was, and still is, exemplified by the modern human/Neanderthal debate: how could two human species have equivalent sized brains, have so much of their lifestyles in common and yet behave so remarkably differently—at least when responding to the environmental conditions of ice age Europe.

The answer I gave drew heavily on two sources. First, the empirical evidence: the contents, patterning and variation in the archaeological record. Second, the theories regarding the nature and evolution of the human mind which came from an assortment of philosophers and psychologists who I thought were telling essentially the same story, although they had their own disagreements and incompatibilities. Most notable was Fodor (1983), Gardner (1983) and the contributors to Hirschfeld and Gelman (1994), especially Boyer, Carey, Cosmides, Pinker, Spelke and Tooby. My answer was essentially a story about mental modularity.

I proposed that the minds of pre-modern humans had a domain-specific structure. The pre-modern humans had essentially modern ways of thinking and stores of knowledge about the social world, the natural world and the material world, but they were unable to undertake significant amount of cross-domain thought. In other words, they lacked the capacity for analogy and metaphor. It seemed to me that this could account for both the high level of expertise evident in their behaviour, whether in tool-making, foraging or socializing, and the apparent absence of creative thought leading to limited, if any, cultural change.

I then argued that the evolution of language provided the means by which such cross-domain thought arose, resulting in what I termed cognitive fluidity. This provided modern humans with the capacity for analogy and metaphor that ultimately underlie art, science and religion. Such cognitive fluidity did not require any increase in brain matter, but merely a change—possibly a minor change—in neural circuitry. It became particularly elaborately expressed in ice age Europe, providing the cognitive means for adaptation. I called this 'the cathedral model' for cognitive evolution because I compared the minds of the Neanderthals to Romanesque architecture, all rather dark with secluded and isolated chapels, while that of modern humans appeared positively high gothic architecture—bright, light open spaces in which ideas and knowledge could freely mingle to create something new and unexpected.

The last decade has not led me to change my overall view that this is indeed the correct interpretation of the archaeological record and cognitive evolution. I did, however, very rapidly recognize weaknesses and inadequacies in the specific model I was proposing, as I will shortly outline. New empirical evidence that may be relevant to the evolution of human cognition has been forthcoming during the last decade, notably the 500,000-year-old Schöningen spears (Thieme 1997), that some proposed as evidence for an advanced cognition, and the possible 300,000-year-old burials from Sima de los Huesos (Arsuaga et al. 1997). But I have found that these and other discoveries, such as the so-called Berekhat Ram figurine (d'Errico & Nowell 2000), can be accommodated within my cathedral model with a sufficiently limited amount of special pleading. More problematic is the *Homo floresiensis* discovery (Brown et al. 2004) and possible associated artefacts (Morwood et al. 2004). However, I do not think that anyone is currently in a position to pronounce on their implications for the evolution of human cognition, and indeed of human evolution in general.

One serious weakness in my cathedral model became apparent to me very soon after publication: the fact that it left material artefacts as the passive outputs from the mind rather than active constituents. The error in doing so became apparent from my reading of Andy Clark's 1997 book *Being there: putting body and world together again* and then more clearly in his 2004 volume *Natural-born cyborgs*. This made me appreciate how material artefacts act as cognitive anchors for cognitive fluid thoughts, such as those about religious entities, and essentially become part of an extended mind (Mithen 1998). Cognitive anchors—paintings, figurines, texts, songs and so forth—are required for religious thoughts because, contra Pascal Boyer (1994), such thoughts are 'unnatural' for the human mind. Hence the brain is insufficient for their repeated conceptualization, manipulation and social transmission (see also Day 2004). Other archaeologists were also reading the work of Andy Clark, especially his key 1998 paper with Chalmers called 'The extended mind', along with related work such as Ed Hutchins' 1995 book *Cognition in the wild*. The value of that approach to material culture has now been widely recognized, this being exemplified, of course, by providing one of the two key themes for the symposium for which this chapter was originally written. So now I would characterize modern minds as even more 'fluid' than I had originally proposed: a mind that flows beyond the confines of the skull into the realm of material culture.

The way I have been tackling the extended mind has not been by seeking to contribute to the theory—that is rather too crowded for me—but simply by using the notion of the metaphorical, extended and distributed mind to influence my archaeological fieldwork. The epilogue of the *Prehistory of the mind* concerned the origins of agriculture. I suggested

that my notion of cognitive fluidity might help resolve some of the out-
standing questions of what I still regard as a Neolithic Revolution. Well,
it has taken me 12 years to reach a position where those ideas might be
realized by having found not only a sufficiently well preserved early
Neolithic site, but also having managed to secure the necessary resources
to undertake an excavation at the required scale.

DISTRIBUTED MINDS IN THE NEOLITHIC

This is at the PPNA site WF16 in Wadi Faynan (Figure 22.1; Finlayson &
Mithen 2007) where the excavation of 2008 has exposed part of a Neolithic
village dating to between 11,600 and 10,200 years ago with an assortment
of structures, burials, middens and a rich material culture (Figure 22.2,
Mithen et al. in press). Ideas about cognitive fluidity, metaphorical,
extended and distributed minds seem essential to its interpretation. Let me
give you a few brief examples.

There is a fluidity in the nature of human bodies at WF16: they had
once lived and worked within this village; they then became transformed
into the material substance of the village by being buried below floors
(Figure 22.3) and within walls, gradually becoming part of the inorganic
substrate. Heads and phalluses were also made in stone, the latter merging
in form with supposedly utilitarian pestles and processors. I have previously argued that such artefacts indicate that a sexual metaphor pervades
the processing of plant foods at WF16 and may have been essential to the
course of plant domestication (Mithen et al. 2005).

Figure 22.4 provides a plan of the exposed structures, with the black
and grey constituting mud pisé walls and platforms that wrap around all
activity within the Neolithic village. Such walls (e.g. Figure 22.5) provide,
in Clive Gamble's (2007) term, containers that encapsulate human activity in a manner that was simply not present in the immediately preceding
hunter-gatherer settlements of the region. Indeed, we find a whole hierarchy of Gamblesque containers at WF16, ranging from the all pervasive
pisé, the walls of individual structures, those surrounding a centralized
area of midden/workshop, those of burials, constructed fireplaces and, of
course, stone vessels themselves. This is a world looking in upon itself.

John Chapman and Bisserka Gaydarska's (2007, ch. 20 this volume)
fragmentation premise also appears to provide a promising route for
interpretation of the activities we find at WF16. One burial for instance,
contained no less than nine fragments of human crania, stacked on top

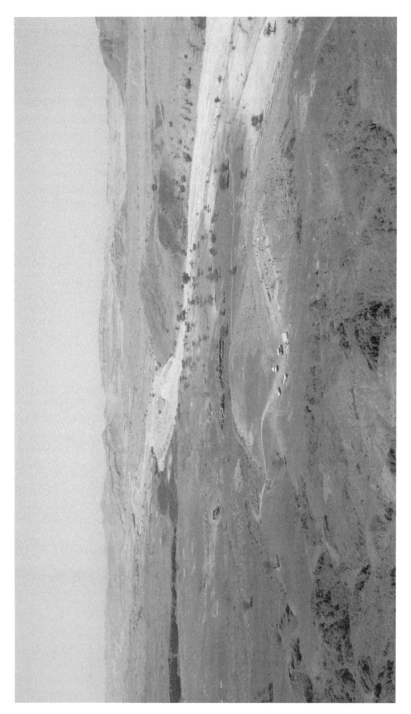

Figure 22.1. Wadi Fayan, southern Jordan, looking west towards the Jordan valley and making the location of the early Neolithic village of WF16 by the site of the 2008 excavation trench (© Steven Mithen)

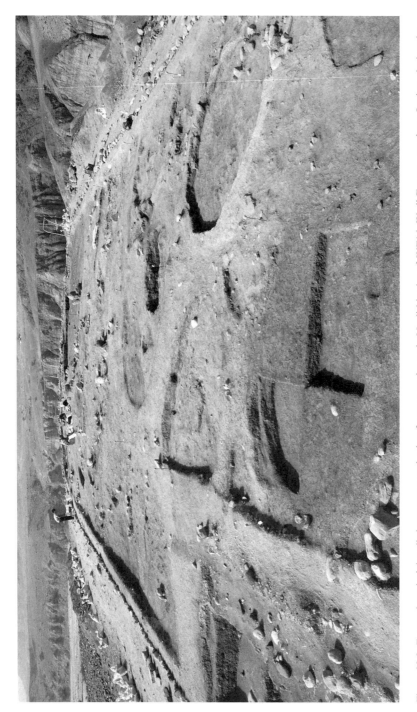

Figure 22.2. Exposed mud-pisé walled structures and other features at the early Neolithic site of WF16, Wadi Faynan, southern Jordan, during the 2008 excavation (© Steven Mithen)

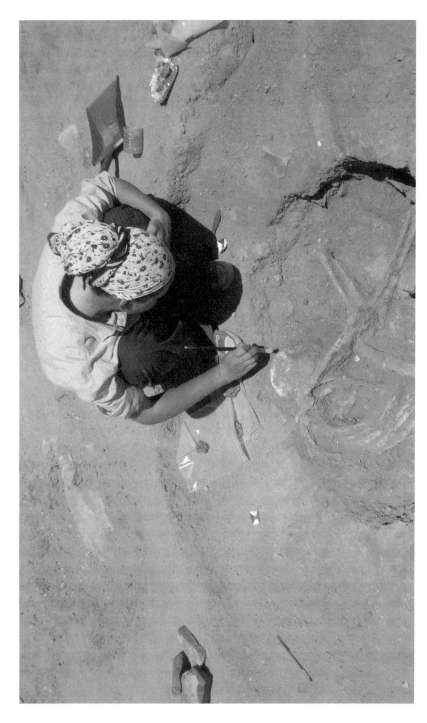

Figure 22.3. Human burial below floor of early Neolithic structure at WF16, Wadi Faynan, southern Jordan (© Steven Mithen)

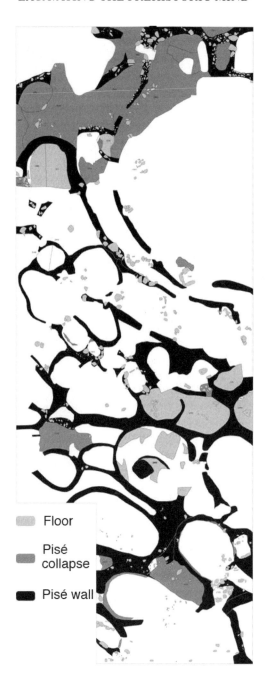

Figure 22.4. Plan of mud-pisé walled structures and other features at WF16, Wadi Faynan, southern Jordan (© Steven Mithen)

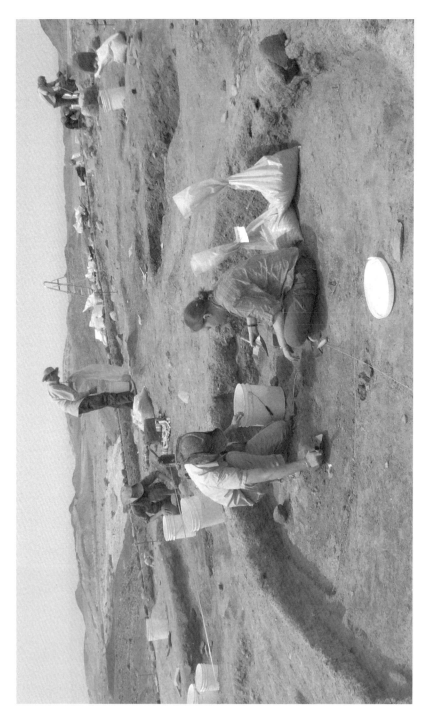

Figure 22.5. Excavation with mud-walled structure at WF16, Wadi Faynan, southern Jordan (© Steven Mithen)

of one another like a set of egg cups. I also wonder whether the extreme fragmentation of the animal bones within the midden (Figure 22.6) can be attributed to post-depositional practices alone; perhaps, as Chapman has argued elsewhere, we are seeing practices of deliberate fragmentation that extends beyond immediate utilitarian needs.

The notion of distributed personhood might also be useful for interpreting the WF16 materials, such as the shell ornaments that originated from either the Red Sea or the Mediterranean. Perhaps also for the finds of objects the like of which have never been seen before in the Neolithic of the southern Levant, such as a highly polished stone point that seems to have been deliberately deposited in the floor of a structure before it was backfilled with mud.

Some, perhaps all, of the Neolithic metaphors will always remain unknown to us. The exquisite object illustrated in Figure 22.7, for instance, bears the same motifs as found on another plaque of stone, one coming from the contemporary site of Netiv Hagdud, located some 200 km away and on the West bank of the Jordan. Objects such as these testify to a cognitively fluid mentality, but one whose specific content will remain beyond our reach.

These few examples are given simply to show how the notions of cognitive fluidity, metaphor, extended and distributed minds might be used to interpret the remains of one particular archaeological site, one that happens to lie at the time of the great cultural transition from hunter-gathering to farming economies. The challenge, however, is to demonstrate that these notions can make a real difference to our understanding rather than amounting to just another description of the archaeological materials, albeit in new terms. For me, this excavation project, which will no doubt take me at least a decade to complete, is a continuation of work started in my 1996 book *The prehistory of the mind*. It is seeking to put the epilogue of that book into practice, and is an acknowledgement that material culture itself must be considered as a key element of human cognition in general, and the state of cognitive fluidity in particular.

CONCERNS ABOUT THE SOCIAL BRAIN HYPOTHESIS

My previous failure to appreciate the active role of material culture in human cognition was one of the weaknesses in my 1996 book. I knew of a second even before it was published, suffering several restless nights after convincing myself that because of this weakness my book would be

Steven Mithen

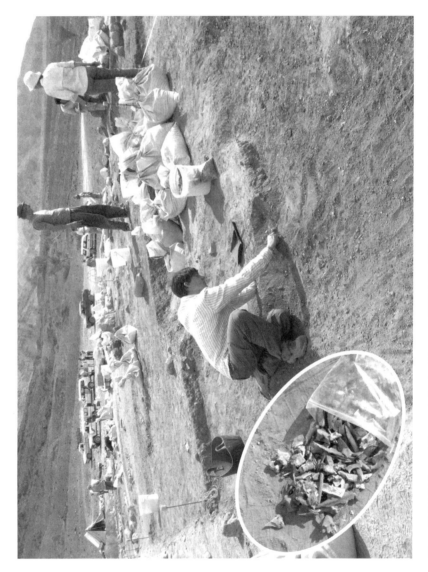

Figure 22.6. Midden and fragmented animal bones at WF16, Wadi Faynan, southern Jordan (© Steven Mithen)

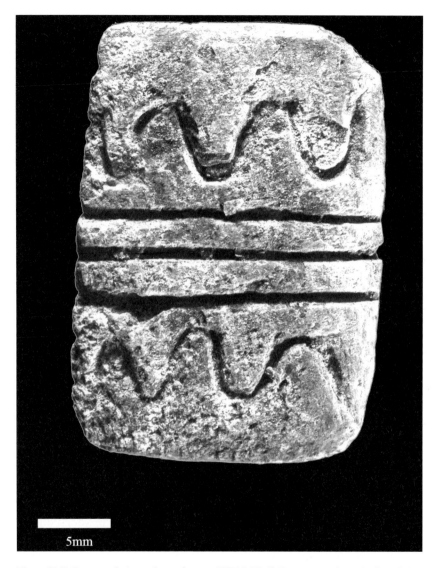

5mm

Figure 22.7. Decorated stone plaque from at WF16, Wadi Faynan, southern Jordan (© Steven Mithen)

dammed in review. This was its appalling neglect of music. Although music is a universal feature of humankind it was ignored in my work, just as it had been ignored in almost every other work published around that time concerning human evolution. I have since tried to make amends for my neglect by focusing on the evolution of music itself, which I soon found required me to also reconsider the evolution of language because I concluded that music and language have a single precursor—a conclusion that several others have reached independently from quite different lines of evidence (e.g. Blacking 1973; Brown 2000). This did in fact resolve—for me at least—a further weakness of the cathedral model concerning the communication systems of pre-modern humans. If they didn't have compositional language, how did they communicate? The answer I gave in my 2005 book *The singing Neanderthals* is that they used a communication system that was *holistic, multi-modal, manipulative, musical* and *mimetic*.

Considering music takes us directly into the social brain hypothesis—because music is essentially about sociality. Robin Dunbar (1993) and his colleagues (Aiello & Dunbar 1993) argued that language evolved as a means of social grooming, but I suspect that he was really thinking about music-like utterances that are so effective at manipulating emotions and building social bonds. While there is this agreeable link with my own views on the origins of musicality and the social brain hypothesis, I nevertheless harbour strong reservations about the latter.

While the social relationships of modern humans are unquestionably far more complex than those of our closest living relatives—whether measured in degree of intentionality, temporal and spatial extent of social networks, complexity of emotions or whatever—it remains unclear why this would necessarily translate into a larger brain size in the manner that Dunbar proposes. The advanced human level of social cognition could be achieved simply by iterations of a small number of neural circuits, suggesting that an expansion in the number of either neurons or neural circuits is unnecessary. Surely there is a lesson here from the development of our material equivalent of a brain: the computer. During the course of the last five decades, the vast increase in computational power has not been matched by an increase in volume (in fact there has been a dramatic decrease). So there is no a priori reason why an increase in social cognition, such as in the number of orders of intentionality that can be comprehended, should have required an increase in brain volume: it could have been accomplished by revisions to existing circuitry.

A second concern with the social brain hypothesis is that while humans have more powerful social cognition than our nearest relatives, they are also far more technically adept. A premise of mental modularity from an evolutionary psychology perspective is that the type of cognition required for solving social problems is not the same as that suited for technical problems (as discussed in Mithen 1996). Consequently, if the expansion of the brain during the Pleistocene is to be accounted for by social intelligence alone, this leaves the advances in technology, such as the Acheulean and Levallois, unexplained.

A third concern is that the social brain hypothesis leaves the modern human/Neanderthal problem untouched. If the size of the brain is equivalent to social intelligence, then we are left with no reason to expect that the Neanderthals were cognitively any different from modern humans. And yet they either lacked material symbolism entirely, or could only engage in it to a limited extent. They also had a limited range of tool-making techniques, sometimes described as cultural stasis. The key problem is that there is a limited correlation between the change in brain size during human evolution, which Dunbar uses as a proxy for social intelligence, and social behaviour as reflected in the material culture of the archaeological record.

MUSIC OF THE MIND

While I have these concerns with the social brain hypothesis, there can be no question that enhanced sociality was a key feature of human evolution and probably linked to the evolution of language, as Dunbar has proposed. But there must have been an intermediary link between the evolution of complex sociality and language: that of music. Inter-disciplinary research into the evolution of music has expanded very significantly during the last few years (e.g. Cross 2001; Wallin et al. 2000). Related to and supporting this are the striking developments in the cognitive neuroscience of music, as led by academics such as Robert Zatorre and Isabelle Peretz (2003) and Larry Parsons (Parsons 2003; Parsons et al. 2005). I want to use music to reflect on how we should be conceptualizing the brain.

One of the striking features of the contributions to the conference from which this volume derived is that the brain was hardly mentioned at all: everyone appeared too embarrassed to mention it, but the brain loomed large as the unspoken elephant in the room. More generally, the majority of emphasis in recent research has been on how we should consider material culture as an extension of our biology, whether framed in terms of memory, mind or simply susceptible to the forces of natural selection (e.g. Collard et al. 2006; Shennan 2002); while this is essential, just as important is that we must come to terms with the brain as a piece of material culture.

The brain of any individual is, of course, an artefact of culture. Its structure and function is a consequence of the complex interplay between genetic inheritance and developmental environment that result in the joint processes of neural constructivism and neural selectionism. A common assumption is that the brain stopped evolving either with the emergence of *Homo sapiens* c. 200,000 years ago, or more recently—as exemplified by Colin Renfrew's (2007) suggestion that molecular genetics cannot help with understanding the evolution of the mind after the origins of farming. There have been several recent studies, however, which have argued persuasively for continuing evolution throughout the Pleistocene and Holocene, with the selective pressures arising from the cultural environment. Most notable is Weaver's (2005) work showing how during the Holocene the cerebellum has become relatively larger and the cerebral hemisphere relatively smaller, so reversing the trend that had existed during the Pleistocene. We should also note the arguments for recent evolutionary changes within two genes that are known to be associated with microcephaly when in their mutant form, but that normally function in facilitating a large brain (Evans et al. 2005; Mekel-Bobrov et al. 2005).

Of equal significance is our growing understanding from advances in neuroscience about how cultural activities impact on the development of the brain within an individual's lifetime, as well as on the long-term evolution of the brain. Indeed it is apparent that we can engage in cultural activities with the deliberate intention of changing the biology of our own brains. Here we shift from viewing the brain not merely as an artefact of the cultural environment, but as a cultural artefact itself.

Several studies have found correlations between structural features of the brain and cultural activity with regard to music. The corpus callosum, that bundle of tissues that connect the two hemispheres, is larger in male musicians than in male non-musicians (Lee et al. 2003; Schlaug et al. 1995). Male musicians also have both relatively and absolutely larger cerebellums (Hutchinson et al. 2003). Then there has been the finding that the posterior hippocampi of taxi-drivers are larger than those of non-taxi drivers, and that there is a positive correlation with the amount of time spent as a taxi driver (Maguire et al. 2000). It is not clear in these studies what is cause and what is effect: are those people with relatively larger hippocampi simply preferentially drawn to taxi-driving, just as those with a large corpus callosum might be drawn to music? Or is cultural activity the cause of their biology? To address this issue longitudinal studies are required—research that monitors changes in the structure of the brain while cultural activities are undertaken. It would be useful to know, for instance, whether the hippocampi of retired taxi drivers revert to their state in pre-taxi-driving days.

One example of a longitudinal study is that by Draganski and his colleagues who compared a suite of brains before and after their owners had spent three months learning to juggle (Draganski et al. 2004). The jugglers were found to have significantly more grey matter in the area of the brain used for visual-motion information. There was a close relationship between the extent of grey matter expansion and juggling performance. After a further three months during which no juggling was allowed the grey matter was found to have decreased in extent. Here an archaeologically relevant study has been provided by Dietrich Stout and Thierry Chaminade (2007). They used PET scans to demonstrate that training in the manufacture of Oldowan-type tools results in enhanced activity within the ventral, lateral and dorsal higher-order visual areas of the brain.

A final case study concerns my own brain (Mithen & Parsons 2008). Being entirely unable to sing, I had an fMRI scan of my brain while undertaking a series of singing exercises in the scanner. I then had a whole year of singing lessons with a professional teacher—a deeply gruelling and often humiliating experience. After that, my brain was scanned for a second time, during which I repeated precisely the same singing exercises as on the first occasion. This identified that the cultural activity I had undertaken, i.e. learning to sing, had resulted in significant changes in my brain activity. Figure 22.8 illustrates the areas in which there had been enhanced activity as measured by increased blood flow within my brain; those areas are indeed the ones where one would expect this to have occurred, as they are known to be involved with secondary auditory processing, the processing of musical structure and enhanced motor control, such as of the vocal apparatus. Figure 22.9 illustrates the areas of my brain where there had been decreased activity, these being generally interpreted as a reduction in working memory.

This singing experiment was merely an exploratory study, largely undertaken to allow me to understand more about how the brain can be considered as a cultural artefact. With the current pace of development in neuroscience it is likely that during the next decade there will be a substantial improvement in our understanding of how the brain works. My point is simply that the further development of the social brain hypothesis, or the notion of domain-specific architecture and cognitive fluidity, or indeed any other notion of cognitive evolution, must pay close attention to these developments in neuroscience and ideally engage in inter-disciplinary research. Acknowledging culture as an influence on the brain's biology is as important as incorporating the biology into material culture.

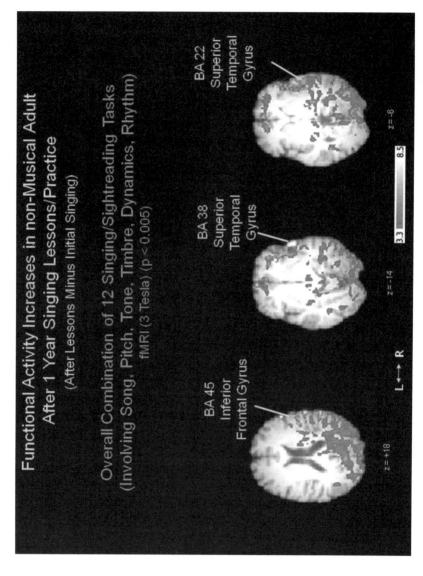

Figure 22.8. Functional activity increases in Mithen's brain after one year of singing lessons and practice

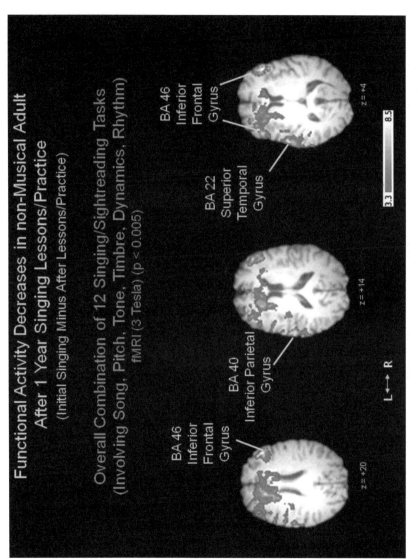

Figure 22.9. Functional activity decreases in Mithen's brain after one year of singing lessons and practice

CONCLUSION: FINDING INTEGRATION

A task facing archaeologists in general is to evaluate the social brain and the distributed mind hypotheses and then integrate their key elements into a unified model for the evolution and nature of the human mind. My own particular task within that undertaking is to bring together my concerns with metaphor, extended and distributed minds which influence my work on the Neolithic with those about neural plasticity and the brain as a cultural artefact that have arisen from my research on music and human evolution in general. In one regard this is straightforward: the brains of those individuals living and dying at the Neolithic site of WF16 would have been moulded by the mud wall structures, burial traditions and farming economy to have been quite different from the brains of their hunter-gatherer ancestors. Also, the brains of Neolithic individuals were connected together into a suite of distributed minds covering extensive geographical areas by new forms and uses of material culture—epitomized in the widespread occurrence of the El-Khiam point, the type artefact of the PPNA. More difficult is using such ideas to make a real difference to our understanding, rather than merely a new type of descriptive narrative, of why and how the momentous transition from mobile hunting and gathering to sedentary farming lifestyles occurred.

Note. I am grateful to Clive Gamble and Robin Dunbar for their comments on an earlier version of this chapter; also to them and John Gowlett for the invitation to participate in the conference and contribute to the publication.

REFERENCES

Aiello, L. C. & Dunbar, R. I. M. (1993). Neocortex size, group size, and the evolution of language. *Current Anthropology* 34: 184–193.
Arsuaga, J. L., Martinez, I., Gracia, A., Carretero, J. M., Lorenzo, C., Garcia, N. et al. (1997). Sima de los Huesos (Sierra de Atapuerca, Spain): the site. *Journal of Human Evolution* 33: 219–281.
Blacking, J. (1973). *How musical is man?* Seattle: University of Washington Press.
Boyer, P. (1994). *The naturalness of religious ideas: a cognitive theory of religion.* Berkeley: University of California Press.
Brown, P., Sutikna, T., Morwood, M. J., Soejono, R. P., Jatmiko, Wayhu Saptomo, E. et al. (2004). A new small-bodied hominin from the Late Pleistocene of Flores, Indonesia. *Nature* 431: 1055–1061.
Brown, S. (2000). The 'musilanguage' model of human evolution. In: N. L. Wallin, B. Merker & S. Brown (eds) *The origins of music*, pp. 271–300. Cambridge, MA: MIT Press.

Chapman, J. C. & Gaydarska, B. I. (2007). *Parts and wholes: fragmentation in prehistoric context*. Oxford: Oxbow Books.

Clark, A. (1997). *Being there: putting brain, body and world together again*. Cambridge, MA: MIT Press.

Clark, A. (2004). *Natural-born cyborgs*. Oxford: Oxford University Press.

Clark, A. & Chalmers, D. (1998). The extended mind. *Analysis* 58: 7–19.

Collard, M., Shennan, S. J. & Tehrani, J. J. (2006). Branching, blending, and the evolution of cultural similarities and differences among human populations. *Evolution and Human Behavior* 27: 169–184.

Cross, I. (2001). Music, mind and evolution. *Psychology of Music* 29: 95–102.

Day, M. (2004). Religion, off-line cognition and the extended mind. *Journal of Cognition and Culture* 4: 101–121.

d'Errico, F. & Nowell, A. (2000). A new look at the Berekhat Ram figurine: implications for the origins of symbolism. *Cambridge Archaeological Journal* 10: 123–167.

Donald, M. (1991). *Origins of the modern mind*. Cambridge, MA: Harvard University Press.

Draganski, B., Gaser, C., Busch, V., Schuierer, G., Bogdahn, U. & May, A. (2004). Changes in grey matter induced by training. *Nature* 427: 311–312.

Dunbar, R. I. M. (1993). Coevolution of neocortical size on group size in primates. *Journal of Human Evolution* 20: 469–493.

Dunbar, R. I. M. (1996). *Grooming, gossip and the evolution of language*. London: Faber & Faber.

Evans, P. D., Gilbert, S. L., Mekel-Bobrov, N., Vallender, E. J., Anderson, J. R., Vaez-Azizi, L. M. et al. (2005). Microephalin, a gene regulating brain size, continues to evolve adaptively in humans. *Science* 309: 1717–1720.

Finlayson, B. & Mithen, S. J. (eds) (2007). *The early prehistory of Wadi Faynan, southern Jordan: archaeological survey of Wadis Faynan, Ghuwayr and al Bustan and evaluation of the Pre-Pottery Neolithic site of WF16*. Oxford: Council for British Archaeology in the Levant/Oxbow Books.

Fodor, J. (1983). *The modularity of mind*. Cambridge, MA: MIT Press.

Gamble, C. (2007). *Origins and revolutions: human identity in earliest prehistory*. Cambridge: Cambridge University Press.

Gardner, H. (1983). *Frames of mind: the theory of multiple intelligences*. New York: Basic Books.

Henshilwood, C. S., d'Errico, F., Yates, R., Jacobs, Z., Tribolo, C., Duller, G. A. T. et al. (2002). Emergence of modern human behaviour: Middle Stone age engravings from South Africa. *Science* 295: 1278–1280.

Hirschfeld, L. A. & Gelman, S.A. (eds) (1994). *Mapping the mind: domain specificity in culture and cognition*. Cambridge: Cambridge University Press.

Hutchins, E. (1995). *Cognition in the wild*. Cambridge, MA: MIT Press.

Hutchinson, S., Lee, L. H., Gaab, N. & Schlaug, G. (2003). Cerebellar volume: gender and musicianship effects. *Cerebral Cortex* 13: 943–949.

Isaac, G. (1986). Foundation stones: early artefacts as indicators of activities and abilities. In: G. Bailey & P. Callow (eds) *Stone Age prehistory*, pp. 221–241. Cambridge: Cambridge University Press.

Lee, D. J., Chen, Y. & Schlaug, G. (2003). Corpus callosum: musician and gender effects. *Neuroreport* 14: 205–209.

Lubbock, J. (1895). *Prehistoric times, as illustrated by ancient remains and the manners and customs of modern savages.* London: Williams & Norgate.

Maguire, E. A., Gadian, D. G., Johnsrude, I. S., Good, C. D., Ashburner, J., Frackowiak, R. S. J. et al. (2000). Navigation-related structural change in the hippocampi of taxi drivers. *Proceedings of the National Academy of Sciences* 97: 4398–4403.

Marshack, A. (1972). *The roots of civilization.* London: McGraw-Hill

Mekel-Bobrov, N., Gilbert, S. L., Evans, P. D., Vallender, E. J., Anderson, J. R., Hudson, R. R. et al. (2005). Ongoing adaptive evolution of ASPM, a brain size determinant in *Homo sapiens. Science* 309: 1720–1722.

Mithen, S. J. (1996). *The prehistory of the mind.* London: Thames & Hudson.

Mithen, S. J. (1998). The supernatural beings of prehistory: the external symbolic storage of religious ideas. In: C. Scarre & C. Renfrew (eds) *Cognition and culture: the archaeology of symbolic storage*, pp. 97–106. Cambridge: McDonald Institute.

Mithen, S. J. (2005). *The singing Neanderthals.* London: Orion.

Mithen, S. J. & Parsons, L. (2008). The brain as a cultural artefact. *Cambridge Archaeological Journal* 18: 401–410.

Mithen, S. J., Finlayson, B. & Shaffrey, R. (2005). Sexual symbolism in the Early Neolithic of the southern Levant: pestles and mortars from WF16. *Documenta Prahistorica* 32: 103–110.

Mithen, S. J., Finlayson, B., Najjar, M., Jenkins, E., Smith, S., Hemsley, S. et al. (in press). Excavations at the PPNA site WF-16: a preliminary report on the 2008 season. *Annual of the Department of Antiquities of Jordan.*

Morwood, M. J., Soejono, R. P., Roberts, R. G., Sutikana, T., Turney, C. S. M., Westaway, K.E. et al. (2004). Archaeology and the age of a new hominin from Flores in eastern Indonesia. *Nature* 431: 1087–1091.

Noble, W. & Davidson, I. (1996). *Human evolution, language and mind: a psychology and archaeological inquiry*. Cambridge: Cambridge University Press.

Parsons, L. M. (2003). Exploring the neuroanatomy of music, performance, perception and comprehension. In: R. J. Zatorre & I. Peretz (eds) *The cognitive neuroscience of music*, pp. 247–268. Oxford: Oxford University Press.

Parsons, L. M., Sergent, J., Hidges, D. A. & Fox, P. T. (2005). The brain basis of piano performance. *Neuropsychologia* 43: 199–215.

Renfrew, C. (2007). *Prehistory: making of the human mind.* London: Weidenfeld & Nicolson.

Schlaug, G., Jaencke, I., Huang, Y. & Steinmetz, H. (1995). Increased corpus callosum size in musicians. *Neuropsychologia* 33: 1047–1055.

Shennan, S. J. (2002). *Genes, memes and human history: Darwinian archaeology and cultural evolution.* London: Thames & Hudson.

Stout, D. & Chaminade, T. (2007). The evolutionary neuroscience of tool making. *Neuropsychologia* 45: 1091–1100.

Thieme, H. (1997). Lower Palaeolithic hunting spears from Germany. *Nature* 385: 807–810.

Wallin, N. L., Merker, B. & Brown, S. (eds) (2000). *The origins of music.* Cambridge, MA: MIT Press.

Weaver, A. H. (2005). Reciprocal evolution of the cerebellum and neocortex in fossil humans. *Proceedings of the National Academy of Sciences* 102: 3576–3580.

Wynn, T. (1979). The intelligence of late Acheulian hominids. *Man* 14: 371–391.
Wynn, T. (1981). The intelligence of Oldowan hominids. *Journal of Human Evolution* 10: 529–541.
Zatorre, R. J. & Peretz, I. (eds) (2003). *The cognitive neuroscience of music*, pp. 247–268. Oxford: Oxford University Press.

Abstracts

2

TECHNOLOGIES OF SEPARATION AND THE EVOLUTION OF SOCIAL EXTENSION

Clive Gamble

Archaeological accounts of cognitive evolution have traditionally favoured an internal model of the mind and a search for symbolic proxies. I argue here for an external model of cognition and use this perspective to develop our understanding of Palaeolithic material culture as based on sensory experience, and hence metaphorical rather than symbolic in form. The chapter explores ways of investigating the evolution of cognition by using the social brain model combined with a theory of distributed cognition. The emphasis is on social extension, which was a necessary step to a global distribution and which was achieved by mechanisms such as focused gaze that amplified the emotional content of bonds. The importance of these mechanisms is examined through three aspects of social extension—ontological security, psychological continuity and extension of self—and examples are provided to show how a metaphorical approach to material culture can investigate these properties.

3

HERTO BRAINS AND MINDS: BEHAVIOUR OF EARLY *HOMO SAPIENS* FROM THE MIDDLE AWASH

Yonas Beyene

The discovery of three late Middle Pleistocene hominid crania, *Homo sapiens idaltu*, at Herto in the Middle Awash research area in Ethiopia in 1997 shed considerable light on this little-known period in Africa. These fossils consist of two adults' and a child's crania. All are morphologically intermediate between geologically earlier African fossils and anatomically modern later Pleistocene humans. The hominid-bearing Upper Herto sediments were dated using Ar40/Ar39 techniques to between 160,000 and 154,000 years old.

Proceedings of the British Academy **158**, 505–518. © The British Academy 2010.

Archaeological excavations and controlled surface collections in the upper Herto localities were carried out to correlate the findings temporally and to understand their geological, geographical, environmental and technological interrelations. The archaeological evidence from the multiple localities has demonstrated the presence of both Acheulean and MSA technological elements. Acheulean hand-axes are represented by cleavers and ovate type bifaces with regular and straight cutting edges demonstrating soft hammer techniques. Together with these were found artefacts demonstrating Levallois techniques, represented by flakes, points, blades and end- and side-scrapers. The discovery in the lake margin paleolandscape of a large quantity of juvenile and adult hippopotamus fossil bones with cutmarks shows that the hominids were very actively engaged in the butchery of these animals.

The three Herto *Homo sapiens idaltu* crania show cutmarks indicating defleshing using sharp-edged stone tools. The post-mortem modifications and manipulation of the crania, demonstrated best on the child and broken adult crania, suggest that *Homo sapiens idaltu* performed ritual mortuary practices of which the dimension, context and meaning might only be revealed by further discoveries. These Herto discoveries are described here, and their technological and behavioural implications discussed in light of the emerging picture of human evolution in the late Middle Pleistocene.

4

SOCIAL NETWORKS AND SOCIAL COMPLEXITY IN FEMALE-BONDED PRIMATES

Julia Lehmann, Katherine Andrews & Robin Dunbar

Most primates are intensely social and spend a large amount of time servicing social relationships. The social brain hypothesis suggests that the evolution of the primate brain has been driven by the necessity of dealing with increased social complexity. In this study, we use social network analysis to analyse the relationship between primate group size, neocortex ratio and several social network metrics. We found that in female Old World monkey grooming networks, neocortex ratio is negatively correlated with clan size and with proportional clan membership when group size effects are controlled for. This indicates that—contrary to expectation—females of species with large neocortices generally belong to only a few, small grooming cliques despite living in closely bonded groups. The finding suggests that social complexity may derive from managing indirect social relationships, i.e. relationships in which a female is not directly involved, which may pose high cognitive demands on primates. We suggest that a large neocortex allows individuals to form intense social bonds with some group members while at the same time enabling them to manage and monitor less intense indirect relationships without frequent direct involvement with each individual of the social group.

5

HUMAN SOCIAL EVOLUTION: A COMPARISON OF HUNTER-GATHERER AND CHIMPANZEE SOCIAL ORGANIZATION

Robert Layton & Sean O'Hara

We compare the social behaviour of human hunter-gatherers with that of the better-studied chimpanzee species, *Pan troglodytes*, in an attempt to pinpoint the unique features of human social evolution. Humans and chimpanzees nonetheless share a fission-fusion type of social dynamic. Although the total size of a typical hunter-gatherer community is greater than that of a chimpanzee community, the size of the action sets that forage together is much the same. One of the most striking differences between hunter-gatherers and chimpanzees, however, is that humans consume much more meat. Thus, although hunter-gatherers and chimpanzees living in central Africa have similar body weights, humans live at much lower population densities due to their greater dependence on predation. Human foraging parties have longer duration than those of chimpanzees, lasting hours rather than minutes, and a higher level of mutual dependence, through (a) the division of labour between men (hunting) and women (gathering), which is in turn related to pair-bonding, and (b) meat sharing to reduce the risk of individual hunters' failure on any particular day. The band appears to be a uniquely human social unit that resolves the tension between greater dispersion and greater inter-dependence. Although hunter-gatherer population densities vary with ecology, band size appears to be stable across different ecological zones and continents. Despite the importance of the band, hunter-gatherers continue to sustain social relations within the wider community, relations that are frequently based on gift exchange, marriage and classificatory kinship. These relations allow individuals to escape local resource shortages and disputes within the band.

6
CONSTRAINTS ON SOCIAL NETWORKS

Sam G. B. Roberts

In both modern humans and non-human primates, time and cognitive constraints place an upper bound on the number of social relationships an individual can maintain at a given level of intensity. Similar constraints are likely to have operated throughout hominin evolution, shaping the size and structure of social networks. One of the key trends in human evolution, alongside an increase in brain size, is likely to have been an increase in group size, resulting in a larger number of social relationships that would have to be maintained over time. The network approach demonstrates that relationships should not be viewed as dyadic ties between two individuals, but as embedded within a larger network of ties between network members. This network can act as a scaffold to the dyadic tie, reducing the time and cognitive costs of maintaining the relationship. Together with relationships based on kinship, this scaffolding may have allowed for larger group sizes to be maintained among hominins than would be possible if such networks were based purely on dyadic ties between individuals.

7
SOCIAL NETWORKS AND COMMUNITY
IN THE VIKING AGE

Anna Wallette

During the Viking Age, the use of private violence was a precondition for social power. Iceland, for instance, was a law-making community but had no executive power to put the laws into effect. Politics throughout the whole of Scandinavia was based on strong personal relations. This was not a society of uncontrolled violence, but, alongside the development of church and kingdom, the attitude towards a legal type of violence changed. The Icelandic sagas are preoccupied with networks; the alliance patterns described can shed light on the relations between both biological and social kin. The texts describe competing loyalties through marriage, fostering, friendship, and pledges of support. Kin and marriage systems are the main organization form for people, and this article discusses alliances and the need for strong bonds with both family and friends at a time when the political and social order was changing.

8

DEACON'S DILEMMA: THE PROBLEM OF
PAIR-BONDING IN HUMAN EVOLUTION

Robin Dunbar

Humans have an unusual mating system—nominally monogamous pair-bonds set within multimale/multifemale communities. In the context of large, dispersed communities, this inevitably places a significant stress on mating strategies, especially for males for whom paternity uncertainty is a real problem. I discuss the nature of this bonding process in terms of the proximate mechanisms that make it possible, and then ask why such a phenomenon might have evolved. I suggest that the evidence for the importance of biparental care (the conventional explanation) is weak, and a more likely explanation is that females attached themselves to males in order to reduce the risks of harassment and infanticide from other males (the 'hired gun' hypothesis). Finally, I ask when pair-bonds of this kind might have evolved during the course of hominin evolution, and suggest that it might have been quite late.

9

THE EVOLUTION OF ALTRUISM
VIA SOCIAL ADDICTION

Julie Hui & Terrence Deacon

Each generation of evolutionary biologists has brought a fresh wave of attempts to answer the evolutionary riddle of altruism, from Darwin's community selection approach to variants on the concept of reciprocal altruism and niche construction effects that influence subsequent genera-tions. All of these have analysed how natural selection could maintain cooperation within a population where non-cooperation is always a risk; however, none describe how such a condition could incrementally evolve from a prior condition of non-cooperation. Here we describe a mechanism that could spontaneously and incrementally give rise to a synergistic codependence among individuals within a social group. We show that prolonged social living in the absence of reproductive cost can mask selection-maintaining traits important for autonomous living, causing them to drift and degrade to the point where individuals can no longer succeed outside the social context. This 'social addiction' will subsequently favour traits that maintain social cohesion (e.g. in ways described by previous selection-based theories) because of the high cost of group dispersion. This mechanism contributes a missing complementary component to existing selection-based explanations of the evolution of pro-social and altruistic behaviours.

10

FROM EXPERIENTIAL-BASED TO RELATIONAL-BASED FORMS OF SOCIAL ORGANIZATION: A MAJOR TRANSITION IN THE EVOLUTION OF *HOMO SAPIENS*

Dwight Read

The evolutionary trajectory from non-human to human forms of social organization involves change from experiential- to relational-based systems of social interaction. Social organization derived from biologically and experientially grounded social interaction reached a hiatus with the great apes due to an expansion of individualization of behaviour. The hiatus ended with the introduction of relational-based social interaction, culminating in social organization based on cultural kinship. This evolutionary trajectory links biological origins to cultural outcomes and makes evident the centrality of distributed forms of information for both the boundary and internal structure of human societies as these evolved from prior forms of social organization.

11

NETWORKS AND THE EVOLUTION OF SOCIO-MATERIAL DIFFERENTIATION

Carl Knappett

Ideas of 'distributed mind' are invaluable to archaeology in explaining the intimate involvement of artefacts in human cognition. Much of the work in this domain, however, focuses on proximate interactions of very limited numbers of individuals and artefacts. The argument developed here is that we need to broaden our understanding of distributed mind to encompass whole assemblages of artefacts spread across space and time; and that these assemblages can be best conceptualized as networks in which both objects and people are enfolded and enacted. While such networks may exist to some extent in the Palaeolithic and indeed Neolithic, it is with the Bronze Age that they really come to the fore, extending the scale of human action beyond the proximate like never before. Examples of this extensive socio-material differentiation are taken from the Aegean Bronze Age, with a focus on the most abundant class of material culture remaining to us, pottery.

12

WHEN INDIVIDUALS DO NOT STOP AT THE SKIN

Alan Barnard

This chapter examines contemporary hunter-gatherer societies in Africa and elsewhere in light of the social brain and the distributed mind hypotheses. One question asked is whether African hunter-gatherers offer the best model for societies at the dawn of symbolic culture, or whether societies elsewhere offer better models. The chapter argues for the former. Theoretical concepts touched on include sharing and exchange, universal kin classification, and the relation between group size and social networks. Reinterpretations of classic anthropological notions such as Wissler's age–area hypothesis, Durkheim's collective consciousness and Lévi-Strauss's elementary structures of kinship are offered. Finally, I outline my own theory of the co-evolution of language and kinship through three phases (signifying, syntactic and symbolic) and the subsequent breakdown of the principles of the symbolic phase across much of the globe in Neolithic times.

13

CLIQUES, COALITIONS, COMRADES AND COLLEAGUES: SOURCES OF COHESION IN GROUPS

Holly Arrow

Research and theory focused on contemporary groups and organizations has identified a variety of bonding agents that hold groups together. Cohesion may be based primarily on interpersonal ties or rely instead on the connection between member and group, while groups may cohere temporarily based on the immediate alignment of interests among members or may be tied together more permanently by socio-emotional bonds. Together, these characteristics define four prototypical group types. Cliques and coalitions are based primarily on dyadic ties. Groups of comrades or colleagues rely instead on the connection of members to the group for cohesion, which reduces the marginal cost of increasing group size. The strong glue of socio-emotional cohesion binds cliques and comrades, while coalitions and groups of colleagues are often based on weaker forms of cohesion. The mix of strong and weak adhesives and the greater scalability offered by the member–group bond provide the building blocks for assembling very large societies without overtaxing the social brain.

14

THE SOCIO-RELIGIOUS BRAIN: A DEVELOPMENTAL MODEL

Daniel N. Finkel, Paul Swartwout & Richard Sosis

Evolutionary approaches to religion and the social brain hypothesis are ripe for functional integration. One conceptual link for such integration lies in recognizing the artificially imposed distinction between religion and most other aspects of culture found in band-level societies. We argue that throughout most of human evolution religion has organized the patterns of belief and behaviour in which the social brain operates. Religious beliefs, myths, symbols and rituals are the means by which emotional bonding, enculturation and identification with an in-group occur. We present a developmental account of socio-religious enculturation in order to clarify the unique role religion plays in social cognition. We propose that the particulars of religious systems are introduced and practised during childhood, sealed in adolescence, reinforced throughout reproductive adulthood and transmitted by post-reproductive adults.

15
SOME FUNCTIONS OF COLLECTIVE FORGETTING

Paul Connerton

Coerced forgetting—forgetting as repressive erasure—has been a hallmark of many of the totalitarian regimes of the 20th century. However, the act of forgetting is not always negative. Three kinds of forgetting are identified and discussed here: prescriptive forgetting, or forgetting as an act of common good; forgetting as constitutive of the formation of a new identity; and forgetting as annulment, a response to a surfeit of information. Far from representing failures, all of these processes may play significant roles in the establishment and enhancement of social bonds.

16
WHAT IS COGNITION? EXTENDED COGNITION AND THE CRITERION OF THE COGNITIVE

Mark Rowlands

According to the thesis of the *extended mind*, at least some (token) cognitive processes extend into the cognizing subject's environment in the sense that they are (partly) composed of processes of manipulation, exploitation and transformation performed by that subject on suitable environmental structures. In contrast, according to the thesis of the *embedded mind*, the manipulation, exploitation and transformation of (external) information-bearing structures provides a useful *scaffolding* which *facilitates* cognitive processes but does not, even in part, constitute them. The two theses are distinct but often confused. The extended mind has attracted three ostensibly distinct kinds of objection, all of which on further analysis reduce to the idea that the arguments for the extended mind in fact only establish the thesis of the embedded mind. This chapter has two goals. First, it argues that these three objections can all be resolved by the provision of an adequate and properly motivated criterion—or mark—of the cognitive.

Second, it provides such a criterion—one made up of four conditions that are sufficient for a process to count as cognitive.

17
FIRING UP THE SOCIAL BRAIN

John Gowlett

The mastery of fire is a great human achievement which has helped shape our species. In modern life, health and safety conscious we build out fire, but even then, 'living flames' and candles hint at its symbolic significance. In this chapter I address the wider importance of fire, arguing that it is part of a fundamental motor of human evolution, deeply tied into our biology as well as economy and technology, and indeed a motor of the social brain. The early record strongly suggests that fire use began as much as 1.5 million years ago. That interpretation would tally with information about human dispersals to northern latitudes, and the attested role of fire in broadening and enriching human diets. Archaeological evidence shows that fire was used continually through the Middle Pleistocene, and that by 400,000 years ago at the latest it was being used in social contexts, as at Beeches Pit. There is however evidence for social collaboration at far earlier dates, as well as the interlinking of different technical routines (e.g. stone to cut wood). It seems likely that fire was involved in this nexus from a very early period, probably back to the time of increases in human brain size in the early Pleistocene, and indeed that it may have been a necessity for the subsequent physical evolutionary and social developments in *Homo*. Fire may be associated so strongly with imagery, imagination and symbolism in the modern world as a result of its primary role in effecting transformation of materials, and acting to link various strands of material culture.

18
A TECHNOLOGICAL FIX FOR 'DUNBAR'S DILEMMA'?

Lawrence Barham

A comparison of the archaeological evidence for symbol-based behaviours with the predictions of the social brain hypothesis has created

'Dunbar's dilemma'. The dilemma lies in a disjuncture between evidence and theory, in this case marked by a long chronological gap between the predicted cognitive potential for syntactic language (500 ka), communal religion (200 ka), and the earliest accepted archaeological evidence for these symbol-based behaviours (~135 ka). One possibility is that the predictions of the social brain hypothesis may simply be wrong and these cognitively demanding behaviours developed with later populations of *Homo sapiens*. Alternatively, the social brain hypothesis may indeed be correct and the dilemma arises from our limited conceptual vision of how to interpret the material record. This chapter makes the case for shifting our analytical focus away from overt expressions of symbol-use towards more indirect indicators of cognitively demanding behaviours as embedded in complex technologies. The hierarchical thought inherent in composite technology may not just resemble the structure of complex language—it may also be founded on the same neural networks that support recursive syntax. The proposed linkage of composite technology with language and its neural foundations provides a framework for examining the archaeological record for evidence of language and the creation of imaginary worlds before their expression in more recognizable forms. The resultant narrowing of the evidential gaps that comprise Dunbar's dilemma highlights the potential analytical insight that can be gained from an integrated approach involving evolutionary psychology, neurobiology and archaeology.

19
THE ARCHAEOLOGY OF GROUP SIZE

Matt Grove

This chapter aims to summarize the results of recent research producing estimates of hominin range areas, population sizes, and land use patterns based on archaeological data. Estimates of such variables are essential to any geographic or demographic discussion of human evolution, yet at present no generally applicable quantitative method is available to link them to the often abundant data of the archaeological record. Such data offer a unique window onto the patterns of adaptation characterizing prehistoric human populations, and developing a generic method to describe trajectories of change will allow researchers to compare range areas, population sizes and land use patterns between different regions and periods from throughout the vast spatio-temporal range of human evolution. Here particular emphasis is given to estimating a trajectory of group size through time from shortly after 2 million years ago until approximately 14,000 years ago.

20

FRAGMENTING HOMININS AND THE PRESENCING OF EARLY PALAEOLITHIC SOCIAL WORLDS

John Chapman & Bisserka Gaydarska

In this chapter, we introduce the fragmentation premise—the idea that the deliberate breakage of a complete object and the re-use of the resultant fragments as new and separate objects 'after the break' was a common practice in the past. We also summarize the main implications of the fragmentation premise for the study of enchained social relations and of the creation and development of personhood in the past. To the extent that the boundaries of the human body can be considered permeable and open to the influences of other persons, things and places, personhood can be conceptualized as 'fractal', with objects emerging out of persons rather than being in contra-distinction to them, and broken objects considered as non-human dividuals. Enchained relations connect the distributed elements of a person's social identity using material culture. These concepts of fragmentation, enchainment and fractality are used to think through some of the earliest remains of objects in the world—the hominin tools of the period 2.7—0.5 million years ago. In contrast to the standard separation of symbolic behaviour by anatomically modern humans after 200,000 years ago from non-symbolic behaviour by early pre-*sapiens* populations, we propose a scenario in which the use of tools and the movement of lithic resources over the landscape led to the emergence of enchained social relations, consonant with increases in brain size following 2 million years ago. Following the philosopher David Bohm, we further support the co-evolution of fragmentation in both consciousness and in objects, and compare Bohm's three-stage ideas to Mithen's model of cognitive evolution and Donald's model of external symbolic storage.

21
SMALL WORLDS, MATERIAL CULTURE AND ANCIENT NEAR EASTERN SOCIAL NETWORKS

Fiona Coward

The cognitive, psychological and sociological mechanisms underpinning complex social relationships among small groups are a part of our primate heritage. However, among human groups relationships persist over much greater temporal and spatial scales, often in the physical absence of one or other of the individuals themselves. This article asks how such individual face-to-face social interactions were 'scaled up' during human evolution to the regional and global networks characteristic of our modern societies. One recent suggestion has been that a radical change in human sociality occurred with the shift to sedentary and agricultural societies in the early Neolithic. This chapter presents the results of a focused study of the long-term development of regional social networks in the Near East, using the distribution of different forms of material culture as a proxy for the social relationships that underpinned processes of trade, exchange and the dissemination of material culture practices. Long-term developments in social networks in the Near East are assessed in robust quantitative terms and their implications for the evolution of large-scale human societies discussed.

22
EXCAVATING THE PREHISTORIC MIND: THE BRAIN AS A CULTURAL ARTEFACT AND MATERIAL CULTURE AS BIOLOGICAL EXTENSION

Steven Mithen

The adoption of an explicitly cognitive approach has become prominent in archaeological research during the last decade, helping to place Palaeolithic archaeology into a driving role in the development of archaeological theory and developing inter-disciplinarity with the cognitive sciences. Two prominent approaches have emerged: the social brain hypothesis and the distributed mind. Precisely how these can be integrated into a single, unified approach for the study of the evolution and nature of the human mind remains unclear, if indeed it is desirable to do so. In this contribution I reflect on the emergence of these approaches within archaeology and comment upon their relative strengths and weakness. This is partly achieved by describing two case studies from my own work, each of which draws on one of these approaches.

Index